THE PRACTICE OF
JAPANESE ACUPUNCTURE AND MOXIBUSTION:
CLASSIC PRINCIPLES IN ACTION

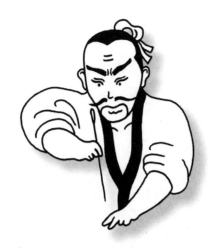

THE PRACTICE OF
JAPANESE ACUPUNCTURE
AND MOXIBUSTION

Classic Principles in Action

IKEDA MASAKAZU

translated by
EDWARD OBAIDEY

EASTLAND PRESS • SEATTLE

Japanese language edition © 1996 by Ido-No-Nippon-Sha, Inc.,
published as *Dentou shinkyuu chiryouhou*

English language edition © 2005 by Eastland Press, Inc.

Translator's Introduction © 2005 by Edward Obaidey

Published by Eastland Press, Inc.
P.O. Box 99749
Seattle, WA 98139 USA
www.eastlandpress.com

International Standard Book Number: 0-939616-43-2
Library of Congress Control Number: 2004118238
Printed in the United States of America

2   4   6   8   10   9   7   5   3

Book design by Gary Niemeier

TABLE OF CONTENTS

Table of Contents

PART TWO:

Table of Contents

Foreword to the English edition

JAPANESE TRADITIONAL MEDICINE has been practiced for over a thousand years. There are four technically distinct categories: herbal medicine, acupuncture and moxibustion, massage, and bonesetting.

All of these were originally based on Chinese medicine but have been partly adapted to suit the sensibilities and constitution of Japanese people, and freshly invented techniques have also been added over the years. Many traditional healers used two or more treatment arts from among the four categories, with herbal treatment as the main one and acupuncture and moxibustion as supplementary treatment, but there were also a certain number of healers who specialized in only acupuncture and moxibustion.

Western medicine in Japan had its beginnings after Francisco Xavier (1506-52) visited Kagoshima in Kyushu Prefecture, the southern part of Japan, in 1549, and introduced Christianity to Japan. In 1583 a Christian hospital was established in Nagasaki, Kyushu, the only town in Japan open to foreigners. At that time Japan had a policy of national seclusion, so that by government policy, foreign culture was excluded, thus the acceptance of Western medicine was a difficult issue. It was under these circumstances that Western medicine infiltrated Japanese society as people were trained in the new methods. While the process was very slow, Western medicine made steady advances aided by its distinctive treatment results.

In 1867 the Edo era ended. This coincided with the end of feudalism, and the curtain rose on modern Japan. The revolutionary government decided to introduce Western civilization into every social system, including politics and the economy, and as a part of this, the Western medical model was adopted wholesale. As a consequence, in one dramatic step Western medicine became the mainstream medical system.

This decision seriously impacted the field of traditional medicine. While the government did not snuff out traditional medicine entirely, in order to coexist with Western medicine there was a strong demand for traditional medicine to become more scientific. In this way, science was grafted onto the basic theories, not only in herbal medicine, but also in the field of acupuncture and moxibustion.

In this process of accommodating the modern thinking, a great number of important general ideas that existed in the classic theory were replaced by new words in the name of scientific interpretation. For example, acupuncture treatment was reinterpreted as 'stimulation therapy,' moxibustion was translated as 'thermotherapy,' and tonification and shunting as 'weak and strong stimulation.'

The concept of meridians is a very important and fundamental part of the traditional medicine that originated in China a few thousand years ago. However, since the existence of meridians had not been proven anatomically, the theory was treated somewhat flippantly, and some Western doctors even asserted that it was superstition. Consequently, the theory of meridian flow was largely discarded and meridian points became reinterpreted as 'stimulative points' for applying needles and moxa.

In this manner, herbal medicine and acupuncture and moxibustion were driven from their position as mainstream medicine to that of an alternative medicine, and the knowledge and practice of classic medical theory and its techniques gradually declined. The art of acupuncture and moxibustion especially, based on the theory of the course of flow in the meridians, went rapidly out of use. 'Stimulative points' therapy became the norm, divorced from the original meridian flow theory.

This perversion of traditional medicine was utterly unacceptable to doctors and healers who studied classical theory, and by the Showa era, which began in 1925 (almost 60 years after the Meiji Restoration), an acute sense of impending crisis prompted a group of young and concerned acupuncture and moxibustion practitioners to take action. Included in this group were Yanagiya Sorei, Okabe Sodo, Takeyama Shinichiro, and Inoue Keiri.

These healers, who had pursued the authentic path of acupuncture and moxibustion, were convinced through their experience in daily clinics and study of the classics that acupuncture and moxibustion could only be truly effective when practiced using classical concepts and techniques. Because sixty years had already passed, they felt a pressing need to find senior healers who were continuing to practice using the exact classical methods. They finally found an old healer, Yagishita Katsunosuke (1854-1946), in a small, poor fishing village in Chiba prefecture.

Yanagiya Sorei wrote: "There are many criticisms of classical traditional acupuncture and moxibustion treatment based on meridian flow theory, claiming, for example, that it isn't scientific. However, the facts cannot be denied. Mr. Yagishita has been getting brilliant results using this theory. The results speak for themselves."

Takeyama had this to say about Yagishita: "When I met him he was 88, but he was very energetic and looked to be only in his 60s. A person of no wants, he is afraid of nothing, and incomparably pure and noble. "

Before the age of 60, Yagishita had practiced acupuncture and moxibustion in addition to his day job of running a haberdashery store. Thereafter he devoted himself entirely to his patients. Acupuncture and moxibustion were, for him, an art for the people and for the world.

Okabe Sodo received Yagishita's treatment directly and also recorded some important information that he received. For example, "For illness of the tongue, use the Heart meridian; for illness of the mouth and lips, use the Spleen meridian; for gout, apply moxibustion to BL-18 as well as GB-31 and LI- 11, and apply needles to GV-20, GB-30, and LI-15; for illness of the ears, use the Triple Burner meridian on the arms and hands, the Gallbladder meridian on the legs and feet, and the Kidney meridian."

In addition to Yagishita, Mori Dohaku is mentioned by Kamichi Sakae, an investigator of the history of modern Japanese acupuncture and moxibustion, as a classical healer who strongly influenced those young lions of the Showa era.

Those who were working for the revival of traditional acupuncture and moxibustion received great encouragement from their encounters with Yagishita and Mori, and from around 1920 to 1930 they worked on developing a neoclassical meridian treatment art based on tradition which was able to stand side by side with the 'scientific' acupuncture and moxibustion art that the government had been advocating. This quest for a new acupuncture and moxibustion system, which involved the rediscovery and animation of the classic art, could be called a renaissance in the history of Japanese acupuncture and moxibustion.

The acupuncture and moxibustion practiced in recent years in Japan can be divided broadly into three schools: the stimulation therapy school, which is the largest; a school which follows the contemporary Chinese style; and finally the neoclassic school, which uses meridian flow theory. In the new century this third group is becoming more influential with the emergence of young healers who demand a deeper and more authentic understanding of the theory and technique of the art of acupuncture and moxibustion.

Ikeda Masakazu, the author of this book, is a well-known person in the field of modern Japanese acupuncture and moxibustion. After graduating from a government accredited acupuncture and moxibustion school, he was initiated into the art of acupuncture and moxibustion by his elder brother, the late Ikeda Takio.

Ikeda Takio was a torchbearer of the second generation who transmitted the spirit and skills of neoclassical acupuncture and moxibustion, and was well known as an excellent healer. He trained and polished his clinical technique under Inoue Keiri, one of the pioneers of the neoclassical art in the Showa era.

After his brother's death, Ikeda Masakazu devoted himself to the study of the Japanese and Chinese classics, developing and elaborating his theory and methods within the framework of the meridian flow theory and the treatment methods of the Showa era pioneers. He also refined the art of pulse diagnosis, and devised some new techniques regarding the use of meridians and their points.

While his brother Takio specialized in acupuncture and moxibustion, Masakazu also studies medicinal herbs and their uses, and his knowledge in this area is profound. He has already written and published many books, including guides to the classics, handbooks on the art of acupuncture and moxibustion, and texts on clinical technique.

This present book covers, in detail, the use of traditional acupuncture and moxibustion in contemporary Japan, with reference to a large number of clinical case studies.

Imura Koji
Director
Nishitenma Clinic of
Acupuncture and Moxibustion

ACKNOWLEDGMENTS

I FIRST STARTED HELPING out at my elder brother's (Ikeda Takeo) clinic when I was 23 years old. I was allowed to actually begin treating people when I was 25 years old. Since that time, thirty-odd years have passed and I have seen a great many patients. I often sigh to myself and think of numerous cases where I failed and think, "If I knew then what I know now, I could have healed that patient." Because of the experience that these and many other patients have allowed me to gain, I have the life that I am able to lead now. When I reflect on this I feel a sense of shame.

The diseases that I have dealt with in this book consist only of those that I have treated personally. There are some diseases which may appear rather unusual, and there are others that I have not mentioned. In any case, I made it a point not to write anything about diseases with which I have no experience.

Looking at the final product that this book represents, I feel a bit unsatisfied. On the other hand, knowing my character, I don't think there would ever have been a time when I would have been completely satisfied with the result. There is literally no end to research on the subject, and I would like to have made a few additions here and there, but this would have delayed the completion of this book indefinitely. If there are any areas of the book that are lacking and need revision, I would be glad to accept them and receive instruction from those willing to do me such a service.

This book was written with great encouragement from Iimura Koji, a man I look up to and respect. He himself is an acupuncturist who is engaged in research on traditional folk medicine on an international scale, especially Tibetan medicine, and was gracious enough to write a foreword for this book.

I must also mention Dr. Ide Toru who helped me with any mistakes with modern medical terms. Dr. Ide, in addition to being the assistant director of the Ide Hospital, is also a fellow student of traditional medicine. The hospital to which I frequently refer patients in the book is, of course, Dr. Ide's. I want to thank him for all his help.

*   *   *

Acknowledgements

It gives me great pleasure to finally see the completion of this English translation by Edward Obaidey. Although Edward is English, his diligent effort has brought him to an understanding of the clinical practice of traditional Japanese acupuncture and moxibustion.

I believe that I first met Edward in 1992, at an international acupuncture and moxibustion symposium in Kyoto. Since that time, owing to the close bonds that have grown between us, we have presented many seminars together in America and Australia. Edward served as my translator at these gatherings, and gradually it became apparent that there was a need to translate one of my texts into English. The book before you is aimed at fulfilling that need.

It is my hope and pleasure that through this text more people will put into practice these traditional methods of acupuncture and moxibustion.

Fortune has smiled on this project because Dan Bensky, a gentleman and a scholar, has been involved in it from the very start. I would therefore like to express my gratitude to both Dan and Edward for their efforts, and sincerely hope that this book will be widely read.

Ikeda Masakazu
October, 2004

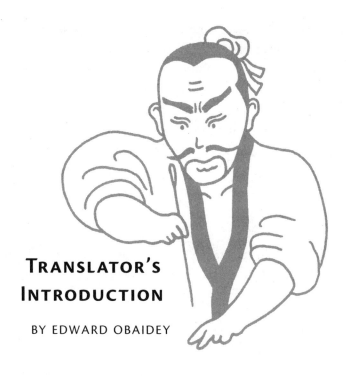

TRANSLATOR'S INTRODUCTION

BY EDWARD OBAIDEY

BACKGROUND ISSUES

Why an Introduction?

THIS IS THE first book to provide a Western audience access to the work of Ikeda Masakazu. Ikeda Sensei has a deep and abiding interest in the classics of Chinese medicine and a firm grounding in clinical practice, including that of his teachers. As a consequence, his approach to medicine, especially with regard to his ideas and terminology, is somewhat different from that of other practitioners. In many ways, the importance of this book is that it *is* different and presents in the guise of a clinical manual a very useful approach to the thought and methodology of classical Chinese medicine. However, the very differences that make the work worthwhile present some difficulties. For this reason, I have prepared an introduction to aid the reader in understanding this material, which I have had the privilege not only of transmitting to a Western audience, but of learning myself, as it is the basis of my own clinical practice.

I will attempt in this introduction to be as clear and straightforward as possible, although this in some ways violates the spirit of the East Asian approach to teaching and learning. As in most traditional paintings, the teacher sketches the outlines of the scenes and presents it with feeling and understanding, and it is up to the student to fill in the blanks. Confucius, perhaps the first known teacher in Chinese history, stated that his goal was to pick up the corner of understanding; the student was supposed to look for himself to see what was underneath. Ikeda Sensei believes that it is important not to give too detailed an explanation, as this will inhibit the function of the discerning mind. Given that, we will address some of the basic approaches in this introduction, if for no other reason than English-speaking readers do not have access to the more than twenty other books that Ikeda Sensei has written in Japanese. Because it is assumed that all readers have a basic grounding in the concepts of East Asian medicine, and because of the constraints of space, this introduction will be brief; it is designed to simply provide the reader with the conceptual tools to understand and use the main text.[1]

Basic Premises

Ikeda Sensei bases his approach on his deep study of the classics of Chinese medicine, not only those usually cited by acupuncturists—the two parts of the *Inner Classic* (*Basic Questions* and *Divine Pivot*) along with the *Classic of Difficulties*—but also the late Han classics of herbal medicine by Zhang Zhong-Jing (whose given name was Zhang Ji), the *Discussion of Cold Damage* and *Essentials from the Golden Cabinet*. He has also done work in the *Divine Husbandman's Classic of the Materia Medica*. His studies of the past and his own clinical practice have made it clear to him that these are not different traditions that should be kept separate, but rather merely different aspects of an integral whole that inform each other. To utilize any of these in one's own clinical practice requires a good understanding of all of them. This synthesis is one of the hallmarks of Ikeda Sensei's approach.

Definitions

JAPANESE ACUPUNCTURE

In the West there has been an attempt to define a so-called Japanese style of acupuncture. To Ikeda Sensei, there is no such thing because there are a plethora of styles and approaches to acupuncture practiced in Japan; it is presumptuous to call any subset of these 'Japanese acupuncture.' However, despite this diversity, there does appear to be one feature that is common to all Japanese styles: the emphasis on touch. And yet there are styles of acupuncture in other parts of the world that also consider touch to be important, so it is incorrect to define all forms of acupuncture that emphasize palpation as being Japanese. Nevertheless, because Ikeda Sensei is Japanese, there are certain aspects of Japanese culture and traditions of acupuncture that inform and influence his work.

....

[1] Note that this introduction includes some material from the handout "From Syndrome to Treatment" by Masakazu Ikeda, translated by Edward Obaidey, for a workshop presented by the Institute of Classical Oriental Medicine and the Japanese Acupuncture and Moxibustion Skills Foundation in Brisbane, Australia, in 2000.

MERIDIAN THERAPY

To Ikeda Sensei, meridian therapy is simply the use of the meridians to diagnose and treat disease, nothing more and nothing less. Some people think that meridian therapy automatically implies shallow needling; it does not. If the treatment requires deep needling, it should be performed. If moxibustion is necessary, it should also be performed. The same can be said of massage, herbs, exercise, and dietary measures. The tools are many and varied, but the emphasis is always on the use of the meridians. If this is kept in mind, the diagnosis and treatment regimens discussed in this book will be more understandable.

In meridian therapy, a disease is interpreted as a pattern of disharmony as viewed through the prism of the meridians, and the same meridians are used to treat the disease with acupuncture and moxibustion. The pattern represents the pathological state of the body, and is understood in terms of the condition of the qi, blood, and fluids of the organ and meridian system; it is assessed in terms of deficiency, excess, heat, and cold. Treatment is carried out by tonifying and shunting (also known as dispersing or draining; see "Meaning and Varieties of Tonification and Shunting" below) the channels. A summary of the parameters, methods of diagnosis, and treatment methods for the various patterns that are used in this book are discussed below.

Organ-Meridian System

The organs and meridians should be viewed as systems of interrelated but frequently complementary functions. To understand physiology and pathology, these interconnected functions and the dynamics that drive them must be clearly understood. The common perception that both the organs and their related meridians have identical functions is not supported by the classics. The organs and meridians comprise a system, not a single entity, which is why Ikeda Sensei refers to them as the organ-meridian system. For example:

- The Liver organ stores the blood, as noted in Chapter 8 of the *Divine Pivot*, and has a spreading, centrifugal function, as noted in Chapter 22 of *Basic Questions*. This spreading function is a consequence of the power of the stored blood. By contrast, the main direction of flow in the Liver meridian is centripetal, as it leads the blood toward the Liver where it is stored. Accordingly, it is the astringent, sour flavor that corresponds to the Liver meridian (*Basic Questions*, Chapter 10). When this centripetal-like action is diminished, there is insufficient blood stored in the Liver. This state is called Liver deficiency, which is another way of saying blood deficiency.

- The Heart organ is always moving and excited; it is therefore yang in nature, and if the Heart stops, the person will die. By contrast, the cooling Heart meridian is full of yin qi. As a result, the lesser yin Heart meridian has the complementary, yet synergistic, effect of preventing the Heart from overworking, tempering its action and keeping it under control. The Heart meridian is a lesser yin meridian, which is the same type or layer as the lesser yin Kidney meridian and therefore similar in its cooling, tempering aspects. This cooling aspect of the Heart meridian can be surmised if one recalls that the Heart meridian is associated with the bitter flavor (*Basic Questions*, Chapter 10).

• The Lung organ is active in the autumn and relates to harvesting and collecting functions (*Basic Questions*, Chapter 22), as well as clarifying and descending functions. The Lung meridian has the offsetting, yet complementary, function of disseminating and spreading the qi throughout the body. This is clear from the connection of the acrid taste to this meridian (*Basic Questions*, Chapter 10), rather than to the organ.

• The Kidney organ is associated with contraction (*Basic Questions*, Chapter 22) while the Kidney meridian acts to ensure that the fluids in the Kidney organ are not overly abundant. Accordingly, the Kidney meridian is associated with the salty flavor (*Basic Questions*, Chapter 10), which has the capacity to move fluids. The overall effect of this storage and contraction of the fluids by the organ and movement of the fluids by the meridian is to ensure that the body stays appropriately firm and hard. This physiological hardness is a consequence of the fluids filling in the structure; it is not the dry and flaky hardness that comes from fluid insufficiency. Both the organ and meridian are mainly associated with cold; they are more active during the winter, and the representative pulse is sunken. This means that the Kidney works silently, and if it becomes too cold, problems with defecation and sexuality ensue. A balance is needed, but in this case it comes from the gate of vitality (命門 *meimon/mìng mén*).

• On the one hand, the Spleen is the peak of yin, and yet it is also placed in the middle—both in the body and in the diagrams of the five phases. The Spleen organ does not do anything that is too yang or too mobilizing. Both the Spleen meridian and Lung meridian are greater yin meridians; as such, both have radiating, discharging, and dispersing actions. This connection in function is reflected in their flavors, as noted in Chapter 5 of *Basic Questions:* "The acrid and sweet qi and flavors discharge and disperse and so are considered yang." However, unlike the Lung meridian, the Spleen meridian cannot perform this function by itself. Rather, it directs the Stomach meridian to do the work, as clearly indicated in Chapter 29 of *Basic Questions*. Therefore, the overall process of obtaining and using food qi requires two steps: the Spleen organ is involved in the production of food qi, while the Spleen meridian is involved in its radiation or dispersal, which is sometimes described as its transportive function.

Deficiency and Excess

The first thing to understand about deficiency and excess is that they are not of equal status; nor should they be considered equal partners in the development of disease. While many believe that if there is deficiency there must also be excess, this is not strictly true.

The presence of true excess as an important aspect of a disease is relatively rare. Therefore, the focus of both diagnosis and treatment should definitely emphasize the deficient aspect of disease, rather than the excessive aspect. With this understanding, it follows that the root of all disease is said to originate from a deficiency of essential qi (精気 *sei ki/jīng qì*) in one of the five yin organs, as noted in Chapter 62 of *Basic Questions*. The most important underlying aspect of the deficient state is that it represents an insufficiency of the upright or normal qi (正気 *shō ki/zhēng qì*).

By contrast, excess is understood as a buildup or excess of pathogenic qi. For our purposes, this is conceptualized as the buildup of heat or blood. This excess manifests primarily in the yang meridians and the yang organs. The one exception is yin excess. Since a yin excess refers to the stagnation and pooling of heat or blood in a yin part of the body, this condition can only occur in the Liver. This can be understood by briefly considering the other yin organs. Only fluids can collect in the Kidneys; this does not result in heat and therefore cannot really be called an excess. The Spleen is where qi, blood, and fluids are produced. If the Spleen were to receive heat, their production would cease, leading rather quickly to death; there is accordingly no state of Spleen excess. Finally, while heat can collect in the Lungs and Heart, they are located in the yang area of the body (above the diaphragm), so any excess that they develop will not be referred to as yin excess.

Similarly, based on this definition of excess, a buildup of cold is not considered to be a condition of excess. When there is a large amount of cold accumulating in yin areas, except for the Liver, it is referred to as an overabundance of yin (陰盛 *insei/yīn shèng*) and not yin excess.

The second thing to understand is that the description of conditions of deficiency is modified by the presence of other factors (described below) to produce various pathological states. In addition, when palpated, the tissues themselves are often classified as deficient or excessive in nature. In this case, deficient tissue refers to tissue which produces a pleasant sensation when pressed, and excessive tissue to that which produces sharp pain when pressed.

Finally, the pulse can also be described in terms of deficiency and excess. A weak, soft, languid pulse is often, but not always, classified as deficient. One counter example is from the *Pulse Classic,* where a deficient pulse is defined as one that is big and soft but disappears on deeper pressure. By contrast, an excessive pulse is often (but not always) seen as being big and forceful. In these cases, the use of the terms deficiency and excess is not directly related to the original pathology, but rather to the secondary stages of the disease, that is, those that are of importance in the branch treatments.

Heat and Cold

Heat is produced when there is a deficiency mainly of the fluids and yin qi, and cold is produced when there is a deficiency of the blood, fluids, and yang qi. Heat can be treated by cooling the body through tonifying the fluids and yin qi. Where it is warranted, shunting can also be carried out. Similarly, cold is treated by warming the body through tonifying the blood, fluids, and yang qi.

BASIC PATTERNS:
DEFICIENCY AND EXCESS,
HEAT AND COLD

Four Basic Patterns

As noted above, all disease begins with a deficiency of essential qi, which is the basis for the functioning of each organ. Because the most important organs are the yin organs, the four basic types of essential qi deficiency are Liver deficiency, Spleen deficiency, Lung deficiency, and Kidney deficiency. Practitioners are often curious why there is no Heart deficiency pattern in meridian therapy. The answer is quite simple and has to do with the fundamental character of the Heart. This organ stores the spirit and is constantly in motion; consequently, the Heart requires a large amount of yang qi. If either the yang or the qi of the Heart becomes deficient, the person is beyond help. (This is explained in Chapter 71 of *Divine Pivot*.) This means that a deficiency in the essence of the Heart cannot be at the root of a disease; it does not mean that the Heart is never affected by disease. The Heart can be affected by influences, good and bad, from other organs, as is often indicated in the symptoms and the pulse.

To reiterate, in meridian therapy these four types of deficiency are the basic patterns. However, while deficiency of the essential qi is *necessary* for the development of disease, it is not a *sufficient* cause. If there is only a deficiency of the essential qi, the person may only complain of fatigue. Before any other symptoms or type of disease appears, a pathological factor of some kind must be present (Fig. I-1). These are the three classes of factors well known to all students of East Asian medicine: internal factors, based on an imbalance of the emotions; external factors, contracted from external pathogens; and other factors, which are categorized as neither internal nor external and include overwork, drug use, or overindulgence in food and/or drink. The combination of one or more of these factors plus a deficiency of essential qi will result in changes in the qi, blood, and fluids stored in the organs, which can manifest in disease.

Buildup of Heat and Cold

Whether the pattern involves the Liver, Spleen, Lungs, or Kidneys, when there is a deficiency of qi, blood, or fluids, some type of pathological heat or cold will be produced. This leads to one of eight patterns:

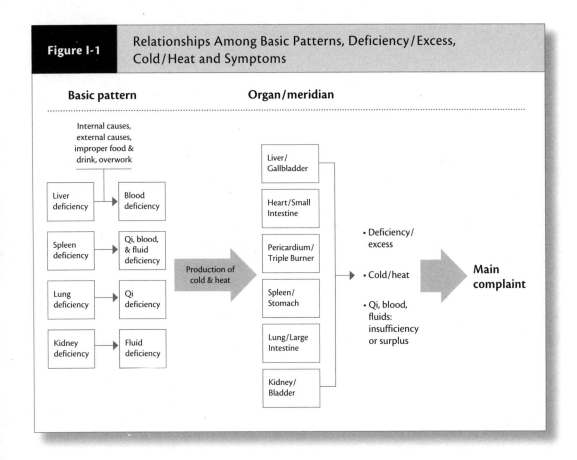

Figure I-1 — Relationships Among Basic Patterns, Deficiency/Excess, Cold/Heat and Symptoms

1. Liver deficiency/heat
2. Liver deficiency/cold
3. Spleen deficiency/heat
4. Spleen deficiency/cold
5. Lung deficiency/heat
6. Lung deficiency/cold
7. Kidney deficiency/heat
8. Kidney deficiency/cold

These basic patterns arise because of the interactions between the pathological factors and the deficiency of essential qi in the organs. The resulting patterns can spread in different ways throughout the organ-meridian system, giving rise to the various combinations of deficiency, excess, cold, and heat that form the basis of sundry diseases.

As noted in Fig. I-1, each yin organ is intimately associated with a set of substances or functions: the Liver with blood, the Lungs with qi, the Kidneys with fluids, and the Spleen with all three. These relationships influence not only how the different organ-meridian systems become diseased, but how those diseases develop and change.

Heat and Cold Patterns

Patterns of heat and cold can be divided into several major groups, each with its own dynamics. Understanding the differences between these groups can be crucial to making a proper diagnosis and treatment.

HEAT PATTERNS RELATED TO DEPLETION OF BLOOD AND FLUIDS

The heat patterns due to deficiency of the yin aspects of the body include Liver deficiency/heat, Spleen deficiency/heat, and Kidney deficiency/heat. In these cases, the heat is produced because of a lack in a structural part or in the fluids; accordingly, this type of heat is also known as yin deficiency heat or simply deficiency heat. In the clinic, we have to be careful about the subtle details of these conditions because when they become chronic, the heat can die down and practitioners can easily misdiagnose them as cold patterns.

HEAT PATTERNS RELATED TO DISRUPTION OF RADIATION OF HEAT

Yang qi is continuously radiated from the surface of the body. When there is a disruption in the production or circulation of the yang qi, or in the outward dispersion of heat by the yang qi, heat symptoms may result. This is true even in cases of yang deficiency, when the deficiency of yang leads to a weakening in the yang function of dispersing. This is turn leads to the entrapment of the remaining yang qi and the production of heat. Patterns where this occurs are Spleen deficiency/heat and Lung deficiency/heat.

Depending on the nature of the factors that precipitate the disease, this buildup of heat from yang deficiency in the outer aspects of the body can be regarded as resulting from either yang excess heat or yang deficiency heat. In addition, over time the heat can move inward and affect the blood. When it does, the result is Liver excess, which is also known as yin excess (see "Deficiency and Excess" above).

COLD PATTERNS RELATED TO BLOOD DEFICIENCY

In this case, the blood insufficiency is such that cold is produced, resulting in a pattern of Liver yang deficiency/cold. However, since the patient is still alive, some yang must still be present. This small amount of heat collects in the chest where it can continue to accumulate. However, this buildup of heat is qualitatively different from the heat seen in yin deficiency patterns, which must be kept in mind when treating these patients.

COLD PATTERNS RELATED TO FLUID DEFICIENCY

Kidney deficiency/cold is characterized by an extreme insufficiency of fluids plus a lack of yang qi coming from the gate of vitality. On the one hand, the fluids are part of the structure of the body; when the structure has diminished it can be construed as yin deficiency. However, because the final result is an increase in cold, and there are aspects of both yin and yang deficiency, it is considered to be a pattern of deficiency cold. Note that even when this cold reaches its peak, some heat signs are still apparent; this state is known as true-cold, false-heat and should not be mistaken for yin deficiency heat or yang excess heat.

Spleen deficiency/cold is characterized by deficient fluids of the Spleen plus faint yang qi of the Stomach. Since the production of food qi has diminished, there is not enough yang qi to carry out the functions of dispersing and collecting, leading to a pattern of yang deficiency cold, or simply deficiency cold.

COLD PATTERNS RELATED TO QI DEFICIENCY

The Lungs are primarily concerned with the yang aspects of the body, that is, with the qi. Lung deficiency can be divided into two types: Lung deficiency that leads to the production of heat, which is called Lung deficiency/yang excess, and Lung deficiency that leads to the production of cold, which is called Lung deficiency/yang deficiency. Basically, in the former condition, the heat makes its way to the periphery of the body but finds itself trapped there, as the pores are closed tight (one sign of Lung deficiency); accordingly, heat accumulates. In the latter condition, the pores are not closing properly (another sign of Lung deficiency), causing any heat that is present to leak out into the environment. This leads to cold, which is also known as Lung deficiency/cold.

Spreading of Heat and Cold

SPREADING OF HEAT FROM YIN DEFICIENCY

Heat from yin deficiency spreads first via the interior-exterior relationship to the yang organ that is paired with the affected yin organ. As the condition becomes more serious, it spreads through the organ-meridian system via the controlling cycle, first affecting the yin organ that is 'downstream' in this cycle. For example, Liver deficiency/heat spreads first to the Gallbladder; if the condition becomes worse, the heat will spread to the Lungs. Kidney deficiency/heat is liable to spread to the Bladder; if the heat reaches the Heart, the condition is very serious. Given the peculiarities of the Spleen and Stomach pair, the heat from Spleen deficiency/heat can spread to the Stomach, from which it can spread to the rest of the yang organs.

SPREADING OF HEAT FROM YANG DEFICIENCY

Heat from Lung deficiency will move to the outer level of the body, which corresponds to the greater yang meridian. From there, it will move to the yang brightness meridian and to the lesser yang meridian, eventually affecting the terminal yin meridian. This pattern was discussed in depth in the late Han dynasty work, *Discussion of Cold Damage*.

Heat secondary to Spleen deficiency will move into its paired yang organ, the Stomach, and end up as Stomach deficiency/heat or Stomach excess/heat. Depending on the patient's constitution and lifestyle, the heat will move from the Stomach to various other organs, where it will cause organ-specific heat symptoms.

SPREADING OF COLD FROM YANG DEFICIENCY

Cold from Liver deficiency has a tendency to sink downward. This leads to a preponderance of cold from the middle burner downward, with the remnants of heat collecting in the upper burner and the organs located there.

With Spleen deficiency/cold, the Stomach organ becomes cold, which leads to the heat being trapped in the yang brightness meridian. There are circumstances when the cold spreads throughout the entire body, producing Kidney deficiency/cold.

Lung deficiency/cold leads to cold in the greater yang meridian. The organs related to this meridian are the Bladder and the Small Intestine. By way of this connection, the cold can enter their related yin organs, resulting in Kidney deficiency/cold or Spleen deficiency/cold. This is an example of cold traveling from the meridian of a yang organ to the related yin organ.

Development of the Main Complaint

As described above, the interaction of an underlying deficiency in an organ with pathological factors leads to the production of cold or heat. The cold or heat then affects the organ-meridian system, and a new pathological pattern emerges. At this time, symptoms begin to appear, either in a systemic fashion or in specific locations that are related to the movement of heat or cold. When there is a specific site to the main complaint, it is called the diseased part and will be the focus of treatment.

DISEASES OF THE ORGANS

When heat and cold enter the organs, the organs themselves can become the diseased part. When this occurs, the problem is considered to be an organ disease. These are relatively serious conditions, for example, the heat from Spleen deficiency/heat can spread to the Stomach, and either Stomach excess/heat or Stomach deficiency/heat may develop.

Another possibility is that the heat or cold goes through various transformations and pathways before it eventually enters an organ. A good example of this is the transfer of Lung deficiency/heat first to the Spleen and the yang brightness meridian, and then eventually to the lesser yang meridian and Liver organ. Naturally, when an organ is affected, the heat or cold can produce secondary problems.

DISEASES OF THE MERIDIANS

When an organ receives heat or cold but is relatively robust, the heat or cold will not enter the organ proper; instead, it spreads to the respective meridian. The meridian then becomes the site of disease, a process that is called meridian disease. For example, we discussed Spleen deficiency/heat spreading to the Stomach. If, however, the Stomach is relatively strong, the heat from Spleen deficiency/heat will not enter the Stomach proper. Instead the heat will be diverted to the meridian, becoming yang brightness excess/heat.

Another possibility is that the meridians receive the heat or cold, which fails to reach the organs themselves. This means that the deficiency, excess, heat, or cold manifests along the meridian, which then becomes the site of the disease. Examples of this are problems affecting the ears, eyes, or nose.

DISEASES OF THE MERIDIAN SINEWS

When a meridian is affected by heat or cold, the meridian sinew (經筋 *keikin/jīng jīn*) related to that meridian may become the focus of the disease. When this occurs, the condition can exhibit signs of deficiency or excess as well as heat or cold. This is known as meridian sinew disease. Most neuromusculoskeletal disorders fall in this category. However, the treatment of these conditions is still based on the diagnosis and regulation of the meridians, which can often be treated successfully without recourse to any of the aspects that are peculiar to the meridian sinews.

FOUR DIAGNOSTIC METHODS

When performing the four diagnoses, it is important to keep in mind the main complaint and the site of disease, which is checked for deficiency, excess, heat, and/or cold. At the same time, we assemble in our mind's eye the basic pattern and determine the extent and location of the spread of heat or cold within the organ-meridian system. Then, of course, we must decide whether the condition is one that can be treated effectively with acupuncture and moxibustion. Sometimes these treatments may be suitable, but we need to proceed with caution.

It is important not only to be intimately familiar with the methods of diagnoses, but also to know the various signs and pathologies. Otherwise the diagnostic process will have no direction and the information gleaned will not be usable. Since it is assumed that the readers of this book know the basics of East Asian medicine, this section will only touch on some of the highlights of the examination process.

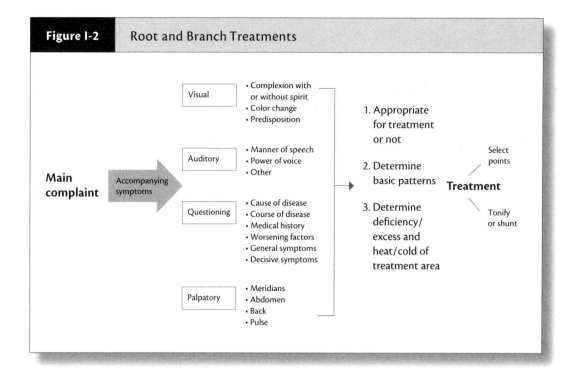

Figure I-2   Root and Branch Treatments

Visual

The appropriate visual signs are presented for each pattern in Part One of the text. Here, we will discuss the general outline of those items to look for.

SPIRIT

Simply put, examining the spirit means looking to see whether or not the patient appears to have vitality. This is primarily done by observing the quality of the facial color and complexion. There should be a healthy luster to the face. If there is a complete absence of luster and a pained or anguished expression, proceed with care or check again whether the patient is suitable for this type of treatment.

COLOR

The body in general, as well as particular areas of the face, are examined for color, which can evidence a disruption in a particular organ-meridian system. For example, if the whites of the eyes have a bluish tinge, there is Liver involvement; if the area between the eyebrows or the tongue itself is redder than normal, the Heart may be involved; if the lips are more pale or red than normal, there may be a problem with the Spleen or Stomach; if the overall complexion is pale, Lung deficiency is a possibility; and if the ears are dark, Kidney deficiency is suggested. There are a myriad of diagnostic clues available on close examination of a patient that are well worth observing.

PREDISPOSING FACTORS

Areas such as the eyes, ears, nose, and mouth are examined for their size and shape. For example, eyes that are large in relation to the rest of the face indicate a predisposition to Liver excess; a relatively large nose suggests a predisposition to Lung deficiency; relatively thin lips a predisposition to Spleen deficiency; and comparatively small ears a predisposition to Kidney deficiency.

The amount and distribution of body hair is also taken into account to assess the predisposition of the patient to a certain pattern. In general, those with more than normal body hair have a constitutional Lung deficiency. Furthermore, localized, particularly dense hair indicates areas where the function of opening and closing of the pores is weak.

Listening and Smelling

SPEECH

Check to see if the patient speaks clearly and cogently. This permits you to assess the emotional state of the individual. Patients who are unable to interact with the practitioner in a reasonable manner may not be mentally deranged, but they may be unsuitable for treatment or need to be approached with great care.

The manner in which a patient talks and the quality of his or her voice should always be assessed. Consider whether the voice is bright and lively or dull and depressed, and whether the individual exaggerates or is self-effacing or speaks in an angry tone. The speech should also be checked to see if it is clear or slurred. For example, a dull, depressed voice expressed in short, clipped sentences is indicative of Liver excess, while exaggerated speech indicates Stomach heat. A generally angry or irritable tone would be indicative of Liver yin deficiency. Along this line, a lively but somewhat unsettled speech pattern is often indicative of yin deficiency heat, with some heat stagnating in the chest.

STRENGTH OF VOICE

Listen to determine whether the voice has power. Those with weak voices need to be watched carefully, as a weak voice indicates yang deficiency, which means that the treatment should be minimal or short to avoid worsening the condition. Also the rate of recovery will be slower than for someone with a stronger voice, regardless of the main complaint.

OTHER FACTORS

Other factors, such as the volume of the voice, body odor, and the way the patient coughs, should all be noted. At the same time, avoid overemphasizing the information obtained in this way because, given all the possible interfering factors, there are times when the information may be irrelevant or very unreliable.

Questioning

MAIN COMPLAINT

The main complaint is the most distressing aspect of the illness to the patient, and its etiology and development should be investigated in some detail. There will be patients with very simple problems, such as fatigue and stiff shoulders, with no other particular complaints. There may be others whose main complaint is a medically-defined disease or syndrome. If there are few symptoms, it is more difficult to determine a pattern, but the pathology can be uncovered by intelligent questioning of some basic symptoms. While the patient's history should only be one part of the diagnostic process, when there is overwhelming evidence of some pathology in the history, it can play a determining role in the analysis.

On the other hand, we sometimes see patients who have so many symptoms that we get lost in the maze of the history to the point that it is difficult to determine the pattern. In these cases, it is important to take the history while keeping in mind the information gleaned from other aspects of the examination, thereby focusing on the salient information and not becoming distracted by the less important facts. Remember that when talking with the patient about the main complaint, the focus is to distinguish the site of the disease, that is, which system, organ, meridian, or meridian sinew is primarily involved, and whether the problem is acute or chronic. With these basic facts in mind, the course of the disease can be ascertained and the appropriate treatment methods applied.

ACCOMPANYING SYMPTOMS

The accompanying symptoms, while not always as important as the main complaint, are useful in classifying the underlying pathology and allowing the pattern to be more readily determined. An example would be checking for the presence of vomiting or dizziness in patients with a main complaint of headache. Relevant details of the questioning aspect of the examination are discussed in connection with individual conditions and diseases in Part Two of this text.

BACKGROUND CAUSES OF DISEASE

Disease can occur for a variety of reasons and with different histories. It can be acute in onset and then subside, develop slowly over time and become chronic, or be a mixture of both. It can arise because of changes in a patient's underlying constitution, work habits, living conditions, or lifestyle. All of this can make it difficult to ascertain the cause of the patient's disease, but once we do find the cause, it is easier to determine the pattern and decide whether or not treatment is appropriate. A good example is lower back pain. If we know that it is caused by physical labor, we may suspect blood deficiency, and can therefore begin to think of a Liver deficiency pattern. If the lower back pain occurs in a woman who also suffers from painful periods, it is more likely to be due to blood stasis.

Of course, living environment and work history also have a strong effect on the types of disease that people get, and on the course of their disease. For instance, there is a big difference in the intensity of physical work performed by an office worker compared with that of a manual laborer. Therefore, even those with pain in identical muscles can have different patterns. Examples of environmental effects would be overeating, which can lead to digestive problems, and spending a lot of time in damp places, which can make an individual vulnerable to wind-dampness.

ONSET AND COURSE OF A DISEASE

It is helpful to be clear on the progression of the patient's problem. We should both be clear as to the present symptoms—how things are at the beginning of the problem—and their subsequent progression. This is somewhat akin to questioning about the cause of the disease. For instance, if a patient has a history of a fever that later receded, then a complaint of pain must be looked at in terms of the fever before deciding on a pattern. Depending on the type of disease, it may be more important to treat the original disease than the present symptoms. A common example is a tooth problem that led to a headache. When this happens, it is better to stop the toothache first before working on the headache.

PAST MEDICAL HISTORY

When reviewing a patient's medical history, we check all the significant problems the person has had and see if there is any connection between them and the present symptoms. A common example is a patient presenting with lower back pain who has a history of a serious traffic accident. This would lead us to suspect blood stasis (Liver excess) as the main causative factor.

Family history can also be important. For example, there are patients with high blood pressure or diabetes who have parents or siblings with the same problem. When there is this type of genetic predisposition, the problem is more difficult to treat.

ADVERSE CONTRIBUTING FACTORS

In meridian therapy, we try to relate the presenting symptoms to things that may adversely affect them. This not only makes diagnosis easier, but also can lead to advice that helps the patient directly. The most common factors that we inquire about are the seasons, time of day, foods, and specific movements and postures that tend to aggravate (or ameliorate) the symptoms. When we check these things, we gather information that is useful in determining the pattern and deciding whether treatment is appropriate. Take the example of a patient whose symptoms tend to worsen in the spring. In that case, we know that this season is dependent upon the blood of the Liver, and so we can reasonably suspect a Liver deficiency pattern.

CHECKING THE AFFECTED AREA

If there is an internal organ problem, the area overlying the organ should be palpated. For example, if there is a muscle or joint problem, then the problem area should be palpated to determine the degree of deficiency, excess, heat, or cold in the local area. (See "Palpation" below.)

GENERAL SYMPTOMS

Irrespective of the nature of the main complaint, a few basic symptoms should be checked, including the state of the stool, urine, appetite, sleep, and degree of fatigue. These symptoms are useful in determining whether the basic pattern pertains to heat or cold, and may be directly connected with the main complaint itself. They are also good markers of the level of general health of the patient. In addition, this information can help us estimate how well the patient will respond to treatment, and the efficacy of treatment.

KEY SYMPTOMS

After questioning and physically examining the patient, we will invariably be led to a tentative conclusion about the nature of the pattern. In order to confirm our conclusions, we check for certain key symptoms that will always be present in the pattern we suspect. For example, a pattern of Liver yang deficiency may be associated with soft stools that are present only at the onset of a period; yang brightness heat may be associated with headaches that worsen in the afternoon; Spleen deficiency may be associated with diarrhea with pain and weakness after evacuation; and Kidney deficiency may be associated with feeling better after an evacuation. This type of information allows us not only to classify the pattern, but also to determine an appropriate treatment.

Palpation

MERIDIAN PALPATION

This is performed on the meridians that are to be treated as well as areas where there are manifestations of deficiency, excess, heat, or cold. We must be aware, however, that not all patients will exhibit tenderness and stiffness on palpation of the diseased area. This is especially true when dealing with patients suffering from cold patterns, or in the very elderly.

ABDOMINAL PALPATION

The abdomen can help us ascertain the pattern and whether an organ is hot or cold. Here again, though, we must also understand that if the disease is meridian or muscular based, the abdomen may not yield any useful information. Also, the abdomen is sometimes a mixture of constitutional factors and the effects of the current disease superimposed on each other; thus, differentiation of the two is important. From the abdomen, an experienced practitioner can identify past illness, the prognosis for the current illness, and the appropriateness of treatment. Abdominal diagnosis is presented for each pattern in Part One.

PALPATION OF THE BACK

The back is examined for dents and bulges, hard and soft areas, and areas of tenderness. Abnormal findings can be used to ascertain the specific organ which is manifesting deficiency, excess, heat, or cold.

PULSE

Most meridian therapists use the pulse to finalize their decision about the pattern. The pulse can be examined last, after the other diagnoses, and then, based on the information the pulse yields, more specific questions can be asked to check the suspected pattern. Another approach is to examine the pulse first, and then go through the other aspects of diagnosis. For example, if a patient with insomnia has a pulse with a sunken, strong quality at the right distal (Lung) position, the patient should be questioned about a history of respiratory problems. While the patient may not mention this himself, thinking it is unrelated to the problem at hand, the heat in the chest can have a direct influence on insomnia. If, as in this case, the pulse is examined first, the practitioner can immediately palpate the chest and check for heat or tension to confirm the presence of the pattern.

The pulse can also be used to determine whether acupuncture is the most appropriate form of treatment. For example, take a patient who comes in with lower back pain and fever and with a history of bladder infections. If the pulse at the left proximal position is sunken, excessive, and rapid, this would indicate that a bladder infection has affected the kidneys. Such a patient would benefit from a quick medical test, and would usually do best with Western medical treatment.

Ikeda Sensei often checks other pulses besides the radial pulse. This tradition goes back at least as far as *Basic Questions,* where it is discussed in detail in Chapter 12. The anterior tibialis and dorsal pedis pulses are noted in *Discussion of Cold Damage,* where they are called the lesser yin pulse (小陰の脈 *shōin no myaku/shào yīn mài*) and the in-step yang pulse (趺陽の脈 *fuyō no myaku/fū yáng mài*) respectively. The lesser yin pulse can be found at the posterior tibialis pulse, and is used to determine the state of the Kidneys; it is palpated at K-3. It should feel sunken and a little firm for those in good health. The in-step yang pulse is used to measure the state of the Spleen and Stomach. It is palpated at the dorsal pedis pulse (around ST-42), and, when healthy, should be floating and a little strong. These pulses can be used to confirm the pulses palpated on the radial artery when things are not clear.

Differentiation between Deficiency and Excess, and Heat and Cold

Performing an examination, making a diagnosis, and determining the basic pattern have far greater implications than just deciding which points are going to be used in the root treatment. A clear and complete diagnosis implies that we understand the following:

- the basic pattern, including whether it generated heat or cold
- the meridians to which the heat or cold have spread
- the type of treatment to be carried out on the back and abdomen
- the type of treatment to be carried out on the diseased part
- the overall degree of tonification or shunting that is required
- the specific techniques that are indicated
- the appropriateness of treatment, and the prognosis.

The root treatment is based primarily on the first two points noted above: an understanding of the basic pattern and a knowledge of which meridians have been affected by heat or cold. The points themselves, and the tonification and shunting techniques, are determined to a great extent by the basic hot or cold pattern; any treatment other than the root treatment is known as a branch treatment. While this is the conventional approach and has much to recommend it, there is no need to be too rigid in applying this definition. The root and branch treatments each represent two parts of the same whole, and no treatment can be considered complete without both. In actual practice, they become one entity, both from the viewpoint of the practitioner and the experience of the patient. (Both the root and branch treatments are discussed in greater detail in the sections entitled "Tonification and Shunting in the Root Treatment" and "Tonification and Shunting in the Branch Treatment" below.)

Simply by determining the pattern, some areas of the body will be favored as sites of treatment, but as far as the diseased part is concerned, nothing has been decided. For this we must look at the meridians of the back and abdomen that have been affected by heat or cold and decide how we're going to treat them.

The methods used to treat the diseased part will vary each time, and are subject to the conditions at the time of the treatment. This lack of a uniform practice can be confusing to the beginner, and for others as well. Here is a sketch of some approaches that I hope will be helpful. Part One discusses some of this materiel in more depth; here I have limited my remarks to background information.

Maintaining a Global Perspective

The core of meridian therapy is its focus on the basic heat and cold patterns. The practitioner must never lose sight of the overall or systemic pathology, and the diseased part should not be looked at independently from the whole. It can be misleading and unhelpful to get into an overly detailed analysis of the diseased part, as this can readily cause one to lose sight of the forest for the trees. An overly rigid focus on the diseased part makes it more difficult to respond with flexibility and in clinically effective ways. It will also stunt the practitioner's technical progress, and, at times, may lead to forgetting the importance of the meridians and concentrating instead on special points to cure diseases.

The basic principle of physiology in meridian therapy is that blood, fluids, and qi circulate through the meridians. Disorders or disruptions of this flow will manifest in deficiency, excess, heat, and/or cold that affect specific areas of the body, what we call the diseased part. The four basic types of problems are:

1. deficiency heat
2. excess heat
3. deficiency cold
4. cold due to blood stasis

The latter term is a synonym for Liver excess since a buildup of blood stasis in the interior of the body results in manifestations of cold in the outer portions.

Because these two states of deficiency and two states of excess are derived from problems of the blood, fluids, or qi, it follows that there is a total of twelve patterns to consider. Many novice practitioners find this a bit daunting; therefore, as far as the treatment of the diseased part is concerned, it is sufficient to classify the problem simply in terms of deficiency and excess. This allows us to proceed with tonification and shunting on a local level.

Initially, the practitioner should develop competency in diagnosing deficiency and excess; thereafter, she can move on to distinguishing heat from cold. With chronic disease, this can be difficult, and is often done only after a patient has failed to respond well to an initial set of treatments. When a lack of response requires a more detailed evaluation, we can assess the qi, blood, and fluids.

Basic Rules for Differentiation of Deficiency and Excess

We should determine how all the points we use affect the basic pattern and the presenting complaint. This applies both to points chosen for root treatment as well as those chosen for the branch treatments. For the root treatment of the yin meridians, however, once the pattern has been determined, the type of stimulation that is applied to the points is more or less decided. Nevertheless, even in this case, there are still times when we palpate the points for deficiency and excess and apply tonification and shunting accordingly. Table I-1 provides a list of the signs used to distinguish between deficiency, excess, heat, and cold in both the affected meridians and acupuncture points.

Table I-1	Signs of Deficiency, Excess, Heat, and Cold in the Meridians and Points	
	Heat	**Cold**
▶ DEFICIENCY		
	Pressure feels good even at hard areas	Pressure or heat feels good
	Swollen, but pressure causes a depression	Mushy and depressed or has slight tension
	Abnormal sensation of heat felt at the surface	Feeling of numbness and/or cold both inside and at the surface
	Floating and deficient pulse	Sunken and deficient pulse
▶ EXCESS		
	Pressure increases the pain	Pressure increases the pain
	Spontaneous pain	Fixed spontaneous pain
	Feeling of heat both inside and at the surface	Feeling of cold at the surface and hard resistant areas inside
	No sweating and reduced urination	Constipation
	Floating and excessive pulse	Sunken and excessive pulse

DIFFERENTIATION BY PALPATION

When a meridian is deficient or excessive, it will exhibit peculiar features on palpation, including pain upon pressure, hard areas, hollow areas, swelling, tightness, increased resistance, cold, heat, moistness, and dryness. Regardless of what else is found, the main method for distinguishing between deficiency and excess is by checking the response to pressure. When the pain increases with pressure, the condition is one of excess; if it feels better with pressure, the condition is one of deficiency. In addition, hard areas are regarded as sites of local blood stasis. Even so, this does not necessarily mean that we shunt these hard areas. They should be checked for pain on pressure before this is done. If the hard areas become less painful with pressure, they should be tonified.

DIFFERENTIATION BY SYMPTOMATOLOGY

This is done by evaluating the symptoms of the diseased part to determine whether it is deficient or excessive. For instance, if it is hot to the touch and there is spontaneous, fixed pain, the condition is one of excess. On the other hand, if it is cold to the touch and there is only intermittent pain with movement, this usually reflects a condition of deficiency. Other symptoms that are generally associated with excess are constipation, inability to sweat, and urinary difficulty. By contrast, diarrhea, spontaneous sweating, and copious urination are regarded as symptoms of deficiency. When it is difficult to differentiate on the basis of the symptoms, we do so by palpating the points.

DIFFERENTIATION BY PULSE

This is particularly important for problems that affect the entire organism, such as an acute febrile disease. In these cases, even if it is clear that heat or cold has already spread through the meridians, the pulse is used to determine the specific nature of the treatment, that is, the pulse is used to determine which meridians will be tonified and which will be shunted. Basically, shunting is used on a meridian if its corresponding position on the pulse is excessive, and tonification if it is deficient. Normally, treatment decisions are based on the pulse and symptoms, as well as the relation between them. If it is still difficult to make a diagnosis, we palpate the points themselves.

APPROACH TO DIAGNOSIS AND TREATMENT

On the most basic level, the treatment strategies used in meridian therapy are quite straightforward: tonify deficiency and shunt excess. Of course, it is not quite that simple and there are a few nuances associated with various patterns. The basic factors to keep in mind when considering the overall treatment include the number of points that will be used, the length of the treatment, the depth of needling, and the number of cones of moxa that will be burned.

To make things clearer for the reader, I will first note some general considerations that affect diagnosis and treatment. Next, I will outline a typical diagnostic and treatment sequence. These can be used as references.

Note that when treating, regardless of the location of the problem, patients should undress down to their underwear. At first, a patient may be reluctant to do so, but the practitioner should explain that whatever the problem, meridian therapy has a traditional approach whereby the whole body should be examined and treated for best results.

General Considerations

AGE AND GENDER

Children should normally be treated very delicately, for example, only a few points should be selected, the entire treatment should be short, needles should not be put in deeply, and only a few cones of moxa should be used. The very elderly are treated in a similar fashion.

It is traditionally thought that the needling should be lighter for men than for women, and that women should be needled more deeply (see Table I-2). This is because women are more likely to suffer from blood stasis.

ACUTE AND CHRONIC DISEASE

When treating an acute disease, use fewer points, shorter treatment time, a shallow needling depth, and only a small number of moxa cones. By contrast, for chronic disease, the needles are generally inserted more deeply, and more moxibustion is applied. As a rule of thumb, the number of moxa cones is equivalent to the patient's age. Naturally, for chronic disease, the treatment time is longer and the number of points used is greater than for acute disease.

Table I-2	Treatment Standards			
Division	Number of Points	Duration of Needling	Depth of Needling	Number of Moxa Cones
Children and elderly	Few	Short	Shallow	Few
Women versus men	Women more	Women longer	Women deeper	Women more
Acute versus chronic disease	Acute fewer	Acute shorter	Acute shallower	Acute fewer
Deficiency cold	Few	Short	Shallow	Few
Deficiency heat	A little more	A little longer	A little deeper	A little more
Excess cold	Many	Long	Deep	Many
Excess heat	Few	Short	Shallow but shuntive	Less but shuntive
Lung deficiency	Few	Short	Extremely short	Extremely few
Spleen deficiency	A little less	A little shorter	Shallow	A little less
Liver deficiency	Quite a lot	A little longer	A little deeper	Many
Kidney deficiency	Many	Long	Deep	Very many
Liver excess	Very many	Very long	Very deep	Very many

HOT AND COLD PATTERNS

Basically, use more needles and insert them rather deeply for hot conditions, and fewer needles and shallow insertions for cold patterns. When we add in the factors of deficiency and excess, we have the following patterns and methods:

- *Deficiency heat.* The treatment is based on tonification but the needling is a little deeper with a larger number of points, and a longer treatment time. Direct scarring moxibustion is performed so that the heat can sink a little deeper into the tissues.

- *Deficiency cold.* Use gentle, shallow needling on a few points over a short period of time. The moxibustion should not be too hot.

- *Excess heat.* Mainly, relatively shallow needling is performed at fewer points over a short period when shunting. When direct scarring moxibustion is used, it is done in a shunting manner; note that heat perception moxibustion can also be used.

- *Excess cold.* Even though the surface is cold, the interior often reflects blood stasis; needling is accordingly deep. Shunting is widely used, and if moxibustion is performed, many cones are applied.

DEPTH OF NEEDLING AND THE BASIC PATTERNS

- *Lung deficiency.* The disease is often found at the level of the skin and body hair. Contact needling is recommended, and even if the needles are inserted, they should be shallower than 1mm.

- *Spleen deficiency.* The disease is often found in the flesh, and the needling is accordingly shallow, that is, around 1mm.

- *Liver deficiency.* The disease is often found at the level of the muscles, and the needling is therefore a little deeper, around 3mm.

- *Kidney deficiency.* The disease is often in the bones, and the needling is accordingly deep. To us, a depth of 5mm is usually sufficient.

- *Liver excess:* Especially when the Liver excess has become chronic and transformed into blood stasis, the needling is deeper still. Generally speaking, the needles are inserted just until resistance from the hard area is encountered. It is not thought to be clinically efficient to needle through the hard area.

FACTORS THAT MAXIMIZE THE EFFICACY OF TREATMENT

An important factor in helping patients get the most from their treatment is the overall atmosphere and cleanliness of the clinic. The clinic should be a place to which the patient feels attracted, and in which he is comfortable. Consider carefully such factors as curtain colors, flowers, and music.

The personality of the practitioner is another important factor. It is important that the practitioner sincerely empathize with the patient, which is the real purpose of practicing a healing art. One common mistake that can be disastrous is to frighten a patient into compliance. This is very disruptive and cannot aid the healing process.

The practitioner should always treat the patient with consideration and gentleness. The pulse should be taken gently and not squeezed too hard. Needles should be gently inserted. The practitioner needs a comforting, gentle touch when palpating a patient. Putting a patient at ease is an important factor in helping them.

Normal Order of Examination and Treatment

EXAMINATION AND TREATMENT OF THE CHEST AND ABDOMEN

After taking the history and checking the pulse, the practitioner should have an idea about the pathology affecting the patient. At this point, the chest and abdomen are examined to see if the findings here confirm the original diagnosis. It is then a good idea to take the pulse again, as it has a tendency to change after palpation of the chest and abdomen.

Following this, needles are inserted and retained at points on the abdomen and chest. Then, if warranted by the main complaint, needles can also be retained anywhere else on the body, including the head, face, legs, and arms. Depending on the pattern, it is possible that the points used for the root treatment are also retained. Needles are generally retained from 15 to 30 minutes; however, depending on the pattern, scatter needling (described below under "Tonification and Shunting in the Branch Treatment") may be performed on the chest, and simple insertion is done on the arms and legs.

Needling of the chest and abdomen normally precedes the root treatment because it makes the pulse clearer. This allows for a more accurate assessment, which is critical for the root treatment. Furthermore, any blockage in the abdomen and chest is removed, improving the efficacy of the root treatment.

ROOT TREATMENT

After treating the chest and abdomen, the pulse is reexamined to confirm the pattern and thereby the points to be used for tonification and shunting.[2] After the root treatment is finished, tonification and shunting are performed on those meridians to which heat or cold have spread (Fig. I-3).

EXAMINATION AND TREATMENT OF THE BACK

....

[2] Guidelines for root treatment can be found in any book on basic meridian therapy. Two such books in English are Shudo Denmei, *Japanese Classical Acupuncture: Introduction to Meridian Therapy* (Seattle: Eastland Press, 1990) and the Society of Traditional Japanese Medicine, *Traditional Japanese Acupuncture: Fundamentals of Meridian Therapy* (Brookline, MA: Complementary Medicine Press, 2003).

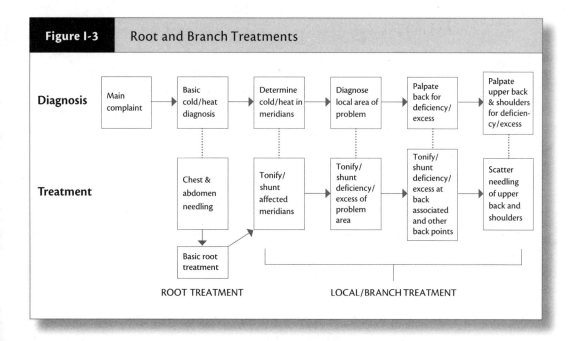

Figure I-3 Root and Branch Treatments

After the root treatment has been administered, the patient is asked to lie face down and the back is examined. The meridians are checked for deficiency and excess, and needles are inserted and retained anywhere on the back, from the upper thoracic area to the sacrum and pelvis. If necessary, needles may also be inserted and retained at areas such as the occiput, back of the neck, and back of the thighs. However, there are times when, depending on the pattern (e.g., Spleen yang deficiency), the needling will consist of simple insertion only.

TREATMENT OF THE UPPER BACK AND SHOULDERS

Last of all, the upper back and shoulders are treated, and the session is brought to an end. Sometimes there is no need to treat the shoulders.

WHEN THE BRANCH TREATMENT SHOULD BE DONE FIRST

When the symptoms are particularly severe, sometimes the branch treatment should be performed first. In this case, the position assumed by the patient should be one that is comfortable, which may not be the usual face-up or face-down position.

MODIFYING THE BASIC ORDER OF TREATMENT

The order of treatment is thought of in terms of yin and yang. For instance, if the diseased part is in the upper part of the body, the lower part is treated first. Conversely, if the diseased part is in the lower part of the body, the upper part is treated first. If the diseased part is in the chest, the upper back is treated first, and if the diseased part is in the lower back, the abdomen is treated first.

TONIFICATION AND SHUNTING

Background

To recapitulate, from the perspective of meridian therapy, the basic principle of physiology is the systemic movement of qi and blood through the meridians. When, for a variety of reasons, there is either a lack (deficiency) or stagnation (excess) of qi and blood, heat or cold will be produced. If this is allowed to continue, it can lead to states that include qi deficiency, qi excess, blood deficiency, blood excess, lack of fluids (dryness), and too much fluid (water stagnation, dampness, or phlegm-thin mucus). We try to understand these states in terms of the basic pattern of deficiency. We then use acupuncture needles and moxibustion to influence the flow and production of qi and blood through the affected meridians in such a way that the body's own healing mechanisms are reinforced and the problem is resolved.

For example, a pattern of Liver deficiency/heat that leads to heat in the Large Intestine meridian can cause a standstill in the flow of qi and blood within the Large Intestine meridian. This leads to stiffness and heat, eventually resulting, for example, in a toothache. In order to treat the toothache, we tonify the Liver to treat the deficiency heat and then apply tonification and/or shunting to the Large intestine meridian, depending on the status of that meridian. At the same time, after differentiating between excess and deficiency at the local level, tonification and shunting can also be applied to the diseased part, which here would include not only the area around the tooth but the neck, shoulders, and any meridian that traverses the problem area. When we actually examine the meridians and points of the diseased part, we will find many changes including stiffness, swelling, depression, numbness, pain on pressure, heat, cold, dryness, and localized edema. Basically speaking, tonification is used when there is pain from deficiency and shunting is used when there is pain from excess. We should remember, however, that the actual techniques of tonification and shunting will vary according to whether the basic pattern is hot or cold, as discussed below.

Meaning and Varieties of Tonification and Shunting

The reader has undoubtedly noticed that in this book we use the term 'shunting' instead of the customary 'draining' for the needling technique and effect. This usage is based on the fact that the Chinese character for this word found in the *Inner Classic* and other classical texts is 寫, which I have translated as shunting, and not 瀉, which came into usage later and is translated as draining. For the sake of completeness, here are the definitions of all three terms as understood by Ikeda Sensei.

TONIFICATION (補 *hō/bǔ*)

- The process used to treat a condition where the qi, blood, and fluids are lacking, thereby causing a reduced flow of these elements.

- The process used to increase the production of qi, blood, and/or fluids.
- The process whereby the yang qi of the qi, blood, and fluids is increased.

DRAINING (瀉 *sha/xiè*)

- The process whereby stagnant qi, blood, and fluids are discharged from the body.
- The process by which qi is radiated out from the body; this can be done using heat perception moxibustion or dispersive scatter needling.
- The process whereby blood is removed from the body to improve its flow; this can be done using pricking to bleed, hook needling, and suppurative moxibustion.

SHUNTING (寫 *sha/xiè*)

- The process used to free the movement of stuck qi, blood, and fluids.
- The process used to resupply areas lacking in qi, blood, and fluids.
- The process whereby the yin qi of the qi, blood, and fluids is increased and the yang qi is decreased or inhibited.

Tonifying and Shunting Methods

1. USING THE BREATH

- *Tonification.* The needle is inserted as the patient breathes out and withdrawn as the patient breathes in. The hole is closed after withdrawal of the needle.
- *Shunting.* The needle is inserted when the patient breathes in and withdrawn when the patient breathes out. The hole can be closed or left open. When there is a large amount of heat, the hole should be left open.
- *Usage.* This method is suitable when needles are retained in the abdomen and back, and also when using a big needle. The technique is performed while observing the patient's breath. The practitioner's breath should also be considered; that is, when used for tonifying, the practitioner should inhale while inserting the needle and exhale while withdrawing it. Similarly, when used for shunting, the practitioner should exhale while inserting the needle and inhale while withdrawing it.

2. USING STABLE PRESSURE WITH OPENING AND CLOSING THE HOLE

- *Tonification.* Pressure is applied along the direction of flow of the meridian in question. Once the point is selected, the left hand is never separated from the point, and the guide tube is dug into the point and clamped into position. The needle is then inserted until the area of deficiency is felt through the fingertips. When the qi is felt to arrive, the needle is withdrawn and the hole is quickly closed.

- *Shunting.* Pressure is applied against the direction of flow of the meridian to scatter areas of heat arising from stagnation. Then the needle and tube are positioned as for tonification, and the needle is inserted. This time, however, the needle is inserted until heat is felt to gather at the tip of the needle; at this point, the needle is withdrawn. This is done slowly with the hole open, and it should feel like a hot air balloon that is slowly discharging its contents externally.

- *Usage.* As a tonifying method, it is used for yin deficiency heat. As a shunting method, it is used for Liver excess/heat, yang brightness meridian excess/heat, or Spleen deficiency/Stomach excess/heat.

3. Using the Direction of Meridian Flow

- *Tonification.* The meridians are gently stroked in the direction of their flow. The left hand is lightly positioned with the feeling that something warm is being added to the system so as to increase the blood flow through the area, and then the needle is inserted. The needles are withdrawn at the same time as the hole is closed.

- *Shunting.* The meridians are rubbed against their direction of flow, and then the left hand is lightly positioned. The needle is inserted so as to increase the blood flow through stagnant areas. When the blood is felt to have begun flowing, the needle is withdrawn and the hole is closed.

- *Usage.* As a tonifying method, it is used for cold patterns, especially Liver deficiency/cold. As a shunting method, it is used for Liver excess/blood stasis.

4. Using the Slow or Fast Technique

- *Tonification.* The needle is inserted and withdrawn slowly, as if you have all the time in the world. The left hand is very gentle, and the patient must experience no pain at all. Contact needling and extremely shallow needling are used.

- *Shunting.* The needle is quickly inserted and quickly withdrawn, as if searching by hand for something that is immersed in hot water.

- *Usage.* As a tonifying method, it is used for cold patterns. As a shunting method, it is used for yang excess patterns and for disease in local areas where there is a large amount of heat.

5. Using the Nails

By *nails* we do not mean just the nails, but also the fingertips. This is because using the fingertips emphasizes the abrasive and splitting functions of the digits.

- *Tonification.* The area around the point is stimulated using the nails of the thumb and fingers, like a gentle scratching of the skin, until the flow of qi is improved; only then is the needle inserted. If the flow of qi is still sluggish, the head of the needle can be vibrated to cause the qi to arrive.

- *Shunting.* The points are pressed until either hard areas, or areas where the thumb and fingers catch, are found. These areas are then pressed with the nails until they soften, at which point they are needled.

- *Usage.* As a tonifying method, it is used for heat patterns. As a shunting method, it is used for Liver excess/blood stasis or where there are hard, stiff areas with localized blood stasis.

6. VARYING THE DEPTH OF NEEDLING

- *Tonification.* The needle is either merely touched to the point or is inserted very shallowly. When the qi arrives, the needle is withdrawn. The left hand is gentle, and when the arrival of yang qi is felt, the qi is sent into the yin areas of the body; that is, when the qi is felt on the surface (the yang qi, by definition), the left hand presses it deeper into the tissues so that it stays in the body. The needle is not inserted deeper at this time. Once this is done, the needle is withdrawn.

- *Shunting.* The point is massaged well and the needle is inserted slightly deeper than for tonification. When the qi is felt in the inside (the yin qi, by definition), it is drawn up to the yang areas and the needle is then withdrawn.

- *Usage.* As a tonifying method, it is used for cold patterns. As a shunting method, it is used for yin deficiency/heat patterns when there is a large amount of heat in the yang areas.

7. USING MOXIBUSTION

- *Tonification method no. 1.* This consists of direct scarring moxibustion, but is performed in such a manner that it is not felt to be hot, but warm. This is done by covering the first cone, leaving an unburnt base on which further moxa cones are burned.

- *Usage.* This is applied at depressed areas that are lacking in resilience, or in chilled areas. It is often applied to the lower abdomen on the Conception vessel.

- *Tonification method no. 2.* The cones are rolled softly, pushed onto the points, and burned. This type of moxibustion should be performed in such a manner that the heat sinks in deeply and feels good.

- *Usage.* This method is most suitable for points that exhibit signs of yin deficiency.

- *Tonification method no. 3.* The cones are again rolled softly and burned directly on the skin. The number of cones burned is equivalent to the patient's age. At first, the cones feel hot, but gradually this sensation subsides. The moxibustion is continued until the heat is felt once again.

- *Usage.* This is performed on hard areas.

- *Shunting method no. 1.* The cones are rolled tightly, and are burned so as to feel extremely hot.

- *Usage.* This is used on hard areas that display pain or heat from excess. Normally, one cone is sufficient.

- *Shunting method no. 2.* The moxa is rolled into big cones, and when the heat is felt, the cones are removed.

- *Usage.* This method is used on hard, hot, or soggy areas where the aim is to disperse the stagnant yang qi.

Tonification and Shunting in the Root Treatment

YIN DEFICIENCY HEAT

The area around the point may be raised as a result of the deficiency heat, and the tendons may be rather taut, making the point difficult to find. In this case, the area should be pressed thoroughly, checking for the point and finding it precisely before needling. Even if the tendons are very tight, the points to be used will manifest as holes the size of the diameter of a guide tube or a finger tip. It is best to use method (2) or (5) for tonification and shunting as needed.

The needles are retained at a depth where they just pierce the skin on the affected meridians. If the heat is very intense, scatter needling shunting is performed using method (4), that is, as if searching for something immersed in hot water. In addition, for this type of problem, it is also possible to shunt by using method (6). The shunting can be used to tonify the yin meridians using the yang meridians; for example, the Liver meridian can be tonified by needling deeply at GB-34.

YANG DEFICIENCY COLD

Depressed and very cold points are selected and extremely shallow needling or contact needling is performed; the left hand must be gentle throughout. Tonifying can be done by using method (4), needling as if you have all the time in the world. It is also appropriate to tonify by carefully utilizing the direction of flow in the meridians, method (3).

Areas to which heat has retreated due to an increase in cold will exhibit hardness. These points should be tonified by inserting and withtdrawing slowly, as the underlying cause is cold and not heat. They will get harder if shunting or draining is used.

YANG EXCESS HEAT

Extremely shallow needling is used on the yin meridians. Since the yang meridians are relatively excessive and very hot, shunting is performed using method (4). Needles are inserted to an extremely shallow depth for the yin meridians, while the yang meridians are relatively excessive and very hot. When there is excessive pain, the area can be pricked and bled (draining technique).

YIN EXCESS HEAT

Hard points are selected, and deep needling is performed against the flow of the meridians, that is, method (3). Both tonification and shunting can be performed, using methods (2) and (5). If there is excessive pain, pricking to bleed a few drops can be very helpful (draining technique).

Tonification and Shunting in the Branch Treatment

At hard areas, insert the needles just to the depth of the hard spot and retain the needles. The needles should not pierce through the hard points, otherwise the hardness will not 'melt' and disperse along the course of the meridian. Areas that experience excessive pain and heat should be shunted using the scatter needling method or heat perception moxibustion.

Shallow retained needles should be applied to areas with deficiency pain and deficiency heat. Tonifying scatter needling or direct scarring moxibustion is also useful. Tonifying scatter needling should also be applied to areas where there are depressions, numbness, or cold.

Shunting using the scatter needling technique is performed in the following manner. The left hand is used to brush or wipe the skin quickly before the scatter needling is done. The right hand is used to bring the needle to the left hand where it is clamped into place with the forefinger and thumb. At this time there is a feeling of convergence of the 'two trinities': the left hand, right hand, and needle, and the patient, practitioner, and universe. In this way, the left hand takes out trapped heat and reduces stiffness and tightness in the tissues.

To tonify using scatter needling, the left hand moves less and contacts the skin lightly and warmly, with no brushing or rubbing movements, moving slowly from point to point. Tonification can also be performed by retaining for only a short time needles that are inserted to an extremely shallow depth, so that the needle just barely manages to stay in the skin. In addition, direct scarring moxibustion that causes only warmth, but not painful heat, is also considered to be tonifying in nature.

Areas that are very dry and lacking in luster respond well to tonifying scatter needling and direct scarring moxibustion. Tonifying scatter needling and heat perception moxibustion are also good on areas where there is a buildup of water.

Note on Certain Techniques

Throughout the text Ikeda Sensei refers to certain techniques which, while commonly used in Japan, may be unfamiliar to practitioners in the West. Below are brief descriptions of some of these techniques and modalities.[3]

知熱灸 *Heat perception moxibustion (chi netsu kyuu)*: A 1cm cone of coarse moxa is applied to the skin and removed as soon as the patient feels that it is hot. Usually, this does not leave a scar.

透熱灸 *Direct scarring moxibustion, penetrating moxibustion (tou netsu kyuu)*: Very fine moxa, formed into rice-grain (or even smaller) sized cones, is applied directly to the skin. It is allowed to burn all the way down, and thus leaves a small scar.

灸頭鍼 *Needle head moxibustion (kyuu tou shin)*: The heat from the moxa is conducted deeply into the tissues through an acupuncture needle. A ball of moxa is affixed to the head of a needle that has been inserted to a reasonable depth, and then lit. Usually, this type of moxibustion does not leave a scar.

導引 *Do In massage:* A term used to differentiate between the type of massage performed with due regard to Oriental medical pathology and physiology, and other forms of massage that do not consider these factors. Generally performed by the practitioner, some aspects of Do In massage can be done by patients themselves as a form of self-care.

Conclusion

Ikeda Sensei always makes a point of saying that what he is doing is not his own approach or style, but that of the classics, and nothing more. While some people insist on calling what he does the "Ikeda style" or some such name, he is not interested in style or making a name for himself. In most cases, he just cannot understand what all the fuss is about when he lectures or demonstrates. He himself describes what he does in the following terms: " I am just practicing medicine as outlined in the classics. I am doing nothing special. It is just that most people nowadays are performing below-average treatment." When receiving or

....

[3] A demonstration of these and many other techniques by Ikeda Masakazu was filmed and is available on DVD from Eastland Press at *www.eastlandpress.com.* The title of the DVD is the *Art of Acupuncture.*

observing Ikeda Sensei's "nothing special" treatments, one immediately gets a keen sense that something crisp and well-ordered is going on.

The diagnosis is flexibly and expertly fashioned around the four methods to garner information that is always greater than the sum of the individual parts. This information is then processed by Ikeda Sensei, using the full weight of classical physiology and pathology, to lead to a diagnosis of the pattern of disharmony. This actually translates into an informed touch and method of communication that varies with the disorder. With this in place, the patient begins to assume a steadily more passive and open state, allowing Ikeda Sensei to easily manipulate the patient's qi. It is in this state that a touch from a needle, a puff of heat from moxibustion, or a kind word—all powered by his intention—have a stunning intensity that leads the person into health. Patient and practitioner are engaged in an exchange of qi that occurs in an honest way that is rarely seen today. This can be thought of as the state before polarity (無極 *mu kyoku/wú jí*), from which yin and yang arise. Once access to this state is gained, the theories and practice of the classics take on an even more profound meaning, and remarkable clinical results can be obtained.

The term 'pattern' is used a lot in this book. Those who practice meridian therapy can often be a bit smug about this term. They cite this as the main difference between their approach and others. They say that treatment according to pattern enables them to treat more effectively than just using points or herbs based on the symptoms or effects of the points or herbs. However, when their methods are examined, we find that they actually spend very little time considering the physiology or pathology of the patient, and determine the pattern based primarily on the relative strength of the pulse; they then use the appropriate five phase points for treatment. In these cases, the 'pattern' devolves into nothing more than the use of four points, which makes a mockery of the concept of using the meridians.

On the other hand, there may be other practitioners who may not use or even be aware of the term 'pattern,' but who treat patients with knowledge of their physiology and pathology with splendid results.

Therefore, it must be said that a master of the caliber of Ikeda Sensei does not treat strictly according to the 'pattern.' His treatments are too fluid and too alive to be limited by an ironclad armor that is made for someone else to wear. What we can say is that his treatments can be viewed very conveniently in terms of the pattern.

It is the responsibility of each practitioner to be as fully informed as possible about the particular patient that he is treating. This is the real meaning of the word pattern (証 *shō/zhèng)* and is inevitably the purpose underlying this entire book. It is not about a style or a particular person. It is an approach toward a fuller understanding of Oriental medicine based on the classics.

The most important thing to understand is that Ikeda Sensei has a flexibility of mind that enables him to grasp, manipulate, and indeed enjoy a number of concepts at the same time. This is very useful in the clinic. So, in addition to learning the approach espoused in this book, it is a good idea to try and divine the mind behind it. Although this may seem to be a rather abstract goal, it is actually the most productive shortcut in terms of results. This is because you will then be able to create your own treatment strategies and approaches; it is what I call the self-generating stage, which takes some time to get to, but is well worth the effort.

Every student of any classical art has to go through this process. In the beginning, there can be no real creativity because technique, basic principles, and sheer learning by rote are of prime importance. In this early stage, the student can feel almost suffocated, or at least bogged down, by the overwhelming weight of observing and incorporating the tradition. Over time, however, the student graduates to becoming less a student of the mechanics and more a student of the energetics. Then, slowly but surely, a very solid type of creativity becomes apparent in the individual; while this vision is based upon classical principles, it nevertheless appears fresh and new.

There is an old Chinese saying, 温故知新 (*on ko chi shin/wēn gù zhī xīn*), which means that reviewing the past allows one to understand the present. Strictly speaking, there probably is nothing new under the sun, but our interpretation of it can be fresh and clinically effective when it is based on tried and tested principles. Contrary to popular opinion, to practice traditional Chinese medicine requires a lively, fluid approach, not a docile follower mentality. If this approach is not in place, treatment will never become the vigorous reality that it should be.

As a final word, I must thank our editors at Eastland Press, Dan Bensky and Louis Poncz. Their dogged determination that this book be of maximum use to a Western audience has significantly improved it. I would also like to thank all the people who help me at my clinic and in my life, especially John Blazevic and Akiko Yoshikawa, who have suffered greatly at my hands and yet have never refused to help me in times of need. Special thanks to Roger Ames for the valuable advice and the little black bits in the eggs and bacon. Foremost thanks to Ikeda Sensei for all his kind and patient teachings, clinical genius, and outrageous humanity.

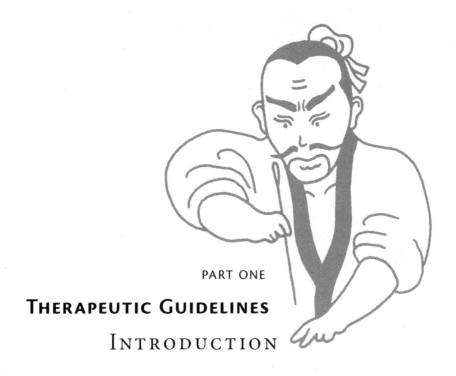

PART ONE

THERAPEUTIC GUIDELINES

INTRODUCTION

Patients will present with various symptoms, some of which may include modern medical terms. How are these patients to be treated using the therapeutic methods of acupuncture and moxibustion? Effective treatment hinges on the correct use of meridians and points, as well as deciding whether acupuncture and/or moxibustion should be applied and to what extent. This is an area of interest for all genuine practitioners.

It is for this reason that I have consulted both classical references and the works of senior colleagues in the field to produce this book. Some practitioners approach treatment from a meridian therapy standpoint while others use modern medical disease classifications as the basis of their treatment. In actual practice, this does not represent much of a divide because the desired result, curing the disease, is the same in all cases. The approach used in this book is to list the disease names, patterns, relevant diagnostic methods, and treatment strategies, including the meridians and points to be used.

I wish to make clear that I am most familiar with classical, traditional acupuncture and moxibustion. Bearing this in mind, the contents of this book may appear biased at times. On these occasions, the reader is invited to refer to the treatment methods of other practitioners. If the practitioner is experienced, then even if his methods are not so traditional, they will always be worth examining.

The so-called meridian therapy method emphasizes pulse diagnosis to determine the meridians which are excessive or deficient. It then bases its treatment on the classics: "For deficiency, tonify it; for excess, shunt it."[1] Point selection is carried out and tonification and shunting applied to these points. This system of identifying the root pattern (証 *shō/zhèng*[2]), which is present in even the most complicated of diseases, and then treating it, is a simple and excellent system of treatment.

It is worth noting that often those trained in the meridian therapy method find it difficult to make use of the information found in old texts written prior to and up through the Edo period (1603-1868). These premodern medical texts were written as part of what was primarily a tradition of oral transmission, where their meaning was explained by the master to the student. As such, they were written in a sort of shorthand. This has caused misunderstandings in two ways. The first has to do with the names assigned to diseases. It is my understanding that in the older texts, the traditional disease name automatically expressed the etiology and pathology of that disease, including the underlying deficiencies. Unfortunately, in the modern meridian therapy system, the technical terms such as Liver deficiency, Spleen deficiency, Kidney deficiency, and Lung deficiency are used without making the relevant pathologies, which are of central importance, clearly understood. This has caused a gap to open up between this system and the older texts such that its practitioners have lost the ability to access the wealth of useful information in those texts. The second misunderstanding is that the information recorded in the older texts is often mostly concerned with the 'branch' or 'local' part of the treatment (標治法 *hyō ji hō/biāo zhì fǎ*), which is aimed directly at the dysfunctional or painful area. There is little, if any, mention of the relevant deficient meridians and of the root treatment (本治法 *hon ji hō/běn zhì fǎ*), which is the part aimed at the root cause of the disease. I believe that this occurred because the root treatment is so obvious that it did not need to be recorded.

With this in mind, I have devoted the first part of this book to a detailed explanation of the etiology, pathology, and symptoms of the basic patterns. The patterns are as important as the disease name in Western medicine, that is, they are an essential piece of information in determining a proper and effective treatment; they are therefore dealt with in some detail in this book. Also, for each of the patterns, the reader will find listed the signs and symptoms that are likely to be uncovered as a result of the questioning and checking of

....

[1] *Classic of Difficulties* (難経), Chapter 69. Probably compiled in the late Han period, this text consists of 81 chapters and details a range of acupuncture theory and practice in the form of questions and answers about difficult passages in other medical classics. The book is traditionally attributed to the legendary healer Bian Que who supposedly lived sometime between 500 and 300 BCE. He is often described as being half bird, half man.

[2] This term is also translated into English as 'presentation' or 'syndrome.' For more information, see Shudo Denmai, *Japanese Classical Acupuncture: Introduction to Meridian Therapy*, and the Society of Traditional Japanese Medicine, *Traditional Japanese Acupuncture: Fundamentals of Meridian Therapy*.

the pulse and abdomen, as well as the appropriate tonifying and shunting techniques for the root treatment. In this way, the contents of Part One will help the practitioner to more fully understand the old texts, and will lay the groundwork for understanding the treatment strategies that are set forth in Part Two.

Traditional medicine is an organic, open-ended system. It is not a rigid way of thinking or working. The basic patterns discussed in Part One cover the vast majority of basic patterns that we see in patients, but the list is not comprehensive, nor is it intended to be. Similarly, all the information about diagnosis, including the presenting pulses and the points chosen, should be seen as general guidelines that must be modified by the specific situation you encounter in the clinic. This will be demonstrated repeatedly in Part Two.

It is important to remember that traditional treatment focuses on tailoring a treatment to suit the individual's condition and needs. Therefore, just like a tailor would do for his customer, we must 'tailor' the basic patterns to the patient in front of us. For example, if the patient presented with a pattern of Liver deficiency/yin deficiency with cough as the main symptoms, the basic pattern would be nudged into a Lung-biased treatment by including the metal points on the Liver and Kidney meridians. Similarly, high blood pressure with the same root pattern would be 'tailored' by including the fire points on the Liver and Kidney meridians. If both patients were given precisely the same root treatment, this would not be treating them as individuals. Rather, returning to our tailor analogy, this would be the equivalent of forcing them into a mass-produced suit which would be much cheaper and more conveniently had at the local department store.

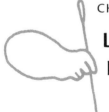

CHAPTER 1

LUNG DEFICIENCY / YANG EXCESS / HEAT PATTERN

肺虚陽実熱証

hai kyo yō jitsu netsu shō/fèi xū yáng shí rè zhèng

YANG QI HAS the basic properties of warmth and movement and thus constantly diffuses and circulates. When for some reason its circulation is interrupted, heat stagnation develops, resulting in a fever. If this occurs in areas connected with yang energy, the result is a pattern of yang excess (陽実証 *yō jitsu shō/yáng shí zhèng*), a process that is often associated with acute fevers.

The yang area can include the yang meridians, the yang organs, and also the relatively yang (or superior) yin organs, the Heart and Lungs. The Heart, however, being a fire organ, will normally have an abundance of heat; if it receives any extra heat, the result would be death. In addition, because the Heart is constantly active, there is no opportunity for the yang qi to stop circulating and stagnate in the Heart. It is for these reasons that in the classic texts, such as Chapter 71 of the *Divine Pivot,* the Heart is compared to the ruler and it is considered impossible for the Heart to become diseased since that would result in death.

Furthermore, because the Kidneys store the fluids, even if they became affected by heat, they would simply dry out, which would not lead to a condition of excess. The Liver stores blood, and if this blood receives heat, it is possible that a condition of excess would arise, albeit one of yin excess. As noted in Chapter 4 of the *Divine Pivot,* the Spleen cannot be in a state of excess, for if heat tries to enter the Spleen it will be pushed out into the Stomach. For these reasons, a pattern of yang excess refers solely to the buildup of heat and stagnation in the yang meridians, the yang organs, and, by default, the Lungs.

BACKGROUND

The Lungs are said to be associated with the qi and with the body hair. The yang qi of the Lungs circulates throughout the body and controls the opening and closing of the pores. This regulation of pore size allows the yang qi to be retained or radiated outward such that the pores themselves act as windows for the entry and exit of qi.

4

The yang qi circulated by the Lungs makes its way to the outermost area of the body, the greater yang meridian. At the same time, the yang qi from the Stomach also travels to the greater yang meridian, and it is these two types of yang qi that come together to protect the body from external pathogens, that is, wind, cold, heat, dampness, dryness, and fire. These pathogens are influenced by changes in such aspects of the environment as the outside temperature, moisture, and atmospheric pressure. The cold will especially be felt when there is a lack of yang qi in the greater yang meridian. Then again, this yang qi can soon be replenished by eating warm food and by exercising. This is because the Lungs work to circulate the yang qi that is delivered by the Stomach.

However, if the lack of yang qi in the greater yang meridian is combined with either undernourishment or overindulgence in food, or with mental or spiritual stress, then the Lungs will be unable to circulate the yang qi properly. When this occurs, the yang qi of the greater yang meridian is not replenished, resulting in chills. Normally, the Lungs react to the chills by attempting to replenish the yang qi in the greater yang meridian. If, however, the Lung qi is deficient, there will not be enough yang qi to clear the chills. Furthermore, there will not be enough power to circulate or radiate the yang qi, causing it to stagnate and give rise to chills with a fever. From our perspective, this stagnation—which is called cold damage or greater yang excess/heat—is considered a yang excess. Nonetheless, it originates from Lung deficiency; thus, either the term Lung deficiency/yang excess/heat or Lung deficiency/greater yang meridian excess/heat can be used to describe this pattern.

Next is the case where the fever trapped in the greater yang meridian begins to seep a little deeper into the yang brightness meridian. As one might expect, this creates a Lung deficiency/yang brightness meridian excess/heat pattern. Tonification of the Lung will resolve the condition in both of these cases.

We can see from this discussion that there are two types of Lung deficiency/yang excess patterns. When there is yang brightness meridian excess/heat, the chills lessen, but are still present. This is due to the fact that the yang qi both warms and radiates heat. With a relative lack of yang qi, both of these functions will diminish. If, as noted above, the heat from the stagnation goes deeper over time, reaching the yang brightness meridian, the chills will then subside, but instead, there will be an increase in body temperature, the neck and head will become stiff and achy, and the eyes and nose will become painful and dry. In addition, since the stagnant heat has not been expelled by sweating and has no place to go except to the Stomach, which is the yang organ of the yang brightness meridian, secondary symptoms may also include vomiting or diarrhea.

Finally, the term miscellaneous diseases (雑病 *zatsu byō/zá bìng*), which goes back to Zhang Zhong-Jing, generally refers to all internal medical diseases that are not directly related to an external pathogen. This type of disease does not usually engender a greater yang meridian excess/heat pattern, but it is a possible outcome. When this happens, problems such as sinusitis, rhinitis, stiff shoulders, upper body pains, skin disease, muscle soreness, and toothaches may readily occur.

It is important to remember that even for cold damage or other disorders linked to external pathogens, the main issue is not the external pathogen itself but the underlying deficiency that allows an external pathogen to invade.

EXAMINATION

Visual

The chills followed by fever cause the face to redden easily and the eyes to be watery. The tongue tends to be dry with little or no coating. Those with a constitutional tendency toward Lung deficiency/yang excess/heat tend to have a relatively dense covering of body hair, as this protects them. They are more susceptible to these Lung patterns because their skin pores do not open and close properly.

Pulse

As a result of the Lung deficiency, the right distal and medial pulses are found to be deficient when pressed firmly. If the overall quality of the pulse is floating and strong, these pulses can then be quite difficult to discern.

The greater yang meridian excess/heat pattern causes the pulse to be floating, rapid, and tight, and the yang brightness meridian excess/heat causes the pulse to become a little larger, floating, rapid, and excessive. The floating and rapid pulse indicates that the yang qi (heat) has become stagnant on the surface. The tight pulse shows that the disease has developed from a cold pathogen and chills are present.

As noted above, when the yang brightness meridian heat stage is reached, the chills will diminish and the heat trapped in the yang brightness meridians will increase. Heat stagnation causes things in general to expand and become more relaxed, in contrast to cold stagnation, which causes things to contract and become tense. This manifests in the pulse here, as the tightness will disappear as the pulse becomes bigger and excessive in nature.

If, however, the yang brightness meridian excess/heat pattern is a miscellaneous disease, that is, not caused by an attack of an external pathogen, the pulse will be floating, big, and powerful. If the pulse is pressed firmly, then it will be slightly rough.*

---

*A rough (渋 shoku/sè) pulse is often described as having the feeling of cutting a piece of bamboo with a small knife that often gets stuck. This pulse indicates poor movement of qi and blood. It is the opposite of a slippery pulse.

Abdomen

In the case of a Lung deficiency/yang excess/heat pattern, the sickness is on the surface so no significant changes will occur in the abdomen. If anything is noted, it will probably be constitutional in nature. This type of sign may reflect a certain vulnerability, but its presence or absence is irrelevant during acute illness.

TREATMENT

First, the Lung deficiency should be tonified; LU-8, LU-9, and HT-7 are common choices (TABLE 1). LU-8 is the metal point on the Lung meridian and LU-9 is the mother, earth point. HT-7 is used as a preventative to keep the cold or heat from entering deeper into the lesser yin meridian.

Next, it is necessary to shunt the stagnant heat in the yang meridians. For the greater yang meridian excess/heat, BL-63, BL-67, and SI-1 are shunted. For yang brightness excess/heat, LI-1, LI-2, and LI-4 can be shunted.

The points mentioned are those that I normally use; other points, however, are also possible. The main idea is to achieve the objective of no deficiency or excess. The yang meridians tend to be areas where symptoms are easily expressed. Therefore, shunting points should be chosen with an eye toward shunting any excess and balancing the qi in those meridians.

Tonification of the Protective Qi

By tonifying the Lung meridian, the protective qi is automatically tonified. This results in increased yang qi, which removes the chills while also dispersing heat from stagnation. In order to further tonify the protective qi, gentle needling is performed by just touching the skin with the needle tip without the use of a guide tube, which might inadvertently disperse the protective qi by pressing against the skin. Only the tip of the needle should be pressed firmly onto the skin. The needle is placed in line with the flow of the meridian and is held firmly in place with the pushing hand (normally the left) until the qi arrives. The arrival of qi is signaled by various phenomena, including warmth along the course of the meridian, the disappearance of chills, or the appearance of slight sweating accompanied by a reduction in fever. When the pattern includes chills or a fever, a systemic treatment should be used that primarily involves tonifying the protective qi. In a miscellaneous (chronic) disease, areas lacking in protective qi are characterized by lack of skin luster and an overall weakness due to low muscle tone. In both of these cases, the needles should not be left in place.

Shunting of the Nutritive Qi

When there is yang brightness meridian excess/heat, it will be necessary to shunt the

Table 1	Lung Deficiency/Yang Excess/Heat Patterns	
	Lung deficiency/greater yang excess/ heat pattern	**Lung deficiency/yang brightness excess/ heat pattern**
PULSE	Overall: floating, rapid, and tight Right distal and medial positions: deficient when pressed firmly	Overall: floating, rapid, excess, and big Right distal and medial positions: deficient when pressed firmly
SYMPTOMS	Chills, fever, headache, cough, wheezing, joint pain, and no sweating	Chills, fever, headache, neck stiffness, nasal discharge, sore throat, no sweating, occasional diarrhea, eye pain, and buildup of pus
TONIFYING POINTS	LU-8, LU-9, HT-7	LU-9, LU-8
SHUNTING POINTS	BL-63, BL-67, SI-1	LI-1, LI-2, LI-4

nutritive qi, which resolves the stagnation, thereby reducing the fever, and increases the flow of blood and fluids. To accomplish this, the site of the stagnant heat or hard mass is selected and needled in the direction opposite to the flow of qi in the meridian. The depth of the needling is determined by the extent of the fever, the pain upon pressure, or the size of any indurations. For example, for a pattern of Lung deficiency/yang brightness meridian excess/heat, a 1- to 2mm painless insertion is sufficient. The emphasis is on the left hand opening the hole and pressing down with the hand when the needle is withdrawn. Finally, the amount of shunting of the nutritive qi is determined by the response of the skin to the needling: The greater the number of red blotches, the more shunting of nutritive qi is required.

For miscellaneous diseases, hard masses on the Stomach meridian are selected and needled down to the center of the mass; the needle is held in place until the area softens. Practitioners feel a sense of heaviness upon entering the hard mass that is released as the mass disappears.

USE OF THICK NEEDLES AND PRICKING THE COLLATERALS

If the use of thin needles does not bring good results, then, depending on the area, thick Chinese needles (equal to or thicker than 0.22mm) are used to bleed areas that are dark, or centers of localized heat, or areas where the blood vessels are discolored. For example, pricking is commonly done on the well points.

SHUNTING WITH MOXIBUSTION

For chronic conditions, hard masses on the upper back or along the Stomach meridian are selected for direct scarring moxibustion. Moxibustion is essentially a tonification method, but when it is used on these hard, tight areas, it is actually 'shuntive' in nature. For these areas, five to seven cones are preferred, but if no heat is felt, the cones should be burned every day. Another method is to burn in a single application up to 20 cones, or even a number of cones equal to the age of the patient. The cones are usually a half rice grain in size.

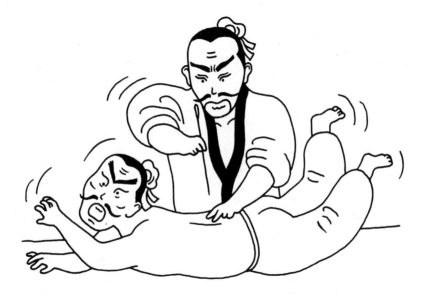

The shunting needling method is performed full-blown

HEAT-PERCEPTION MOXIBUSTION (知熱灸 *chi netsu kyū/zhī rè jiǔ*)

This type of moxibustion is applied to the surface of hard masses or areas where there is stagnant heat. The cone has a 1cm diameter and is 1cm tall, and it is removed as soon as it is felt to be hot.

RETAINED NEEDLES (置鍼 *chi shin/zhí zhēn*)

When there are chills or fever, the needles are usually not retained. However, this is not the case for the branch treatment of chronic conditions where retaining the needles can be used for both tonifying and shunting. (Retaining the needles is not used for root treatment purposes.) I maintain that the root treatment should be the most lively and active part of the treatment, where the patient's balance is restored to health. This is one reason that I do not usually retain needles for the root treatment. In addition, many premodern texts state that needles are to be stimulated for only a certain number of breaths. This is not supportive of the idea of retained needles, particularly in the root treatment.

When the nutritive qi is to be tonified and the needles are to be left in place, I use 0.1mm needles that are 1.3 units in length and insert the needle to a depth ranging from 0.1 to 1mm. When the nutritive qi is deficient in a particular area, that area may be hard and bulging, but a hole opens when the area is pressed. It is in this hole that the needle is inserted and left in place. When the nutritive qi is to be shunted and the needles are to be left in place, the needle is inserted a little deeper, about 2 to 3mm; alternatively, a thicker needle can be used with a more shallow insertion. The important points are summarized in Table 1.

Herbal Treatment

Deficiency of Lung qi with heat trapped in the greater yang meridian can cause chills and a fever without sweating. In this case, a formula containing both Cinnamomi Ramulus (*kei shi/guì zhī*) and Ephedrae Herba (*ma ō/má huáng*) can be used. A typical formula would be Ephedra Decoction (麻黄湯 *ma ō tō/má huáng tāng*).

When the heat trapped in the greater yang meridian increases, it can spread to the great brightness meridian. In this case, the flow of qi in the greater yang meridian should be increased by using Puerariae Radix *(kakkon/gé gēn)*. A typical formula would be Kudzu Decoction (葛根湯 *kakkon tō/gé gēn tāng*).

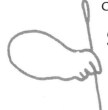

CHAPTER 2

Spleen Deficiency / Yang Excess / Heat Pattern

脾虚陽実熱証

hi kyo yō jitsu netsu shō/pí xū yáng shí rè zhèng

Yang excess, as explained above, is defined as stagnant heat occurring in any or all of the yang meridians, the yang organs, or the Lungs. When making this diagnosis, the practitioner should determine the foci of the nonradiating heat, as this is where the stagnant heat is found. In this chapter, yang excess caused by Spleen deficiency is examined.

Background

Looking at Spleen disorders gives us a brief and very useful overview of how the various systems of the body work together. The Spleen is the central or middle organ and is one of the key points in the body for a variety of transformations. The Spleen and Stomach are considered one unit, so whatever affects the Spleen affects the Stomach. Similarly, the Stomach is associated with one of the two yang brightness meridians, the other being the Large Intestine. Often, a problem with one of the yang brightness meridians will affect the other, and Large Intestine problems often end up affecting its paired yin organ, the Lungs. Another reason why Spleen and Lung problems often occur together is that the Lung meridian begins in the middle burner, and so if the Spleen is deficient, it cannot produce enough qi for the Lungs, as earth is the mother of metal in the generative cycle of the five phases. These influences go both ways, that is, heat in the greater yang meridian, which formed as a result of Lung deficiency, can stagnate over time and penetrate to the yang brightness meridians. All these connections must be kept in mind when approaching problems where Spleen deficiency is the root.

The transformative functions of the Spleen underlie the activity that leads to digestion of foods and liquids by the Stomach and Intestines, which produce qi, blood, and fluids. The qi that is produced from this process is circulated throughout the body by the Lungs. The blood is circulated by way of the blood vessels, while the Liver also stores some of it.

The fluids are delivered to the Kidneys and stored. The blood and fluids are then used to produce body hair, blood vessels, flesh, muscles, bones, organs, and other aspects of the body that have a form. Fleshy components comprise a large portion of these, thus the Spleen is said to control the flesh. The impurities in ingested food and liquids are processed through the Small and Large Intestines and eliminated by way of the Large Intestine and Bladder. Finally, as noted in Chapter 8 of *Basic Questions*, the Gallbladder works to maintain the overall balance of the body.

When there is deficiency of the Spleen, there will automatically be a problem with the Stomach meridian, the flesh, and all the other organs. Depending on the individual's constitution and other factors, such as whether there is deficiency of blood or fluids, this can turn to either heat or cold. Usually, individuals with blood deficiency tend toward cold while those with fluid deficiency tend toward heat. When the deficiency turns to heat, there are a variety of manifestations, including stagnant heat in the yang brightness meridian, the yang organs, and the Lungs. This pattern is known as Spleen deficiency/yang excess/heat.

When there is deficiency in the Spleen coupled with excess heat in the yang brightness meridians, fluid collects in the flesh. In this state, should an external pathogen like wind or cold also be present, it will lead to damp diseases.

The Stomach receives instructions from the Spleen and produces yang qi, which makes its way to the surface of the body where it is discharged (radiated outward). This discharge is in part achieved by the Lungs, but, as noted above, also by the Stomach itself. This is reflected in the fact that hot meals can induce sweating, which is a form of yang qi discharge. However, if the Spleen is deficient, the yang qi of the Stomach is constrained at the level of the yang brightness meridian and does not spread as far as the greater yang meridian. In this state, sweating cannot occur, and fluids that are to be distributed to the flesh collect there instead. With the addition of external pathogens, the yang qi becomes stagnant, resulting in heat and fluids combining to produce such symptoms as swelling in the flesh or joints and/or pain. Of course, reduced urination, chills, and fever may also be present, and this pattern is defined as Spleen deficiency/yang brightness meridian excess/heat. This pattern is often present with acute or chronic arthritis and/or skin diseases.

Next, let us consider the previously mentioned Lung deficiency/greater yang or yang brightness meridian excess/heat patterns. If the Spleen is deficient, the heat from these patterns can enter and damage the digestive system. Based on the admonition in Chapter 69 of the *Classic of Difficulties* to tonify the mother when there is deficiency, both the Spleen and the Lungs are tonified for patterns of Lung deficiency. If the heat enters the Stomach and the Intestines, it could also invade neighboring yang organs and yin meridians, resulting in a depletion of yin qi and fluids and even greater fever. At the same time, heat would lodge in the Gallbladder and Bladder, giving rise to the pattern known as Spleen deficiency/yang organ excess/heat pattern. Another possibility is that the Lungs are also invaded by this heat, in which case it would be called Spleen deficiency/Lung excess/heat pattern.

When there is heat in the yang organs, the chills and aversion to cold disappear, leaving only fever marked by an aversion to heat. Another possibility is that there may be fever that increases in the afternoon. Other symptoms are a feeling of fullness in the abdomen, constipation, sweating from the hands and feet, and incoherent speech, all of which arise from heat accumulating in the Stomach and Intestines.

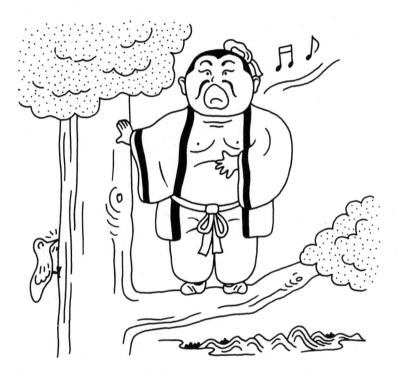

Those with Stomach excess climb to high places and start singing

The earliest clear description of excess heat in the yang organs is found in the *Discussion of Cold Damage*, where the treatment of choice is purgatives. This problem often arises from acute febrile diseases, and when the heat takes a hold at this level of the body it is difficult to shift. This type of pattern is not often seen in the average Oriental medical clinic today. It will definitely not respond to treatment unless there is a strong emphasis on discharging the heat through the stool.

If the individual's constitution or a chronic illness is causing the Spleen deficiency/yang organ excess/heat pattern, there will be a tendency to overeat. There are even cases where the person will eat glass. The voice is abnormally loud, with a fondness for singing, and there is an intolerance of heat, with a desire to strip naked when possible. These patients tend to have strong hands and feet and are very active, often overeating and overdrinking.

The second pattern, Spleen deficiency/Lung excess/heat, is referred to as knotted chest (結胸 *kekkyō/jié xiōng*) in the *Discussion of Cold Damage*. This obviously describes the tight feeling experienced in the chest with this pattern, which can readily develop in disease states such as pneumonia with symptoms such as a stiff neck and back, and tight chest with wheezing. This pattern can sometimes be a result of constitutional factors that lead to chronic asthma. However, acute fevers that have lingered and end up causing further damage are the most common cause.

Finally, it should be remembered that neither Liver deficiency resulting in Gallbladder meridian excess nor Kidney deficiency resulting in Bladder meridian excess are referred to as yang excess. This is because in these cases, yin deficiency, that is, deficiency of fluids, is the main component. This is different from cases of Lung deficiency, discussed in Chapter 1, where the deficiency is of that organ's yang qi, which in turn leads to excess in the related meridians.

EXAMINATION

Visual

Those with either a chronic Spleen deficiency/yang organ excess/heat pattern, or who have a constitution that favors that pattern, usually have large lips and tend to be overweight. With a pattern of Spleen deficiency/yang brightness meridian excess/heat, there will be joint swelling with spontaneous pain and a reddish sheen to the skin. This joint swelling is a form of swelling from excess.

Spleen deficiency with either a yang organ excess/heat pattern or Lung excess/heat pattern can result in an acute fever with a red face and a feeling of intense feverishness. Because of the fever, the patient will often avoid the use of blankets, and when the fever is particularly high, speech will be incoherent. The tongue will be dry with a yellow coating, and the lips will be dry and sometimes cracked.

Pulse

Over time, the pulse associated with an excess heat pattern will become sunken because the heat, which is not being radiated outward, instead moves deeper into the body. However, for yang brightness meridian excess/heat, the pulse will often be floating, as this condition is just a little deeper than the greater yang level, and some heat is still being produced. Pressing firmly will reveal that the left distal and right medial pulses are deficient, while pressing lightly at the right medial position reveals a strong, easily-felt pulse. Excess heat in the yang brightness yang organs will result in a sunken, excessive pulse. Of course, if there is a fever, the pulse will be rapid. If pressed firmly, the right medial position, rather than the left distal position, will display overt deficiency. Should this become a chronic condition, the left proximal pulse will often become deficient as the heat from the yang organs consumes the fluids of the Kidneys.

Lung heat manifests as a sunken, rapid, excessive pulse, but a large pulse is often prominently felt. The prominence of the large pulse makes it seem to be floating in nature. If pressed firmly, the left distal position will be deficient, but the right distal position will be excessive.

For chronic Lung excess/heat, the pulse will be sunken, wiry, and rapid, and, when pressed firmly, both the left and right distal positions will be excessive. On the other hand, the left and right proximal pulses will be deficient because the excess heat from the Lungs affects the Heart, and, at the same time, dries out the Kidney fluids.

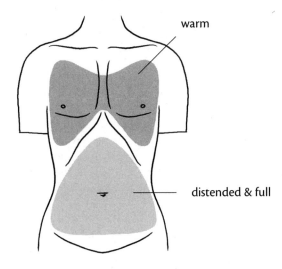

warm

distended & full

Fig. 2   Abdominal signs for Spleen deficiency/yang excess pattern

Abdomen

The abdomen is swollen overall, and when pressed, will show resilience (FIG. 2). The patient will often complain of abdominal distention. When there is Lung heat, there will be a feeling of heat throughout the chest. This can easily be checked by delicately touching the chest with the palm of the hand. The affected area will feel as if it is emitting heat upward through the hand.

TREATMENT

When there is either a yang brightness meridian excess/heat pattern or a yang organ excess/heat pattern, PC-8 and SP-2 are tonified (TABLE 2). For Lung excess/heat, HT-4, HT-5, and LU-10 are tonified. The reason for tonifying the Heart meridian is to increase the yin qi of the lesser yin meridian so that the fever in the chest can be removed. This is effective because, while the Heart organ is related to fire, and is thus yang in nature, to maintain balance, the Heart meridian is yin and therefore cooling. The point LU-10 is the fire point of the Lung meridian; tonifying it increases the bitter principle, which tonifies the fluids, and thus clears Lung heat.

Table 2	Spleen Deficiency/Yang Excess/Heat Patterns		
	Spleen deficiency/yang brightness meridian excess/heat pattern	Spleen deficiency/ yang organ excess/ heat pattern	Spleen deficiency/ Lung excess/ heat pattern
PULSE	Overall: (a) sunken, thin, rapid, and excess; or (b) floating, rapid, and excessive Left distal and right medial positions: deficient when pressed firmly	Overall: sunken, rapid, and excessive Right medial position: deficient when pressed deeply Left proximal position: becomes deficient over time	Overall: sunken, rapid, excessive, and big Left distal position: deficient All other positions: excessive, with right distal position especially sunken and excessive
SYMPTOMS	Chills, fever, joint pain (especially in the afternoon), swollen joints, urinary difficulty	No chills but only fever, sweating of hands and feet, delirium, high fever in the evenings, bloated stomach, constipation	Pain and fullness in the epigastric region, wheezing, fever, stiff neck, constipation
TONIFYING POINTS	PC-8, SP-2	PC-8, SP-2	HT-4, HT-5, LU-10
SHUNTING POINTS	ST-36, SI-6, LI-2	BL-54, ST-36, ST-37, ST-39	LU-6, LU-7, LI-4

For a pattern of yang brightness meridian excess/heat, points such as ST-36, SI-6, and LI-2 are used for shunting. For a yang organ excess/heat pattern, points such as BL-54, ST-36, ST-37, and ST-39 are used for shunting. The reason for dispersing BL-54 is to remove the heat from the Bladder meridian caused by the fever from the Stomach and Intestines that is drying up the Kidney fluids. By removing the Bladder heat, the Kidney fluids are increased and the Stomach and Intestines are cooled down. For the Lung excess/heat pattern, LU-6, LU-7, and LI-4 are dispersed. LI-4 on the yang meridian is used to dispel yin meridian heat.

Tonification of Nutritive Qi

For patterns of Spleen deficiency/yang excess, first, tonify the nutritive qi. This will improve the circulation of blood and fluids, and thereby reduce the fever. The area to be needled is kneaded thoroughly—Chapter 78 of the *Classic of Difficulties* states that the fingernails should be used in an "angry manner"—but the important point is to bring blood to the area. For point selection, one should select the areas that are hard but have a dent in them; one should needle the dent.

For points that are located relatively proximally, such as KI-7 and PC-6, it will be found that kneading the flesh will cause depressions about the size of an insertion tube to appear. The left hand is firmly applied to these points, and the needle is inserted in the same direction as the flow of qi in the meridian. At first, a depth of 2 or 3mm is sufficient, at which point the practitioner should be able to feel the qi sensation. If no sensation is detected, the needle is inserted a little deeper. Another method is to vibrate the needle or rotate it toward the midline until the qi sensation is felt. The needle is then withdrawn and the hole is pressed shut to prevent any leakage of qi from the point.

For areas located more distal to KI-7 and PC-6, kneading will reveal tight, thin bands of tissue to which needling can be applied. When this is done properly, the area around the points as well as the involved meridian will warm up and start to pulse slightly. Sensitive patients may also feel a sensation like warm bubbles or very light tingling moving along the meridians in these areas. These sensations differ from the muscular contraction or heavy pressure associated with deep needling.

Shunting of Nutritive Qi

In order to disperse fever from the yang brightness meridian, the yang organ, or the Lungs, the dispersive method described in Chapter 1 can be used, namely, using the dent in the hard areas. If the fever is particularly strong, deeper needling is performed more often and sometimes blood letting may be necessary.

Herbal Treatment

Spleen deficiency that leads to heat and dampness trapped in the yang brightness meridian is treated with formulas containing both Ephedrae Herba (*ma ō/má huáng*) and Gypsum fibrosum (*sekkō/shí gāo*). This will expel heat and dampness by means of urination. A typical formula would be Maidservant from Yue Decoction plus Atractylodes (越婢加朮湯 *eppi ka jutsu tō/yùe bì jiā zhú tāng*).

When the yin qi of the Spleen is deficient and heat increases and becomes trapped in the Stomach and Intestines, a formula containing both Rhei Radix et Rhizoma (*daiō/dà huáng*) and Natrii Sulfas (*bōshō/máng xiāo*) is used to expel heat by way of the feces. A typical formula would be Major Order the Qi Decoction (大承気湯 *dai shō ki tō/dà chéng qì tāng*).

CHAPTER 3

Lung Deficiency / Yang Deficiency / Cold Pattern

肺虚陽虚 寒証

hai kyo yō kyo kan shō/fèi xū yáng xū hán zhèng

Yang deficiency refers to a lack of yang qi. Because the yang qi is hot in nature, yang deficiency indicates a cold condition. Of course, the deficiency of yang qi can occur in both the yang meridians as well as the organs themselves.

As noted in Chapter 1, the Lungs and Heart are the yin organs that are relatively yang, due in part to their position above the diaphragm. As such, they have a large amount of yang qi. The blood stored by the Liver also contains yang qi. The Spleen itself has no yang qi, but the Stomach is brimming with it. As noted in Chapter 76 of the *Divine Pivot* and Chapter 36 of the *Classic of Difficulties*, the Kidneys have their own yang qi, but also receive some from the Heart by way of the Pericardium, which descends and becomes the fire at the gate of vitality.

The various yang qi of the yin organs are collectively known as ministerial fire (相火 *sō ka/xiāng huǒ*), and the most important of these is the fire at the gate of vitality, also known as the source qi of the Triple Burner. The ministerial fire serves to make the yin organs function and is also present in the connected yang organs and their corresponding yang meridians. In addition, the Stomach produces and sends yang qi to the yang meridians. This is why on the yang meridians the source points—where the Triple Burner source qi and the ministerial fire are accessed—and the earth points are distinct.

When the term yang deficiency is used here, it refers to a simultaneous depletion of the yang qi of both the yin organs and the yang meridians. This can also be explained in another way by considering that all disease begins with a deficiency of essential qi (精気 *sei ki/jīng qì*) in the yin organs. Normally, when there is a deficiency in the yin aspect, heat increases in the yang aspect. However, if the patient's constitution is one that has little yang qi, or if a mistaken method of treatment was previously attempted, there may be an absence of heat in the yang aspect even though the yin is deficient. This indicates a deficiency of the yang qi in both the yang meridians and the yin organs themselves, and this is why this state is sometimes referred to as a double deficiency of the yin and yang.

Normally, with Lung deficiency the pulse is felt easily on light pressure but disappears under heavy pressure. This indicates yin deficiency with the qi collecting in the yang areas. However, in the case of yang deficiency, the pulse becomes sunken and weak, or floating and weak. The difference between the two states can be explained by the fact that, in the case of stagnation, the qi is somewhat blocked from moving internally, so even more of it radiates outward. By contrast, in the case of yang deficiency, there is not enough qi to radiate outward. The symptoms are mostly cold-based; however, there are cases where heat is also present. Therefore, a yang deficiency/cold pattern means that both the yin and yang must be tonified, otherwise a cure is impossible. There are a number of types of yang deficiency. In this chapter, we will explain the Lung deficiency/yang deficiency patterns.

BACKGROUND

When the body is exposed to wind it produces fever. Classically, this was known as fever and irritability because it was caused by the constraint of yang qi in the outermost aspects of the greater yang meridian or stage. When the yang qi is stagnant, fever will be produced. If the yin qi is also deficient, this will adversely affect the contracting function of the greater yang meridian, which is evidenced by profuse sweating. The yin qi has the function of contracting, and when it is deficient, sweating will be profuse. If the yin qi is deficient and the only other problem is that of the greater yang meridian, the pattern can be cured in a couple of hours by restoring normal function to the Lungs, which circulate the yang qi and control the opening and closing of the pores.

However, there are also instances where the Lung qi is deficient and the yang qi does not circulate properly, resulting in pores that do not close as tightly or as well as they should. In this state, there will be continued sweating. At the same time, the yang qi that has ceased to circulate becomes stagnant, leading to fever. Exposure to wind and drafts while sweating will cause such symptoms as chills, headaches, and general malaise. Therefore, the term Lung deficiency/yang deficiency/cold pattern or Lung deficiency/greater yang meridian deficiency/cold *can* be used to describe this pattern (see, however, below). In the same way, Lung deficiency can lead to the yang qi becoming blocked in the yang brightness meridian. Since in that case heat is produced, the term Lung deficiency/yang brightness meridian deficiency/heat *can* be used to describe this pattern.

Where chills are dominant, the term yang deficiency/cold *may* be used. By contrast, where stagnant heat symptoms are dominant, the term yang deficiency/heat *may* be used. However, it should be noted that both of these states are derived from a common pathway where the chills come first and the fever follows. In addition, in this book, it is necessary to differentiate between these two patterns and the more serious yang deficiency/cold pattern. For this reason, both of the two patterns above will be classified here as yang deficiency/heat patterns.

The two Lung deficiencies discussed above should be treated by tonifying the Lung meridian and the yang meridians; otherwise, a cure will not be possible. Also, even if the pulse is floating and there is a fever, the pattern is that of yang deficiency. In *Discussion of Cold Damage* it is known as wind attack (中風 *chū fū/zhòng fēng*) of the greater yang.

In the early stages of Lung deficiency the pulse is floating. If improper treatment is given, the Lungs will become even more deficient, leading to a more pronounced deficient pulse. Furthermore, the fever will be replaced by chills, heavy sweating will occur or urination will increase, and the legs will become chilled and cramped. This type of development is seen in chronic rheumatism and neuralgia.

There is a continuum among the various types of Lung deficiency from greater yang meridian deficiency/heat to yang deficiency/cold to Lung cold. It is sometimes difficult to differentiate among them, but it is important. If Lung yang deficiency continues to worsen, the pulse will become sunken and weak, and the sweating will cease; instead of fever, chills become the main problem, and symptoms such as sore throat, chilled legs, coughing, and copious urination become evident. This is known as a Lung deficiency/yang deficiency/cold pattern. This pattern can be found among the miscellaneous diseases, but there are no chills or fever, just a feeling of a long, drawn-out cold with such symptoms as coughing and nasal congestion. Depression that is a result of qi deficiency of the Lungs is another symptom that is often seen; it belongs under the rubric of Lung deficiency/yang deficiency. If the yang deficiency continues to progress even further, the Lungs themselves will become chilled, which results in very stubborn coughs, a whole body sensation of cold, and extreme lassitude. This pattern is known as Lung deficiency/Lung cold.

EXAMINATION

Visual

When a fever is present, the face is obviously red in coloration, and as the fever disappears and chills become evident, the face begins to lose its color. As the yang deficiency progresses, the face eventually becomes pale and lifeless. Further progression of yang deficiency leads to the loss of skin luster of the whole body. The tongue is generally moist with teeth marks.

An individual with a constitution of Lung yang deficiency will have pale skin and a propensity to sweat easily. Also, women with this tendency often have relatively profuse, fine body hair.

Pulse

Obviously, as we are dealing with Lung deficiency, the right distal and right medial pulses will be deficient on firm pressure. For the greater yang meridian deficiency/heat pattern, the pulse will be floating, rapid, and deficient. If the fever has progressed as far as the yang brightness meridian, the pulse will become slightly bigger. When the condition reaches that of the Lung deficiency/yang deficiency/cold pattern, the previously floating pulse begins to sink and the deficient pulse becomes more deficient, changing to a weak pulse. Of course, if there is a fever, the pulse will be rapid.

When the qi of the Lungs is deficient, the pulse will be sunken, deficient, rough, and thin. The rough pulse indicates that the flow of qi is constricted and circulating poorly. When the Lung deficiency/Lung cold pattern is reached, the pulse becomes completely sunken and thin.

Abdomen

Since the symptoms associated with Lung deficiency/yang deficiency patterns are mostly superficial, there will be little if any change in the abdomen. Such changes as are present would be indicative of a different pattern, or of constitutional factors that are not relevant (TABLE 3).

TREATMENT

For the Lung deficiency/greater yang meridian deficiency/heat pattern, LU-8, LU-9, and BL-58 are tonified (TABLE 3). For the Lung deficiency/yang brightness meridian deficiency/heat pattern, LU-9, SP-4, and LI-11 are tonified; in addition, the protective qi at ST-44 is shunted if there are headaches and stiff neck and back, and the skin is lightly stroked after the needling. Needling of BL-58 and LI-11 is performed to tonify their respective yang meridians and to strengthen the yang qi overall. This will allow heat to radiate out. SP-4 is the connecting point on the Spleen and can therefore tonify both of the connected yin and yang meridians. This is important in yang deficiency patterns because yang deficiency contains an element of deficiency of both the yin and the yang. For the Lung deficiency/yang deficiency/cold pattern, LU-9, HT-7, and SP 5 are tonified. For the Lung deficiency/Lung cold pattern, LU-8, SP-5, and LI-11 are tonified.

For Lung deficiency/yang deficiency patterns, it is easy to unwittingly disperse the protective qi. To avoid this, treatment must be performed very carefully. The entire root treatment should be focused on tonifying the protective qi.

The overall treatment should involve gentle contact needling with no needles left in place. Normally a distinct lack in resilience and luster will be evident around the Lung points on the back. If this is the case, some light moxibustion until warmth is felt at BL-13 and BL-42 will be beneficial. Moxibustion should be performed until there is a slight redness around the points. For chronic Lung qi deficiency, needles can be retained in the upper back with the insertions shallow enough that the needles end up lying flat on the back.

Table 3	Lung Deficiency/Yang Deficiency/Cold Patterns	
	1. Lung deficiency/greater yang meridian deficiency/heat pattern	**2. Lung deficiency/yang brightness meridian deficiency/heat pattern**
PULSE	Overall: floating, rapid, deficient Proximal position: deficient Right distal and middle positions: deficient when pressed firmly	Overall: floating, rapid, deficient, and big Right distal and middle positions: deficient when pressed firmly
SYMPTOMS	Chills, aversion to wind, fever, headaches, sweating, nasal discharge	Chills, aversion to wind, fever, stiff and painful neck, sweating, wheezing, coughing, rhinitis
TONIFYING POINTS	LU-9, LU-8, BL-58	LU-9, SP-4, LI-11
SHUNTING POINTS	None	ST-44
	3. Lung deficiency/yang deficiency/cold pattern	**4. Lung deficiency/Lung cold pattern**
PULSE	Overall: (a) floating and weak or sunken; (b) weak and rapid; or (c) sunken, rough, and thin Right distal and middle positions: deficient when pressed firmly	Overall: sunken, thin, rough, and deficient Right distal and middle positions: deficient when pressed firmly
SYMPTOMS	Sweating or no sweating with chills, aversion to wind, and cold feet	Coughing, copious urine, excessive saliva, cold hands and feet
TONIFYING POINTS	LU-9, HT-7, SP-5	LU-8, SP-5, LU-11
SHUNTING POINTS	None	None

Herbal Treatment

When there is heat trapped in the greater yang meridian and there is sweating and a soft pulse, Cinnamomi Ramulus (*keishi/guì zhī*) and Paeoniae Radix (*shakuyaku/sháo yào*) should be combined in a formula. This will improve the opening and closing of the skin pores and cause the sweating to stop. A typical formula would be Cinnamon Twig Decoction (桂枝湯*kei shi tō/guì zhī tāng*).

When there is heat trapped in the yang brightness meridian and there is sweating and a soft pulse, Puerariae Radix (*kakkon/gé gēn*) should be used. A typical formula would be Cinnamon Twig Decoction plus Kudzu (桂枝加葛根湯 *kei shi ka ka kon tō/guì zhī jiā gé gēn tāng*).

For deficiency of yang qi in the greater yang meridian leading to symptoms that include chills and spontaneous sweating—one form of the Lung deficiency/yang deficiency/cold pattern described above—a typical formula would be Cinnamon Twig Decoction plus Prepared Aconite Accessory Root (桂枝加附子湯 *kei shi ka bu shi tō/guì zhī jiā fù zǐ tāng*). However, when the qi of the greater yang meridian is exhausted, sweating stops, and there are mainly cold-based symptoms—one form of the Lung deficiency/Lung cold pattern described above—a typical formula would be Ephedra, Asarum, and Prepared Aconite Accessory Root Decoction (麻黄附子細辛湯 *ma ō bu shi sai shin tō/má huáng xì xīn fù zǐ tāng*).

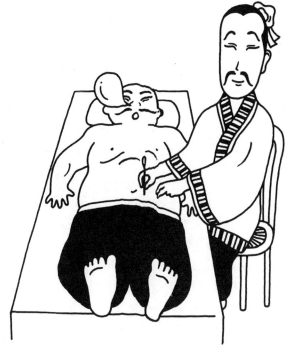

Tonification of defensive qi is performed gently

When there are no chills or fever and the main problem is a result of Lung qi deficiency, a typical combination would be Cyperus and Perilla Leaf Powder (香蘇散 *kō so san/xiāng sū sǎn*). When the Lung qi is deficient to the extent that cold has spread as far as the Lungs themselves, a typical formula would be Gleditsia Fruit Pill (皂莢丸 *sō kyō gan/zào jiá wán*).*

....

* This formula comes from Chapter 7 of the *Essentials from the Golden Cabinet* and is made up of ground Gleditsiae Fructus (*so kyo/zào jiá*) and honey.

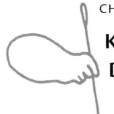

CHAPTER 4

KIDNEY DEFICIENCY / YANG DEFICIENCY / COLD PATTERN

腎虚陽虚寒証

jin kyo yō kyo kan shō/shèn xū yáng xū hán zhèng

BACKGROUND

As explained in Chapter 1 with regard to Lung deficiency/yang excess/heat patterns, if the circulation of Lung qi is poor, the amount of Stomach yang qi will become insufficient. Should this occur, it will be impossible to replenish the yang qi of the greater yang meridian, and chills will result. If the Lung deficiency is particularly marked, the disease will progress in its chilled state. If, however, the Lungs improve, the yang qi will circulate, and the patient will warm up.

This chilled state occurs when the Lung qi becomes deficient and the yang qi of the greater yang meridian fades, leaving its paired lesser yin meridian full of yin qi. It is because of this relatively large amount of yin qi that the disease is marked by sensations of cold. This state can also occur through mistaken diagnosis and treatment of a Lung deficiency/greater yang meridian excess/heat pattern or a Lung deficiency/greater yang meridian deficiency/heat pattern. Patterns of Lung deficiency/yang deficiency/heat or Lung deficiency/yang deficiency/cold are especially prone to evolving into a pattern of Kidney deficiency/yang deficiency/cold.

When the Kidney yin qi increases, cold will become more marked. In its extreme state, the whole body will become cold, and the patient will even be loathe to move. In the acute stage, the patient will often just doze off, waking only to pass large amounts of clear urine. At the same time, the small amount of yang qi that is left in the lesser yin meridian begins to push upward, causing pain in the throat. Since it is essential in such cases to tonify the yang qi of the Kidneys to affect a cure, this state is known as Kidney deficiency/yang deficiency/cold. In the *Discussion of Cold Damage* it is known as lesser yin disease (少陰病 *shō in byō/shào yīn bìng*).

24

This phenomenon occurs because of the interplay of a couple of processes. The Kidneys store the fluids, including the yin qi, which normally rises to the Heart. Meanwhile, the yang qi from the Heart, also known as the ministerial fire of the Triple Burner, passes through the Pericardium and moves downward into the lower burner. In the lower burner, this yang qi forms the fire at the gate of vitality, preventing the yin qi in this area from becoming overabundant. However, if for some reason the fluids of the Kidneys become deficient, the yang qi from the Pericardium will not descend. Because of this, there will be no warmth circulating downward to the lower burner, and the yin qi that remains will, paradoxically, become overabundant.

Kidney deficiency/yang deficiency/cold patterns can also arise from miscellaneous diseases, usually as a result of cold lower extremities, which end up causing internal cooling. The cold entering from the environment causes the fire at the gate of vitality to become deficient, leading to a chilled lower back and legs and lower back pain. In addition, the cold increases both the frequency and volume of urination, which leads to hard stools and a loss of appetite. Impotency and spermatorrhea can also occur.

EXAMINATION

Visual

Kidney deficiency/yang deficiency/cold pattern will always be felt subjectively as a sensation of cold, even if the thermometer indicates a fever. The face, therefore, does not feel hot, and even if there is a fever, it is not usually very high. The tongue is moist and white.

Sometimes there is a redness present in the cheeks that appears to be a sign of health. This, however, is not the case as it is actually the yin qi of the Kidneys becoming so overabundant that it pushes the yang qi that is present inside the body out to the surface, thereby creating the color. This is known in the *Discussion of Cold Damage* as a face made up with yang (面載陽 *men sai yō/miàn dài yáng*) or, more commonly, as true-cold, false-heat.

Pulse

When there is a fever, the pulse will be overall sunken, tight, thin, and rapid. When they are pressed firmly, the right distal and both the left and right proximal pulses will be deficient. When there is no fever, the pulse will be sunken, wiry, and always slow.

Abdomen

The lower abdomen will look like the bottom of a ship in the way it is sunken and curved. In addition, there will be creases and the abdomen will be weak, that is, when it is pressed firmly, there is very little resistance. When the abdomen is pressed firmly and deeply, it is often possible to feel the internal organs in these patients. Another possibility is that the abdomen balloons up, but on firm pressure is found to be lacking in resilience. These signs are evident when this pattern results from a miscellaneous disease. However, when it occurs as part of an acute febrile disease, the abdomen is not a reliable indicator.

TREATMENT

First and foremost, KI-3 should be tonified (TABLE 5, see page 30).* Normally, this alone is enough to regulate the pulse because it is the earth and source point of the Kidney meridian. Tonification of this point leads to an increase in fluids and strengthening of the Triple Burner's source qi.

For painful throats, KI-6 is used together with KI-3 to great effect. The "leg Triple Burner meridian" is also tonified. The area to be used for this purpose is found one finger width lateral to BL-58. Note that the "leg Triple Burner meridian" emerges from BL-39 (the lower uniting point of the Triple Burner) and clinically is said to end at BL-59. It runs between the Gallbladder and the Bladder meridians in this area. This meridian is alluded to in Chapters 2 and 4 of the *Divine Pivot*; in the *Inner Classic*, the Triple Burner and Bladder are frequently mentioned together.

In the Kidney deficiency/yang deficiency pattern, both the yang qi and the fluids are deficient, and thus it is necessary to tonify the nutritive qi. The method of tonification is slightly different, however, from that mentioned in Chapter 2 with respect to Spleen deficiency. The tips of the fingers are used to lightly touch the skin and find those areas along the Bladder meridian where the qi is lacking. These areas are soft and mushy to the touch, and so are easy to discern. The tip of the needle is lightly applied to these areas with a slight feeling of penetration. At the same time, the left pressing hand contracts and grips the needle slightly. If there is any penetration at all, it is on the order of 1mm, and there should be no accompanying pain whatsoever. The needle should then be held in place until the qi arrives, which is usually marked by a warm feeling along the course of the meridian. This warming can occur quite quickly if the practitioner takes a few breaths while waiting.

If there is a fever, contact needling should be performed over the entire length of the Bladder meridian. If there is no fever, the needles can be retained but deep needle retention should not be performed. The most important thing is to warm the lower half of the body.

In chronic cases it is also good to perform direct moxibustion on the lower back and

....

*Note that in this table the Kidney deficiency/yang deficiency/cold pattern is being compared to the Spleen deficiency/Kidney deficiency/cold pattern, the subject of Chapter 5.

abdomen, but the patient should not feel hot as a result. Rather, for best results, the moxibustion should result in a feeling of warmth and the skin around the treated point should become red. Pleasantly warm, tonifying, direct moxibustion can be achieved by placing the tips of the thumb and index fingers around the burning moxibustion cone. As the half rice-grain sized cones burn down toward the skin, the position of the fingers is changed slightly in order to regulate the intensity of the heat.

This pattern is very common among the elderly who also sometimes suffer from constipation. In these cases, laxatives should never be used. It is better to warm the lower body, which will result in a reduction in urination, thereby causing the constipation to clear up by itself.

Herbal Treatment

In each of the following there is a preponderance of yin qi in the lesser yin meridian, which is evidenced by sensations of cold. If, in addition, there is throat pain from heat collecting locally, a typical formula to use would be Platycodon Decoction (桔梗湯 *ki kyō tō/jié gěng tāng*). If there is a complete absence of yang qi in the Bladder meridian there will be general lassitude, chills, joint pain, cold hands and feet, cold abdomen, and no dryness in the mouth. A typical formula for this would be Aconite Accessory Root Decoction (附子湯 *bu shi tō/fù zǐ tāng*). Finally, if there is a chronic lack of yang qi in the lower burner, a typical formula to use would be Poria, Ginger, Atractylodes, and Licorice Decoction (苓姜朮甘湯 *ryō kyō jutsu kan tō/líng jiāng zhú gān tāng*).

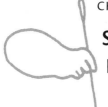

CHAPTER 5

Spleen Deficiency / Kidney Deficiency / Cold Pattern

脾虚腎虚寒証

hi kyo jin kyo kan shō/pí xū shèn xū hán zhèng

Background

THE QI AND blood made in the middle burner migrate to the chest to become the yang qi of the Heart and Lungs. The yang qi of the Heart travels first to the Pericardium, becoming the ministerial fire. From there, it goes down to the Kidneys where it becomes the fire at the gate of vitality. When the fire at the gate of vitality is strong, the Spleen and Stomach above it are warmed and function well, producing large amounts of qi and blood. If, however, the yang qi of the Kidneys becomes deficient, that is, the fire at the gate of vitality has diminished and a pattern of Kidney deficiency/yang deficiency/cold has emerged, the resultant extra load placed on the yang qi of the middle burner will cause it to decrease, adversely affecting the Spleen and Stomach. As a result, the production of blood and qi is diminished and the yin qi of the body is increased. This leads to cold both on the inside and outside of the body, a pattern known as Spleen deficiency/Kidney deficiency/cold.

The patient will have chills, extremely cold hands and feet, no appetite, undigested food in the stools, and no vitality whatsoever. Other symptoms include dizziness, nausea and vomiting, abdominal pains, and urinary difficulty. In some cases, the diarrhea can be so severe as to cause fear for the patient's life. Yet even in this state, if the Triple Burner's source qi is still present, the patient will not immediately die. This state is known as true-cold, false-heat and occurs often. As noted in Chapter 4, it is a result of the inside having an abundance of yin qi, which gives rise to extreme cold. In addition, the tiny amount of yang qi that is left makes its way out to the surface of the body, giving the appearance of a heat pattern. The patient may have a dry throat (but will not actually drink very much) and may feel hot (but likes to stay covered up in bed). The patient does not feel thirsty and does not want to get out from under the covers. If for some reason she does, she becomes cold and develops goose pimples.

In addition, these patients may exhibit irritability and restlessness to the point where they just cannot remain still. In practice, it is unusual to encounter a patient with such advanced symptoms. However, many patients will be found to fall within the stages leading up to these symptoms. This pattern is often seen in patients with rheumatism, Menière's disease, low blood pressure, chronic colitis, and heart disease. The cause is often owing to mistaken treatment of colds and influenza, or inappropriate treatment of acute or chronic gastrointestinal disorders. Those with constitutionally weak digestive tracts are particularly prone to this pattern.

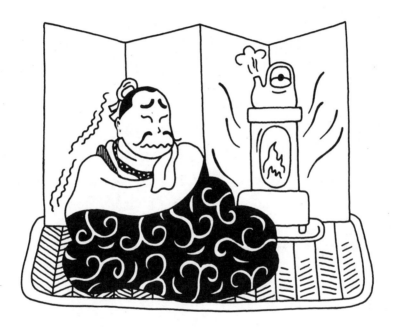

Yang deficiency simply means being chilled

EXAMINATION

Visual

The facial complexion is either white or conversely red in color, as explained above. Owing to constitutional factors or chronic disease, such patients are thin and their flesh is weak. Their lips are often pale, with a moist tongue and a white coating.

Pulse

The pulse is sunken, thin, rapid, and weak, or alternatively sunken, tight, and rapid. Another possibility is that it is sunken, slow, and weak or fine. A tight pulse, or a feeling of fever accompanied by a slow pulse, are signs of a poor prognosis.

A deficient left proximal pulse indicates Kidney deficiency. However, in order for it to be classified as a *pattern* of Kidney deficiency, there should be a simultaneous deficiency at the right distal pulse. Similarly, a deficient right medial pulse implies Spleen deficiency, but if there is no deficiency occurring simultaneously at the left distal pulse, it cannot be termed a *pattern* of Spleen deficiency. To be considered a pattern of Spleen deficiency/Kidney deficiency, both the left proximal and right medial pulses should be simultaneously deficient, but the left and right distal pulses should not be deficient.

Abdomen

The abdomen feels cool overall and is lacking in resilience. Normally, the patient is not sweating, but if there is sweating, it is a result of a severe yang deficiency/cold pattern. This is known as white sweating (白汗 *haku kan/bái hàn*) because when it occurs it leaves the body cold and pale. In this state, there will also be cramping of the arms and legs. If a pattern of Spleen deficiency/Kidney deficiency occurs as a result of improper treatment of an acute febrile disease, the abdomen will not yield any useful information.

Table 5	Spleen Deficiency/Kidney Deficiency/Cold Patterns	
	Kidney deficiency/yang deficiency/ cold pattern	Spleen deficiency/Kidney deficiency/ cold pattern
PULSE	Overall: (a) sunken, tight, thin, and rapid; or (b) sunken, thin, weak, and slow; or (c) wiry and slow	Overall: (a) sunken, thin, rapid, and weak; or (b) sunken, tight, and rapid; or (c) sunken, slow, and weak
	Right distal and left and right proximal positions: deficient when pressed firmly	Left proximal and right medial positions: deficient when pressed firmly
SYMPTOMS	Chills, headaches, sore throat, coughs, nasal discharge, joint pain, general lassitude	Chills, indigestion, diarrhea, chilled hands and feet, cramping of hands and feet, dizziness, vomiting, red face
TONIFYING POINTS	KI-3, KI-6, BL-58	KI-3, KI-4, TB-4, ST-42
SHUNTING POINTS	None	None

TREATMENT

KI-3, KI-4, TB-4, and ST-42 should be tonified (TABLE 5). KI-4 is the connecting point on the Kidney meridian and is therefore useful in tonifying both the yin and yang. By tonifying TB-4, the source point of the Triple Burner, the tight and rough pulses, which result from deficiency of yang qi, can be smoothed out and normalized. ST-42 is the source point of the Stomach meridian and is therefore a good point for making the Stomach qi full and abundant, which helps normalize the speed of the pulse.

In addition to the root treatment, the abdomen and the back should be treated with very light contact needling to build up the protective qi. Also, direct moxibustion on the lower abdomen at points that include CV-4, CV-5, and CV- 6 may be performed to put qi into the lower burner.

Herbal Treatment

As discussed above, deficiency of the yang qi at the gate of vitality causes a lack of yang qi in the middle burner, generating a pattern of Spleen deficiency/Kidney deficiency/cold. A typical combination for this would be True Warrior Decoction (真武湯 *shin bu tō/zhēn wǔ tāng*). When a pattern of Spleen deficiency/Kidney deficiency/cold becomes more serious and exhibits the symptoms of true-cold, false-heat, then Frigid Extremeties Decoction (四逆湯 *shi gyaku tō/sì nì tāng*) can be used. Finally, when a pattern of Spleen deficiency/Kidney deficiency/cold arises as part of a miscellaneous disease in someone with chronic Spleen deficiency, a typical formula would be Pinellia, Atractylodis Macrocephalae and Gastrodia Decoction (半夏白朮天麻湯 *han ge byaku jutsu ten ma tō/bàn xià bái zhú tiān má tāng*).

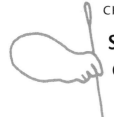

CHAPTER 6

Spleen Deficiency / Yang Deficiency / Cold Pattern

脾虚陽虚寒証

hi kyo yō kyo kan shō/pí xū yáng xū hán zhèng

BACKGROUND

THE SPLEEN RECEIVES fire from the Pericardium and fluids from the Kidneys. It then directs the Stomach and Intestines to produce blood, qi, and fluids. The fire from the Pericardium is essential for normal Spleen function, and so when the Spleen is deficient, it is the Pericardium meridian that should be tonified first. Another way of looking at this is that by tonifying the Pericardium meridian, the fire at the gate of vitality is strengthened, which in turn warms the Stomach.

A deficient Spleen will produce either cold or stagnant heat or fluids in the Stomach itself, thereby impairing the function of the Stomach and Intestines. This state of cold, or of both cold and stagnation of fluids, is characteristic of a pattern of Spleen deficiency/yang deficiency/cold.

When the Stomach becomes cold, the hands and feet also become cold and there is a tendency toward diarrhea, which can lead to exhaustion. In addition, the epigastrium becomes full and distended. There is no real appetite, and so if food is taken, it is only eaten in small amounts. Fortunately, its flavor can be appreciated because the sense of taste is not affected. In addition, the amount of saliva increases, urination is excessive, the patient feels nauseous, and there is rheumatic pain in the joints. In the *Discussion of Cold Damage* these symptoms are known as greater yin organ cold (太陰臓寒 *tai in zō kan/tài yīn zàng hán*).

The causes can be mistaken treatment of a fever-based disease, the inappropriate consumption of cold food, or chilling of the body. These are known as internal cold or cold-attack (中寒 *chū kan/zhòng hán*) in the *Discussion of Cold Damage*; this is an example of an approach that focuses on the pathogen rather than any underlying deficiency. Other possible causes are chronic overconsumption of food and excessive worry over a long period of time. Finally, there is, of course, the constitutional tendency toward Spleen deficiency/yang deficiency, which will predispose the person to the above symptoms.

If an appropriate treatment is not carried out, the production of blood and fluids will diminish and the fire at the gate of vitality will dim; thus, the yang qi of the Stomach becomes even more deficient. There is the possibility that, as a result, both the Kidneys and the Spleen will become deficient, which would lead to the pattern of Spleen deficiency/Kidney deficiency/cold discussed in the previous chapter.

Comparison of the Four Cold Patterns

All told, we have discussed four cold patterns so far: Lung deficiency/yang deficiency, Kidney Deficiency/yang deficiency, Spleen deficiency/Kidney deficiency, and Spleen deficiency/yang deficiency. From this we can see that the cold produced by these yang deficiency patterns affects more than the areas directly influenced by the organs in question. There is also a tendency for the cold to spread throughout the body, which would mean death if it was complete and if there was no yang qi, no matter how little, remaining.

Clinically speaking, the patient's main complaints often correspond to the areas that are cold. On the other hand, there is also the possibility of the yang qi being pursued by the cold into one small area where it stagnates and gives rise to the various symptoms comprising the main complaints. The organ-meridian system needs to be examined to determine the location of the heat or cold, and treatment must focus on tonifying the yang qi.

So, for instance, even if the patient has a pattern of Spleen deficiency/yang deficiency/cold that causes cold in the Stomach itself, the Stomach meridian can still harbor heat, giving rise, for example, to headaches. This is because the Stomach has become cold to the point where there is no exchange between the qi in the Stomach meridian and the Stomach itself. When the heat in the Stomach meridian increases, it can cause fever, vomiting, and diarrhea, all of which indicate a great deal of heat.

Another scenario would be a patient who presents with a mix of cold and hot symptoms as well as a sensation of stagnant heat in the chest area upon abdominal examination. Accordingly, the symptoms may include a lack of thirst and marked fatigue after diarrhea (which indicate that the Stomach has become cold), as well as fullness and pain under the rib cage, vomiting, belching, distention and pain in the abdomen, borborygmus, and the urge to evacuate immediately after a meal (which are all indicative of heat). This patient may therefore have a mix of cold in the Stomach, Spleen deficiency, and stagnant heat in the chest area from heat in the Heart and Small Intestines. Since heat always has the tendency to spread upward and outward, the heat in the Small Intestines is, in this case, responsible for the fullness and pain under the rib cage, vomiting, belching, distention and pain in the abdomen, borborygmus, and urge to evacuate immediately after a meal. The heat in the chest may also affect the patient's sleep, causing the patient to wake often in the middle of the night.

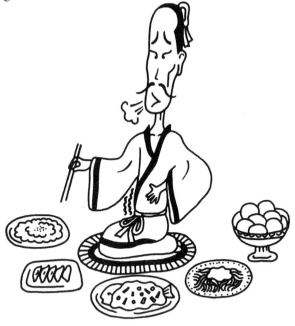

If the Stomach is chilled, food cannot be eaten

EXAMINATION

Visual

One thing to pay attention to is the lips. If the Stomach is cold, even if there is a fever, the complexion and lips will usually be pale. However, if there is heat in the Stomach *meridian*, the lips will be red, which is easily confused with Stomach heat. Also, if there is heat in the chest, the complexion may become red, which can also be misconstrued as Stomach heat. As a check, if there is heat in the chest as a result of Stomach heat, the tip of the tongue will be red and the tongue will lack a coating. Finally, if the Stomach is cold, the tongue is moist.

Pulse

If the yang deficiency is light, the pulse will be sunken and wiry. If there is a more marked deficiency, the pulse will either be fine and weak, or sunken, thin, and deficient. If there is a fever, the pulse will be slightly floating and rapid. However, the usual pulse for this pattern is a combination of sunken, thin, weak, deficient, wiry, and slow. The left distal pulse and the right medial pulse are deficient when firmly pressed. When there is heat in the Stomach meridian, the right medial pulse can be felt upon light pressure, but it will not be an excessive pulse. Likewise, when there is heat in the Small Intestine, the left distal pulse is also easily felt with light pressure, but, again, it will not be an excessive pulse.

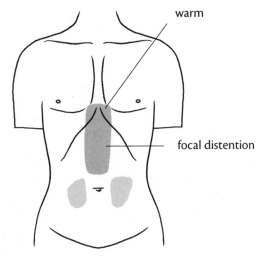

warm

focal distention

Fig. 6   Abdominal signs for Spleen deficiency/yang deficiency/cold pattern

Abdomen

With Spleen deficiency, there will be a feeling of fullness in the center of the abdomen below the apex of the ribs and around the Heart alarm point (CV-14) area. This is sometimes known as epigastric focal distention (心下痞 *shin ka hi/xīn xià pǐ*). The degree of fullness and the resistance to pressure in this area of focal distention will vary depending on the amount of fluids and on the extent of stagnation of heat or cold.

Resistance to pressure near CV-14, and sometimes as far down as CV-12, may indicate stagnation of fluids in the Stomach. The resistance to pressure can also be indicative of internal heat trying to make its way out to the surface; subjectively, the internal heat feels like fullness or distention. Normally, if the Stomach is quite cold, the whole abdomen will display an absence of any feeling of fullness or resistance to pressure. If, however, there is a small amount of heat, it will manifest as fullness in the center of the abdomen and below the ribs. For example, heat in the Small Intestine presents not only with fullness below the ribs but also resistance to pressure as well as heat from the bottom of the sternum to CV-17. This heat is sometimes subjectively felt by the patient, but in any case, it is readily felt by the practitioner with light palpation.

TREATMENT

The basic approach is to tonify the yang qi of PC-7 and SP-3 (TABLE 7, see page 40). If there is fluid stagnation in the area below the ribs, ST-42 should be added. If there is heat in the Stomach meridian, ST-36 is tonified and ST-44 is shunted. For Small Intestine heat, SI-4 is tonified.

ST-36 is used to clear heat by tonifying the nutritive qi, thereby tonifying the fluids: An abundance of fluids can cool the Stomach meridian. Another way of looking at it is that ST-36 tonifies the yin qi of the Stomach meridian, which then results in a reduction of heat. This means that the type of needling used to tonify the nutritive qi in this case needs to be slightly deeper to achieve a type of 'indirect shunting,' that is, to realize a net (indirect) cooling of the heat in the Stomach meridian by tonification of the cooling element and not by direct shunting of the excess heat. If this still does not result in cooling of the Stomach meridian, ST-44 is shunted at the protective qi level, that is, very superficially, as this level most influences the yang and here we want to tonify the yang.

Overall, treatment is aimed at tonifying the yang deficiency; accordingly, the needling is extremely shallow. It is alright to leave the needles in place on the abdomen and on the back, especially when there is fullness below the rib cage. If there is a large amount of heat in the chest, heat perception moxibustion can be applied to the hottest areas. Small scarring moxibustion can also be performed on the back to the Spleen back-associated point (BL-20) or the Stomach back-associated point (BL-21). Small scarring moxibustion that leaves only a 1mm scar, and is not painful when properly done, is tonifying in its effect.

Herbal Treatment

When the yang qi of the Stomach and Intestines is diminished, marked by increased production of saliva, cold hands and feet, diarrhea, and a reduced appetite, a typical formula would be Ginseng Decoction (人参湯 *nin jin tō/rén shēn tāng*), which is the decocted form of Regulate the Middle Pill (理中丸 *ri chū gan/lǐ zhōng wán*). When the yang qi of the Stomach and Intestines is diminished and there is fluid stagnation and phlegm, Six-Gentleman Decoction (六君子湯 *riku kun shi tō/liù jūn zǐ tāng*) would be an appropriate formula.

When the Stomach and Intestines are cold and there is heat in the yang brightness meridians marked by nausea, vomiting, headaches, and fever, Evodia Decoction (呉茱萸湯 *go shu yu tō/wú zhū yú tāng*) can be used. When the Stomach is cold and there is heat in the Small Intestine marked by epigastric focal distention, borborygmus, heartburn, either diarrhea or constipation, and large swings in appetite, a typical formula is Pinellia Decoction to Drain the Epigastrium (半夏瀉心湯 *han ge sha shin tō/bàn xià xiè xīn tāng*).

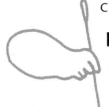

CHAPTER 7

Liver Deficiency / Yang Deficiency / Cold Pattern

肝虚陽虚寒証

kan kyo yō kyo kan shō/gān xū yáng xū hán zhèng

Background

IN THIS PATTERN both the fluids and the fire at the gate of vitality are deficient. At the same time, the blood stored by the Liver is diminished, causing the appearance of cold-related symptoms.

With respect to qi, the blood—which can, from one perspective, include the fluids—is yin. Furthermore, considering the two major divisions into qi and form, blood pertains to yin since it is needed to produce form. However, the nutritive qi makes the blood circulate, and nutritive qi is yin when compared to protective qi, but yang when compared to blood. A lack of nutritive qi in the Liver and Kidneys will therefore cause an insufficiency of blood and fluids, thereby producing cold symptoms.

Since the nutritive qi is yang and circulates the blood, and since blood is considered yin, a deficiency of blood will result in a relative abundance of the yang nutritive qi. A yin deficiency pattern will therefore manifest with various heat symptoms because of the relative abundance of yang. However, these symptoms will be fundamentally different from the heat symptoms present when there is an abundance of protective qi, as in a pattern of Lung deficiency/yang excess (see Chapter 1). Therefore, when there is an abundance of nutritive qi, it is never termed 'yang excess' regardless of the amount of heat produced.

In addition, the Liver deficiency/yang deficiency pattern and yin deficiency patterns represent opposite states. Although a deficiency of nutritive qi may be thought of as leading to a relative increase in the amount of blood, this does not happen. Instead, since the nutritive qi moves the blood, a nutritive qi deficiency leads to a reduction in blood flow, thereby producing blood stasis and a range of cold symptoms (as discussed above); this deficiency of both yin blood and yang nutritive qi leads to the Liver deficiency/yang deficiency pattern. The cold produced by this yang deficiency can spread to various areas and can even consume the entire body, which is a terminal condition. However, most of the time, the cold spreads to the lower and middle burners, with the remaining yang qi found in the upper burner (Pericardium). In the *Discussion of Cold Damage* this state is known as terminal yin disease (厥陰病 *ketsu in byō/jué yīn bìng*).

The factors that most often lead to this pattern include childbirth, miscarriage, abortion, emotional exhaustion, physical overwork, sexual overindulgence, physical trauma, internal cold, or a bout of acute vomiting and diarrhea. In addition, women with poor dietary habits or living conditions, as well as a constitutional predisposition, are also associated with this pattern.

Symptoms include cold hands and feet, lower abdominal pain, and a tendency toward soft stools or diarrhea (for women this is especially evident during menstruation). Other symptoms include lack of appetite, but once a meal is begun, it can be finished. These patients often develop problems such as dizziness upon standing, vertigo, fatigue, weak eyes, eye twitches, joint pain, lower back pain, irregular menstruation, infertility, anemia, low blood pressure, and numerous gynecological conditions.

In acute cases when this pattern is accompanied by vomiting and diarrhea, the condition can be severe. It may be necessary to send the patient to an urgent care center to be evaluated by a modern biomedical physician.

EXAMINATION

Visual

The complexion is usually that of a pale anemic look; however, there can also be flushed red cheeks. This redness is known as 'face made up with yang,' which, as discussed in Chapter 4, means that the color is not caused by an excess of yang. Rather, the last bit of remaining yang has been pushed up and out to the face by the presence of increased yin. This type of pattern is typically found among thin people, but there may be some obese patients with it as well. Although the obese patients may look stronger than their thin counterparts, they are every bit as exhausted. This is important to remember when treating these patients.

Pulse

The overall pulse is sunken, rough, thin, and deficient, which is in agreement with the pulse described in the *Pulse Classic* where it is written that when the nutritive qi is deficient, the pulse will be sunken, and when the blood is deficient, the pulse will be rough as a result of the weak blood flow. The left medial and proximal pulses are deficient when pressed firmly. The right medial pulse is rough and thin when pressed firmly, but not deficient. If the patient is very tired and has a fever, the pulse will also be rapid.

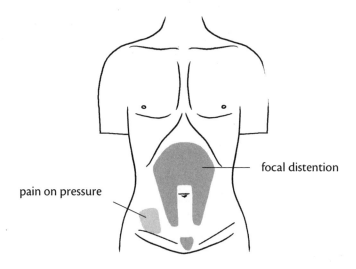

focal distention

pain on pressure

Fig. 7   Abdominal signs for Liver deficiency/yang deficiency/cold pattern

Abdomen

The upper part of the abdominal musculature will be tight and tense but will lack resistance on pressure (Fig. 7). By contrast, pressure exerted on the area around the appendix results in resistance and pain. This abdominal presentation is known as long-term cold (久寒 *kyū kan/jiǔ hán*). The inguinal area and the pubic symphysis are painful on pressure, and the pain and tenderness from the inguinal region can spread and end up affecting the lower back.

TREATMENT

The basic treatment involves tonification of KI-3, LR-3, SP-1, and GB-40 (TABLE 7). If the pulse is rapid, KI-7 and LR-4 are also used. These points are used to tonify the nutritive qi, but deep needling is not administered. The needle is touched on the surface of the skin and, at the very most, penetrates the skin very slightly. The needle is held firmly in place with the left hand until the qi arrives, which is felt as warmth along the meridian. Overall, needles should be retained in the upper part of the abdomen, but moxibustion should be applied to the lower part. It is acceptable to retain the needles in the back, but the needling must be extremely light because of the yang deficiency. The moxibustion should also be applied carefully so that the patient feels tonifying warmth rather than dispersive heat.

Herbal Treatment

When the yang qi is just about to completely disappear with abdominal cramps, diarrhea, and cold hands and feet, a typical formula would be Tangkuei Decoction for Frigid Extremeties plus Evodia and Fresh Ginger (当帰四逆加呉茱萸生姜湯 *tō ki shi gyaku ka go shu yu shō kyō tō/dāng guī sì nì jiā wú zhū yú shēng jiāng tāng*). When there is mainly

The Practice of Japanese Acupuncture and Moxibustion: Classic Principles in Action

cold but still some heat in the upper burner manifesting as dry lips, flushed palms, and irregular menstruation, a typical formula would be Warm the Menses Decoction (温経湯 *un kei tō/wēng jīng tāng*).

Table 7	Liver Deficiency/Yang Deficiency/Cold Patterns	
	Spleen deficiency/yang deficiency/ cold pattern	Liver deficiency/yang deficiency/ cold pattern
PULSE	Overall: sunken, thin, wiry, and weak; if there is a fever, the pulse is rapid Left distal and right middle positions: deficient when pressed firmly	Overall: sunken, rough, thin, and deficient; if there is tiredness or fever, the pulse may be rapid Left medial and proximal positions: deficient when pressed firmly Right medial position: thin and rough
SYMPTOMS	Excessive urination, cold hands and feet, diarrhea, epigastric focal distention and firmness, lack of appetite, headaches, borborygmus, vomiting	Cold hands and feet, diarrhea during menstruation, dizziness upon standing, no appetite but once a meal is started, it can be finished, irregular menstruation
TONIFYING POINTS	PC-7, SP-3, ST-42	KI-3, LR-3, SP-1, GB-40
SHUNTING POINTS	None	None

When there is more heat in the upper burner marked by cold limbs and trunk, occasional nausea, and chronic diarrhea, a typical formula would be Mume Pill (烏梅丸 *u bai gan/wū méi wán)*. When there is an abundance of heat in the upper burner that spreads to the lower burner there will be diarrhea with severe cramping, a dry mouth, and dark urine. For this problem a typical formula would be Pulsatilla Decoction (白頭翁湯 *haku tō ō tō/bái tóu wēng tāng)*.

When there is a sudden cessation in the exchange of yin and yang between the upper and lower burners, the symptoms will include a lack of vitality, severe vomiting and diarrhea, and vomiting directly after meals. A typical formula for this pattern would be Dried Ginger, Coptis, Scutellaria and Ginseng Decoction(乾薑黄連黄芩人參湯 *kan ky ō ō ren ō gon nin jintō/gān jiāng huáng lián huáng qín rén shēn tāng)*.

CHAPTER 8

Spleen Deficiency/Liver Excess/ Heat Pattern

脾虚肝実熱証

hi kyo kan jitsu netsu shō/pí xū gān shí rè zhèng

A STATE OF EXCESS is characterized by the stagnation and pooling of yang qi (heat) or blood in parts of the body. Stagnation of blood is known as blood stasis. Stagnation of fluids or yin qi is not referred to as a state of excess because this stagnation is caused by yang deficiency. To get the fluids to move, the yang must be tonified; if one tries to directly drain the fluids, the yang deficiency will worsen.

The term 'yin excess' refers to the state where heat or blood stagnates and pools in a yin section of the body. Since this can only occur in the Liver, any reference to yin excess must be referring to the Liver. And because the Liver stores blood, a Liver excess would automatically produce blood stasis. Therefore, the two terms Liver excess and blood stasis are interchangeable. In this chapter we will first consider the case of acute Liver excess, that is, the Spleen deficiency/Liver excess/heat pattern. The Spleen deficiency/Liver excess/blood stasis and Lung deficiency/Liver excess/blood stasis patterns are considered in Chapters 9 and 10, respectively.

BACKGROUND

As noted in the *Discussion of Cold Damage*, Liver excess often occurs in the context of the six-meridian (also known as six-stage) progression scheme. First, Lung deficiency leads to yang qi stagnation (yang excess), which in turn produces heat. As the process continues, the Spleen becomes more deficient and heat enters the yang brightness meridians. If it continues still further, it can enter the lesser yang meridians, and as the Gallbladder and Liver are both affected, this can lead to Liver problems. Alternatively, the progression can lead from the lesser yang meridian to the yin meridians to reach the terminal yin (Liver) organ directly. Invasion of the Liver can occur when there is a preexisting deficiency of Liver essence. This preexisting deficiency of the Liver essence can cause heat to enter the blood being stored in the Liver, affecting its flow and giving rise to a condition of excess. There are also other factors that can lead to the development of Liver excess heat such as inflammation of an internal organ, overconsumption of alcohol, postpartum exhaustion, and constitutional factors. Then, in accordance with the controlling cycle of the five phases, the Spleen becomes weakened and deficient as the heat from the Liver consumes the fluids of the Spleen. This state is known as the Spleen deficiency/Liver excess/heat pattern, which corresponds to a lesser yang problem. In the *Discussion of Cold Damage* it is known as heat entering the chamber of the blood (血室 *ketsu shitsu/xuè shì*).

Heat that enters the chamber of the blood often precipitates a fever, which frequently results in an unresolved condition of Liver excess even after the acute febrile episode is over. The symptoms that accompany an acute fever are alternating chills and fevers or a fever that increases in the afternoon, menstrual-related fever, loss of appetite (even when there is no fever), stomachache, dry mouth with constipation, sometimes nausea, cough, wheezing, urinary difficulty, joint pains, headache, stiff shoulders, and ear pain.

EXAMINATION

Visual

There is no characteristic facial complexion. In almost every case the tongue is dry, sometimes with a white coating. Thus, even if there are other signs that point toward the presence of this pattern, the lack of a dry tongue mitigates against this diagnosis.

Pulse

Overall the pulse is sunken, wiry, and excessive. It can also be sunken, rough, and excessive. When there is a fever, a rapid pulse will of course be evident. The wiry pulse occurs when there is heat in the Liver that is unsuccessfully trying to move upward and outward. The rough, excessive pulse is also attributable to the heat that remains, despite all efforts, stuck in the Liver. The left distal pulse and the right medial pulse are deficient when pressed firmly. The left middle pulse is found to be wiry and excessive or rough and excessive.

Abdomen

In this pattern there is pain on pressure just above and below the apex of the rib cage, fluid stagnation, and resistance to pressure beneath the ribs (Fig. 8). The combination of all three symptoms is known as a sense of discomfort and fullness in the chest and ribs, but it should literally be translated as suffering from fullness in the chest and ribs (胸脇苦満 *kyō kyō ku man/xiōng xié kǔ mǎn*); this term can only be applied to the combination of all three symptoms. Note, however, that a patient can have Liver excess heat without having these abdominal symptoms.

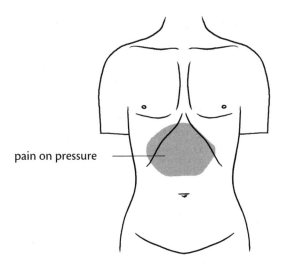

pain on pressure

Fig. 8   Abdominal signs for Spleen deficiency/Liver excess/heat pattern

TREATMENT

The root treatment involves the tonification of PC-7 and SP-3 and the shunting of LR-2, TB-3, GB-41, and other areas along the Gallbladder meridian that are tight (TABLE 10, see page 50). The tonification and shunting should be directed toward the nutritive qi, so the needling should be done up to a depth of 3mm for the root treatment and a bit deeper when needling on the back. LR-2 is the fire point of the Liver meridian, and consequently this point is suitable for dispersing the heat in the Liver. TB-3 and GB-41 are used because the heat that overflows from the Liver excess spreads to the lesser yang meridians. As a general rule, heat is first shunted from the connected yang meridians, and the Liver meridian is directly shunted *only* if this is insufficient.

As an overall treatment strategy, retaining the needles is indicated. In addition, LR-14, GB-24, BL-17, BL-18, and BL-19 should be shunted. When there are alternating chills and fever, moxa head needling or direct scarring moxa (with a large number of cones) should be applied at LR-14. Note, however, that the moxibustion techniques should be administered only when the patient is not feverish.

Moxa Head Needling Technique

I use the Imura method of moxa head needling, which is named after Koji Imura, my good friend and associate. The type of needle used is normally a 1.3 unit (40mm length) No. 3 or 4 (0.16cm to 0.18cm) gauge needle.

The amount of moxa to be placed on the needle head is about three times the normal amount. Therefore, tissue paper is used to prevent it from falling off the needle head. The moxa is rolled tightly in the tissue paper to form a reasonably hard mass, which is then placed on the head of the needle. In order to prevent burning of the skin, a thick piece of cardboard is placed on the skin around the needle.

With this method, the point is being warmed not only by the heated needle but also by the piece of cardboard, which becomes warm during the process and thereby prevents the skin from cooling rapidly even after the moxa has finished burning. Moxa head needling is warming in nature, which implies that it is basically tonifying in nature. However, depending on the depth and location of the insertion, the technique can be used to treat areas of either deficiency or excess. For instance, an excess point responding with pain on pressure with an internal hard area would receive moxa head needling to 'melt down' the hard area, thus shunting it. On the other hand, an area that feels open and is hollow on pressure could receive moxa head needling to tonify the deficiency of nutritive qi.

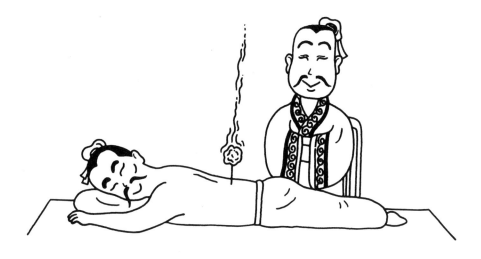

Moxa head needling

Herbal Treatment

When there is a pattern of Spleen deficiency/Liver excess/heat with a loss of appetite, a typical formula would be Minor Bupleurem Decoction (小柴胡湯 *shō sai ko tō/xiǎo chái hú tāng*). If, in addition, there is joint pain and headaches, a typical formula would be Bupleurem and Cinnamon Twig Decoction (柴胡桂枝湯 *sai ko kei shi tō/chái hú guì zhī tāng*). If the patient has Spleen deficiency/Liver excess/heat as well as Stomach excess heat, a typical formula would be Major Bupleurem Decoction (大柴胡湯 *dai sai ko tō/dà chái hú tāng*).

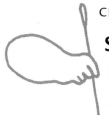

CHAPTER 9

Spleen Deficiency / Liver Excess / Blood Stasis Pattern

脾虚肝実瘀血証

hi kyo kan jitsu o ketsu shō/pí xū gān shí yū xuè zhèng

Background

THERE ARE TWO types of Spleen deficiency/Liver excess/blood stasis patterns. The first is characterized by blood stasis under the right rib cage, and the second is characterized by blood stasis in the lower abdomen.

Blood Stasis under the Right Rib Cage

This results from a history of fevers from tonsillitis, influenza, or other similar infections. In these cases, the Spleen deficiency/Liver excess/heat pattern is a very common outcome because Liver heat leads to poor blood flow, and even after the heat has dissipated, the blood stasis remains. Another possible cause is an accident involving a collision of some sort that results in internal bleeding. Since the Liver stores the blood, the internal bleeding ends up pooling in the Liver, forming blood stasis.

This condition can also result from internal causes. People who are frequently angry but always hold it inside can also develop blood stasis. When anger is present, the yang qi of the Liver becomes excessive, and if it is not dispersed (through expression of that anger), it causes the blood to stagnate internally, once again giving rise to blood stasis. Blood stasis below the ribs is accompanied by stiffness around the medial aspect of the scapula that reaches all the way up to the neck. When this stiffness becomes chronic, the result is chest wall pain and coughing. If these problems persist, they can predispose the individual to the development of cancer. In addition, as the yang qi of the blood of the Liver is not radiating outward properly in these cases, problems such as depression, loss of libido, stomachache, heartburn, and stomach and duodenal ulcers are more likely to occur.

Blood Stasis in the Lower Abdomen

This is caused by a variety of mostly gynecological diseases. These include irregular periods, postpartum carelessness, and miscarriage. Of course, heavy bruising and traffic accidents can lead to blood stasis. Blood stasis in the lower abdomen can lead to chills and flushing, stiff shoulders, headaches, neurosis, high blood pressure, arteriosclerosis, infertility, irregular periods, postmenopausal syndrome, and other gynecological diseases. Also hemorrhoids, constipation, rashes, and other skin diseases occur more easily in these people. Stubborn pain patterns, chronic internal organ diseases, sties, and inverted eyelashes (entropion) are also commonly linked to blood stasis.

EXAMINATION

Visual

Individuals with blood stasis beneath the ribs generally have a dark reddish tinge to their faces. By contrast, blood stasis in the lower abdomen results in a large number of liver spots and pimples. The tongue in both of these cases is typically larger than usual, with a good color.

Pulse

Overall, the pulse is sunken, rough, and excessive. The pulse does not have the strength to repel the finger away from the artery, and some people therefore believe that it should not be labeled as an excessive pulse. However, bearing in mind that the pulse for blood stasis is sunken, it will of course not repel the fingers. Within this state, it will be found that with firm pressure, the pulse does not disappear; rather, the firmer the pressure, the tighter the pulse will be. When there is blood stasis in the lower abdomen, the pulse is even thinner, more sunken, rough, and excessive. This means that it is easy to miss this type of blood stasis in the pulse. The pulse may also be slow because the large amount of blood stasis causes poor blood flow.

To summarize, there is a sunken, rough pulse that does not disappear when it is pressed firmly. The pulse is slow despite the absence of cold either externally or internally. Many of the symptoms are therefore the opposite of those found in cases of yang deficiency.

Finally, in both blood stasis beneath the right rib cage and in the abdomen, the left distal and right medial pulses are found to be deficient on firm pressure. This would suggest Spleen deficiency, but since the left medial pulse is sunken, rough, and excessive, the overall diagnosis is that of Spleen deficiency/Liver excess/blood stasis.

Abdomen

In cases of blood stasis under the right rib cage, the area below the right ribs displays muscular resistance to pressure as well as pain on pressure, or perhaps fluid stagnation (FIG. 9). This abdominal presentation is sometimes known as Lung accumulation (肺積 *hai shaku/fèi jī*). It should not be confused with the abdominal pattern known as suffering from fullness in the chest and ribs, described in Chapter 8. For blood stasis of the lower abdomen, there will be pain on pressure around the navel. However, the most common area for pain on pressure is on the left from the area of ST-25 downward, and also extending laterally from the area of SP-14 to SP-13. If this also appears on the right side of the abdomen, it indicates that the blood stasis is of a more longstanding nature. If it also extends to below the navel, it indicates that there is a large amount of blood stasis.

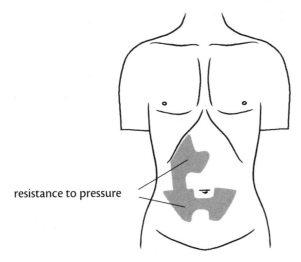

resistance to pressure

Fig. 9   Abdominal signs for Spleen deficiency/Liver excess/blood stasis pattern

TREATMENT

The root treatment consists of tonifying PC-7 and SP-3 followed by shunting SP-6, SP-10, or LR-8, whichever is the most tender on pressure (TABLE 10, see page 50). Of course, because we want to affect the yin and blood, this treatment should be administered at the nutritive qi level, which means slightly deeper needling (2 to 3mm). If the area under the right side of the ribs is found to be hard, moxa head needling is done on the right LR-14. In addition, moxa head needling can be performed on the hard and painful areas below the navel.

As usual, the needles on the back can be left in place. If there is blood stasis in the lower abdomen, the area around BL-25 will probably be hard. Moxa head needling should be applied to the hard areas.

Herbal Treatment

When the blood stasis is located principally beneath the rib cage, a typical formula would be Frigid Extremities Powder (四逆散 *shi gyaku san/sì nì sǎn*). When the blood stasis is located principally in the lower abdomen, a typical formula would be Cinnamon Twig and Poria Pill (桂枝茯苓丸 *kei shi buku ryō gan/guì zhī fú líng wán*).

47

CHAPTER 10

LUNG DEFICIENCY/LIVER EXCESS/ BLOOD STASIS PATTERN

肺虚肝実瘀血証

hai kyo kan jitsu o ketsu shō/fèi xū gān shí yū xuè zhèng

BACKGROUND

THIS PATTERN IS the same as that described in Chapter 75 of the *Classic of Difficulties* as a yin excess pattern (陰実証 *in jitsu shō/yīn shí zhèng*). It occurs when both the circulation of Lung qi becomes poor, causing Kidney fluids to become deficient, and heat and blood stasis increases in the Liver, causing heat to spread as far as the Heart. Normally, a Kidney deficiency would also lead to a Liver deficiency. In this case, however, the fluid deficiency of the Kidneys leads to a drying out of the Liver blood, resulting initially in poor circulation of the blood and finally in blood stasis. This pattern is particularly common in women who are middle-aged or older, especially if they have a large amount of blood stasis from other causes and become Kidney deficient as a result of the aging process. In general, by the time this condition has developed, there is blood stasis in both the upper and lower parts of the abdomen.

When the fluids of the Kidneys dry out, deficiency heat is created; the deficiency heat normally spreads outward. As a result, Kidney deficiency often leads to symptoms such as uncomfortably hot and flushed hands and feet and profuse sweating. If, however, this state becomes chronic, the yang qi required for this process is simply not available anymore and so surface fluid stagnation results. All this, of course, implies that the Lung qi circulation is already poor, and the combination of the two states leads to cold sensations and obesity. Furthermore, the deficiency heat derived from the Kidney deficiency heats the Stomach, causing a tremendous increase in appetite, which obviously will add to the obesity problem. In this situation, an individual who already has a degree of blood stasis is likely to develop the Lung deficiency/Liver excess pattern.

48

The problems connected with this pattern can include constipation, stiffness in the shoulder and upper back, chills with hot flashes, palpitations, depression, gynecological problems, prostatic hypertrophy, high blood pressure, diabetes, heart disease, chronic hepatitis, trigeminal neuralgia, serious eye problems, and various types of cancer. As noted above, the appetite is extremely strong.

A Lung deficiency/Liver excess pattern can also occur suddenly. The acute type occurs when Lung qi circulation becomes poor, leading to the production of Liver excess heat, which causes the Kidney fluids to dry up. This acute form can lead to problems such as palpitations, shortness of breath, slight fever, constipation, diarrhea, hepatitis, insomnia, neurasthenia, thyroid disease, heart disease, and high blood pressure. Finally, a Lung deficiency/Liver excess pattern can also be the result of constitutional factors, for instance, children with atopic eczema or asthma are genetically prone to developing blood stasis and tend to be rather thin, probably as a result of unbalanced diets, and to have frequent fevers.

EXAMINATION

Visual

These patients fall into one of two extremes. They are either obese, or they are thin and sinewy. The tongue is dry, and if there is constipation, there will be a relatively thick tongue coating.

Pulse

Overall, the pulse is generally sunken and forceful. The left proximal pulse is deficient when firmly pressed. If the left medial pulse is also found to be deficient, the diagnosis is Liver deficiency. However, in the patients with a pattern of Lung deficiency/Liver excess/blood stasis, the left medial pulse is sunken, rough, and excessive. At the same time, the left distal pulse is sunken, wiry, and forceful, while the right distal pulse is not deficient when pressed firmly. In addition, the right medial pulse is wiry and powerful, and the right proximal pulse is wiry and deficient.

Abdomen

There is heat in the chest and the area around the underside of the right rib cage is found to be hard on palpation (FIG. 10). Blood stasis is to be found on either side of and below the navel, which manifests as resistance and pain on pressure. The area around the appendix shows resistance to pressure. The area on the inguinal fold and above the pubic symphysis displays pain and resistance to pressure.

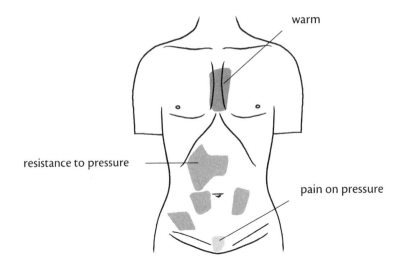

Fig. *10*   Abdominal signs for Lung deficiency/Liver excess/blood stasis pattern

Table 10	Spleen Deficiency/Liver Excess Patterns		
	Spleen deficiency/Liver excess/heat pattern	**Spleen deficiency/Liver excess/blood stasis pattern**	**Lung deficiency/Liver excess/blood stasis pattern**
PULSE	Overall: sunken, wiry, and excessive; or (b) sunken, rough and excessive; if there is fever, pulse is rapid Left distal and right medial positions: deficient when pressed firmly Left medial position: wiry and excessive when pressed firmly	Overall sunken, rough, and excessive; sometimes thin and slow Left distal and right medial positions: deficient when pressed firmly Left medial position: rough and excessive	Overall: sunken and forceful Left proximal position: floating and deficient Left middle position: rough and excessive Left distal position: sunken and wiry Right distal position: may be strong, depending on amount of heat
SYMPTOMS	Alternating chills and fevers, loss of appetite, nausea, constipation, dry mouth, chills, hot flushes	Stiff shoulders, stomachache, heartburn, chest pains, irregular menstruation, chills and hot flushes	Shoulder and upper back stiffness, palpitations, chills and hot flushes, depression, constipation
TONIFYING POINTS	PC-7, SP-3	PC-7, SP-3	KI-7, KI-10
SHUNTING POINTS	LR-2, TB-3, GB-41	SP-6, LR-8, SP-10	LR-8

TREATMENT

KI-7 or KI-10 are tonified and LR-8 is shunted (TABLE 10). Normally, KI-10 is a good choice since it is the water point and is used to move fluids via the Kidneys to restore the dried out blood in the Liver. However, if the pulse is overall rapid and thin, then KI-7 is used since it is the metal point and thereby helps regulate the rapid pulse. LR-8 is used to shunt the Liver excess. I have tried various points for shunting the Liver, but the best results appear to be associated with using LR-8.

As part of the overall treatment, moxa head needling is done at SP-6 and ST-36. SP-6 tonifies the yin, which is often painful on pressure as a result of the blood stasis. ST-36 is used to tonify the fluids. Also, areas of blood stasis on the abdomen and hard areas below the Kidney back-associated points should be treated by moxa head needling.

Herbal Treatment

When the pattern is the result of a miscellaneous disease with blood stasis under the rib cage and in the lower abdomen, a typical formula would be Bupleurum Powder to Dredge the Liver (柴胡疎肝湯 *sai ko soku kan tō/chái hú shū gān tāng*), originally created at the famous herb shop in Japan called Ikkandō (一貫堂) during the Edo period.[1] When there are also signs and symptoms connected with the Heart and there is nervousness, insomnia, and hypertension, typical formulas include Bupleurum, Cinnamon Twig, and Ginger Decoction (柴胡桂枝乾姜湯 *sai ko kei shi kan kyō tō/chái hú guì zhī gān jiāng tāng*) and Bupleurum plus Dragon Bone and Oyster Shell Decoction (柴胡加竜骨牡蠣湯 *sai ko ka ryō kotsu bo rei tō/chái hú jiā lóng gǔ mǔ lì tang*). When the patient also has an allergic constitution, a typical formula would be Bupleurum Decoction to Clear the Liver (柴胡清肝湯 *sai ko sai kan tō/chái hú qīng gān tāng*),[2] again from the famous Japanese herb shop Ikkandō, or Schizonepeta and Forsythia Decoction (荊芥連翹湯 *kei gai ren gyō tō/jīng jiè lián qiáo tāng*).

....

[1] The formula consists of:

    Angelicae sinensis Radix *(tōki / dāng guī)* 3g

    Paeoniae Radix alba *(byakushaku/bái sháo)* 3g

    Chuanxiong Rhizoma *(senkyū/chuān xiōng)* 3g

    Rehmanniae Radix *(shōjiō/shēng dì huáng)* 3g

    Persicae Semen *(tōnin/táo rén)* 3g

    Moutan Cortex *(botanpi/mǔ dān pí)* 3g

    Bupleuri Radix *(saiko/chái hú)* 3g

    Cinnamomi Ramulus *(keishi/guì zhī)*............. 3g

    Citri reticulatae Pericarpium *(chinpi/chén pí)* 3g

    Aurantii Fructus immaturus *(kijitsu/zhǐ shí)* 1.5g

Carthami Flos *(kōkaa/hóng huā)* 1.5g

Glycyrrhizae Radix *(kanzō/gān cǎo)* 1.5g

Rhei Radix et Rhizoma *(daiō/dà huáng)* 1.5g

Natrii Sulfas *(bōshō/máng xiāo)* 1.5g

[2] The formula consists of:

Bupleuri Radix *(saiko/chái hú)* . . . . 2.0 g

Angelicae sinensis Radix *(tōki/dāng guī)* . . . . 1.5 g

Paeoniae Radix alba *(byakushaku/bái sháo)* . . . . . . 1.5 g

Chuanxiong Rhizoma *(senkyū/chuān xiōng)* . . . . . 1.5 g

Rehmanniae Radix *(shōjiō/shēng dì huáng)* . . . . . . 1.5 g

Forsythiae Fructus *(rengyō/lián qiào)* . . . . 1.5 g

Platycodi Radix *(kikyō/jié gěng)* . . . . 1.5 g

Arctii Fructus *(gobōshi/niú bàng zǐ)* . . . . 1.5 g

Trichosanthis Radix *(tenkafun/tiān huā fěn)* . . . . . 1.5 g

Menthae haplocalycis Herba *(hakka/bò hé)* . . . . . . 1.5 g

Glycyrrhizae Radix *(kanzō/gān cǎo)* . . . . 1.5 g

Coptidis Rhizoma *(ōren/huáng lián)* . . . . 1.5 g

Scutellariae Radix *(ōgen/huáng qín)* . . . . 1.5 g

Gardeniae Fructus *(shishi/zhī zǐ)* . . . . 1.5 g

Phellodendri Cortex *(ōbaku/huáng bái)* . . . . 1.5 g

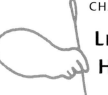

CHAPTER 11

LIVER DEFICIENCY / YIN DEFICIENCY / HEAT PATTERN

肝虚陰虚熱証

kan kyo in kyo netsu shō/gān xū yīn xū rè zhèng

THE YIN QI and fluids have several basic characteristics, including stillness, cold, contraction, and lubrication. When the yin qi becomes deficient, the result is the production of heat. This heat is produced in yin areas—the yin organs and the yin meridians—and thus it is called a yin deficiency heat pattern. Within the yin organs, the Kidneys, Liver, and Spleen contain the fluids. When the Heart and the Lungs become deficient in yin qi, heat is produced. However, because this heat is produced in a yang area, both distal pulses become stronger, and this situation is not called yin deficiency. Here we will consider the Liver deficiency/yin deficiency/heat pattern.

BACKGROUND

The pattern of Liver deficiency/yin deficiency/heat is the result of a deficiency in the fluids of the Kidneys, which in turn causes the fluids in the blood of the Liver to become deficient. The heat that is produced as a result of Kidney fluid deficiency causes the hands and feet, or just the feet, to become hot and uncomfortable. Also, the heat tightens the Liver meridian—a process known traditionally as bulging disorders (疝 *sen/shàn*)—and thus the lower abdomen or the testicles develop painful cramps. The tightness and pain can also radiate to the lower abdomen and back. Finally, since the blood of the Liver is affected, patients with this condition become irritable when they fail to do their work to their own satisfaction.

There are many causes of this pattern, including excessive physical labor, overindulgence in sex, pregnancy, childbirth, or having an abortion or miscarriage. In fact, anything that causes the fluids in the blood to dry up and produce heat can lead to this pattern. If pathogenic wind is also present, fevers will readily develop, a condition described in the *Discussion of Cold Damage* as wind attack (中風病 *chū fū byō/zhòng fēng bìng*).

Heat produced from Liver deficiency/yin deficiency moves to the surface by way of the Gallbladder meridian, and the patient will feel feverish as a result. This sense of feverishness may or may not be accompanied by an increase in body temperature. However, since the heat is the product of deficiency, it will not last very long, and after radiating outward, the body cools off, which is subjectively felt as chills. This coming and going of hot and cold is typical of this pattern and is known as alternating fever and chills. If the heat radiation is inadequate, problems such as migraines, stiff shoulders, insomnia, and neurasthenia will occur. The deficiency heat can also go to the Heart, Lungs, or Bladder directly or spread to the meridians, slowing down their circulation and thereby causing hard areas. As a consequence, problems such as a variety of neuralgias, joint inflammations such as frozen shoulder, facial and other types of paralysis and lower back pain are more likely to occur. Other problems include heart disease, high blood pressure, hardening of the arteries, hemiplegia, cataracts and other eye diseases, and gynecological diseases such as menopausal problems and cystitis.

EXAMINATION

Visual

The faces of patients who have a significant amount of heat from yin deficiency tend to be red. Those with a constitutional tendency to develop Liver deficiency/yin deficiency have relatively narrow and long eyelids. By contrast, those with small eyes tend to develop Liver deficiency/yang deficiency, while those with large eyes are prone to blood stasis. Finally, the edge of the ear (the antihelix) tends to stick out further than the rest of the ear in Liver deficient types.

Pulse

The pulse will be floating and big, and when firmly pressed it will reveal itself to be lacking in force. Because the pulse is big, it will feel as if it is floating, but if the pulse is examined by applying varying levels of pressure (light, medium, and firm), the practitioner will find that sunken pulses are quite common. In this way the big, deficient pulse will compress like a sponge and will actually feel more like a submerged pulse. Furthermore, a big pulse can range from being forceful and big to weak and big. This variance is a consequence of the variable amount of deficiency heat produced in different individuals. It is also commonly wiry or tight, which is a sign of more advanced disharmony.

When lightly pressed, the left medial pulse will be found to jut out from the rest. When firmly pressed, the left medial and proximal pulses will be found to be deficient. This pulse pattern is typical of Liver deficiency/yin deficiency. Note, however, that sometimes the pulse is found to be hard to the touch when it is firmly pressed. This is because in these individuals the deficiency heat is unable to make its way to the outside and causes internal dryness.

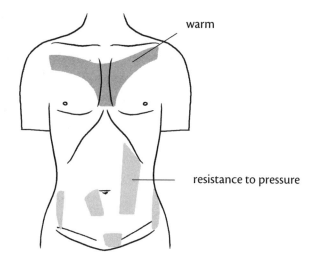

warm

resistance to pressure

Fig. *11*　Abdominal signs for Liver deficiency/yin deficiency/heat pattern

Abdomen

The chest will feel warm, and there will be muscular tightness and resistance on the left side, from the ribs downward; this pattern is known as Liver accumulation (肝積 *kan shakū/gān jī*) (Fig. 11). In addition, a pulsing can be felt on the left side of the navel as well as pain on pressure in the inguinal area, which usually radiates to the lower back, and around the pubic symphysis. Finally, the sides of the abdomen are tight, and the area around the navel will display resistant areas, which are a result of blood stasis.

TREATMENT

As a basic rule, KI-1, KI-10, LR-1, and LR-8 are tonified (Table 13, see page 63). KI-10 and LR-8 are the water points, which help to cool the body by moving fluids into the Kidneys and Liver, respectively. LR-1 and KI-1 are the wood points and help to tonify (and, in the process, cool) the Liver by tonifying the nutritive qi. The next step is to shunt the Gallbladder meridian. This is done at either the protective qi level or the nutritive qi level, depending on the extent of deficiency heat present.

Overall, many needles should be left in place, and moxa head needling can be performed on hard, resistant areas. On hot, tight areas, heat perception moxibustion is performed. In areas where there is paralysis and pain, Do In massage can be performed to good effect.

Herbal Treatment

When the symptoms are principally connected with menopause, a typical formula would be Augmented Rambling Powder (加味逍遥散 *ka mi shō yō san/jiā wèi xiāo yáo sǎn*).

For irritability and anger with increased blood pressure, a typical formula would be Restrain the Liver Powder (抑肝散 *yoku kan san/yì gān sǎn*). For signs and symptoms principally connected with the Heart and Lungs that are indirectly caused by a pattern of Liver deficiency/yin deficiency/heat, a typical formula would be Honey-Fried Licorice Decoction (炙甘草湯 *sha kan zō tō/zhì gān cǎo tāng*).

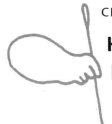

CHAPTER 12

Kidney Deficiency / Yin Deficiency / Heat Pattern

腎虚陰虚熱証

jin kyo in kyo netsu shō/shèn xū yīn xū rè zhèng

Background

THIS PATTERN OCCURS as a result of a deficiency of fluids stored by the Kidneys. As a consequence, heat is produced, which rises out to the surface and is dispersed. It is for this reason that in the *early stages* of Kidney deficiency there are symptoms such as uncomfortable heat in the hands and feet and sweating, especially from the ankles downward. The face is oily, and because there is so much sweating, the patient is usually thin but has a large appetite.

When the Kidney deficiency becomes *chronic,* heat does not make its way out to the surface in such large quantities. This results in an inability to eliminate fluids from the surface. This will cause superficial edema that can be cleared if the Lung qi is sufficiently strong. In Kidney deficiency, however, it is very common for both the Lungs and Kidneys to be simultaneously deficient, producing symptoms such as water retention, obesity, hands and feet that readily chill, and extreme sensitivity to both hot and cold. If the deficiency heat decreases even more, the condition will approach a Kidney deficiency/yang deficiency/cold pattern.

The deficiency heat from the Kidneys can easily jump to the Spleen or Heart. If the heat lodges in the Spleen, the fluids normally transformed and transported by the Spleen begin to dry up and more heat is produced. The heat will also lodge in the Stomach, which begins to work harder as a result, causing a huge increase in appetite. Also the Kidney deficiency affects the contractive ability of the Kidneys to hold things in; when this is combined with the tendency toward a large appetite, the outcome is often obesity, a process that can lead to diabetes.

The presence of deficiency heat from the Kidneys in the Heart is known as deficient yin with disturbed fire (陰虚火動 *in kyo ka dō/yīn xū huǒ dòng*). This state results in such problems as palpitations, shortness of breath, high blood pressure, and a higher likelihood of heart disease.

Of course, there are other areas to which the deficiency heat can spread, but there are a few standard symptoms that are common to the Kidney deficiency/yin deficiency pattern. These include lower back pain, weak legs, a decline in sexual performance, nocturia, urinary difficulty, edema, peptic ulcers, and a decrease in hearing. The most common causes of Kidney deficiency/yin deficiency/heat are overindulgence in sex and being physically overworked.

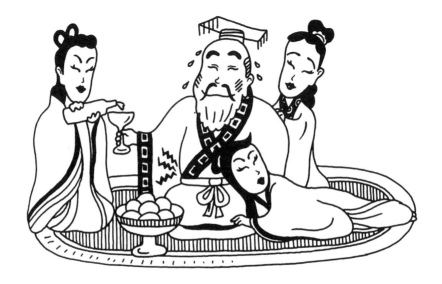

Kidney deficiency is brought on by overindulgence in sex

EXAMINATION

Visual

The faces of patients who have a large amount of deficiency heat display a grayish color and have an oily texture. The ears should be inspected carefully because they provide important information. Typically, they will be darker than usual. Finally, patients with especially large ears are constitutionally prone to developing Kidney deficiency/yin deficiency, particularly if the helices come forward.

Pulse

If there is a substantial amount of deficiency heat, the pulse will be floating and bigger. However, when there is only a small amount of deficiency heat, fluid is retained at the surface, causing the pulse to be sunken and difficult to discern. One other factor in this pattern is the ability of the deficiency heat to radiate outward; if this is impaired for any reason, the Kidneys themselves will receive the heat. This results in a sunken, hard pulse.

On firm pressure, the left proximal and the right distal pulses will be deficient. By contrast, if there is a large amount of deficiency heat, the left proximal pulse will be very evident even on light pressure. In conditions such as nephritis, if the pulse at the left proximal position is sunken and tight, the prognosis is not good.

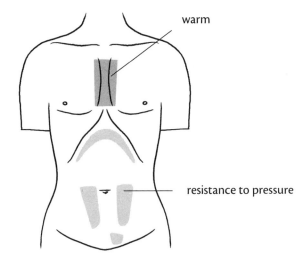

Fig. 12   Abdominal signs for Kidney deficiency/yin deficiency/heat pattern

Abdomen

In cases of Kidney deficiency, the area of the abdomen below the navel along the Conception vessel feels weak (FIG. 12). When the *entire* lower abdomen feels week, this is *not* indicative of Kidney deficiency/yin deficiency, but rather of Kidney yang deficiency. When there is yin deficiency, the heat produced will try to make its way outward. This results in tension in the abdominal muscles, which is most evident in the Stomach meridians of the lower abdomen. Also there is sometimes hardness in the epigastrium around CV-14. Moreover, yin deficiency heat will tend to create a sensation of heat in the chest.

TREATMENT

The basic treatment is to tonify LU-5, the water point of the Lungs, and KI-7, the metal point of the Kidneys (TABLE 13, see page 63). If there is a large amount of deficiency heat, KI-2 (fire point) and KI-10 (water point) can also be used. In all cases, the nutritive qi is being tonified; shunting is not so important. However, moxa head needling should be performed as this technique is both tonifying and warming, and tonifies the yin qi as well. For chronic Kidney deficiency, direct moxibustion at the Kidney back-associated point, BL-23, is very effective. Also Do In massage to KI-1 and KI-2 is recommended.

Herbal Treatment

When there is a deficiency of fluids giving rise to a large amount of deficiency heat, a typical formula would be Six Ingredient Pill (六味丸 *roku mi gan/liù wèi wán*). Outside of Japan, this formula is more commonly known as Six Ingredient Pill with Rhemania (六味地黃丸 *liù wèi dì huáng wán*).

When there is deficiency heat internally but the patient presents with cold symptoms because of a lack of yang qi at the surface of the body, a typical formula would be Eight Ingredient Pill (八味丸 *hachi mi gan/bā wèi wán*). Outside of Japan, this is more commonly known as Kidney Qi Pill from the *Golden Cabinet* (金櫃腎氣丸 *jīn guì shèn qì wán*).

When the deficiency heat is negligible and there is water collecting near the surface of the body, a typical formula would be Stephania and Astragalus Decoction (防已黄耆湯 *bō i ō gi tō/fáng jǐ huáng qí tāng*). Finally, when the deficiency heat has moved inward and has affected the Kidney meridian itself, a typical formula would be Coptis Decoction to Resolve Toxicity (黃連解毒湯 *ō ren ge doku tō/huáng lián jiě dú tāng*).

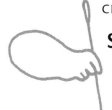

CHAPTER 13

Spleen Deficiency / Yin Deficiency / Heat Pattern

脾虚陰虚熱証

hi kyo in kyo netsu shō / pí xū yīn xū rè zhèng

Background

T HE BLOOD, QI, and fluids of the body are all contained in the Spleen. A deficiency of mainly the fluids is referred to as a pattern of Spleen deficiency/yin deficiency. This obviously creates a type of deficiency heat that can spread very easily to the Stomach and Intestines. Also the flesh, joints, and the entire organ-meridian system are susceptible to an attack by the deficiency heat.

Constitutional factors leading to the development of this pattern are very common. It also frequently occurs after the resolution of a febrile disease. Other causes can include overexertion (especially in the use of the hands and feet), overindulgence in food and drink, and excessive deliberation.

The symptoms are mainly those involving deficiency heat of the Stomach and Intestines such as gastric fullness, abdominal pain, constipation or diarrhea, along with a feeling of lassitude in the arms and legs or of the entire body, and hypersomnolence. Other symptoms include fatigue, lack of vitality, and a lack of stamina. When the patient is tired, the body lacks the ability to push heat outward, so it moves inward and leads to such symptoms as dry mouth, lack of appetite, and joint inflammation. If heat spreads to other parts of the organ-meridian system, a variety of problems may appear, depending on which part is affected. These include middle ear infection, skin rashes, toothache, insomnia, hepatitis, heart disease, cough, wheezing, nocturia, cystitis, and nephritis.

This situation can be understood when we see that deficiency heat entering the Bladder can cause, for example, a decrease in urination or diarrhea with cystitis-like symptoms. Alternatively, if the deficiency heat spreads to the Liver and Gallbladder, it can result in, say, jaundice, and if it spreads to the Lungs or Kidneys, it can lead to coughing or nephritis, respectively.

EXAMINATION

Visual

The face, or at least the area around the mouth, usually has a yellow pallor. The lips themselves are usually either too red or too pale, depending on the amount of Stomach heat present. Similarly, the tongue is moist but may or may not have any coating.

Pulse

The pulse is sunken and wiry. When pressed firmly, the left distal and right medial pulses are deficient. In this case, the wiry pulse is indicative of heat in the Stomach and Intestines. At times, the right medial pulse can be felt to jump out even under light pressure. Also the left medial pulse may be wiry, leading to the conclusion that the pattern is one of Liver excess. This can sometimes be the case, so careful consideration of the symptoms, abdominal signs, and tongue are necessary to determine the correct pattern.

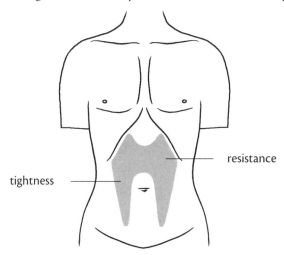

resistance

tightness

Fig. *13*   Abdominal signs for Spleen deficiency/yin deficiency/heat pattern

Abdomen

The left and right rectus abdominus muscles are tight, and there is resistance and pain on pressure in the epigastrium (FIG. 13). The lower abdomen may be distended, but more often than not, the lower abdomen is found to be soft and weak on pressure.

TREATMENT

The basic treatment is to tonify PC-7 and SP-3, the earth points of the fire and earth yin meridians, respectively (TABLE 13). If there is abdominal pain, SP-4, the connecting point of the Spleen meridian, is added. If there is a large amount of yin deficiency heat, SP-9—the water point—is added. To tonify, the treatment is administered at the level of the nutritive qi. There is no real need for shunting unless there is a large amount of deficiency heat. When that occurs, points such as ST-36 and ST-37 may be used to shunt or redistribute the heat. The overall treatment should consist of many retained needles, and moxibustion to the back is also good.

Table 13	Yin Deficiency/Heat Patterns		
	Liver deficiency/yin deficiency/heat pattern	Spleen deficiency/yin deficiency/heat pattern	Kidney deficiency/yin deficiency/heat pattern
PULSE	Overall: (a) floating and smooth; or (b) sunken and wiry or tight Left proximal and medial positions: deficient when pressed firmly	Overall: sunken and wiry Left distal and right medial positions: deficient when pressed firmly	Overall: (a) floating, big, and deficient; or (b) sunken, smooth, and tight Right distal and left proximal positions: deficient when pressed firmly
SYMPTOMS	Alternating chills and fever, irritability, migraine, stiff neck muscles, lower back pain, cramping pain in the testicles	Generalized feeling of lassitude (especially in hands and feet), abdominal distention, abdominal pain, constipation or diarrhea, lack of appetite	Uncomfortable heat in hands and feet, surface retention of fluid, large increase in appetite, nocturia, lower back pain, palpitations, weakness in legs
TONIFYING POINTS	KI-10, LR-8, LR-1, KI-1	PC-7, SP-3, SP-4, SP-9	LU-5, KI-7, KI-10, KI-2
SHUNTING POINTS	GB-41, GB-38	ST-36, ST-37	None

Herbal Treatment

When the heat that results from deficiency of the Spleen's yin qi moves internally and leads to deficiency heat of the Stomach and Intestines, a typical formula would be Cinnamon Twig Decoction plus Peony (桂枝加芍薬湯 *kei shi ka shaku yaku tō/guì zhī jiā sháo yào tāng*). When there is deficiency of the Spleen's fluids with deficiency heat in the Stomach and Intestines that manifests as fatigue from overwork (especially of the limbs), a flushed feeling affecting different parts of the body, dry mouth, abdominal pain, excessive urination, and constipation, a typical formula would be Minor Construct the Middle Decoction (小建中湯 *shō ken chū tō/xiǎo jiàn zhōng tāng*).

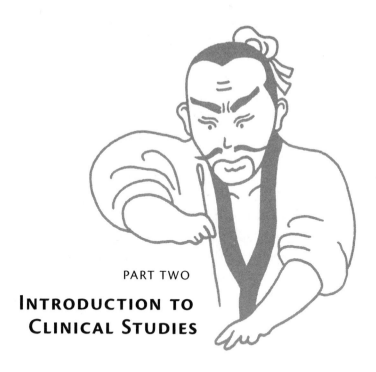

PART TWO

INTRODUCTION TO CLINICAL STUDIES

T HE REMAINDER OF this book discusses the treatment of specific complaints, diseases, and patterns. Only those diseases that I am personally familiar with and have treated effectively will be covered.

The disease states have been listed by their modern medical name to facilitate ease of reference. To obtain the best clinical results, the contents of each section should be read with a firm understanding of the thrust of the preceding chapters in Part One, which describes the root treatments for the various patterns. Each section contains diagnostic information, including the modern medical name for the disease and very general classification methods, and the points and methods to be used in the branch treatments. Detailed information on these subjects can be found by consulting the appropriate medical texts. Next, the classical name, pathology, and pattern as described in the premodern texts are discussed. Some of the disorders are merely simple complaints, in that they have neither a modern medical name nor are they mentioned in the classical texts; only their pathology and associated patterns are discussed. The choice of points and methods used for the branch treatment were influenced not only by the classical texts, but also by senior practitioners with whom I have been privileged to study. Most of the points and methods, however, evolved after having proven their worth in the clinic.

It is difficult to describe, by means of the written word, the process of treatment. This is because in the clinical situation, one's hands will move instinctively to reactive areas without thinking of the name of the points. Moreover, I have forgotten the names of many of the points! Notwithstanding these minor problems, it is hoped that the thirty years of experience that are the foundation for this book will be of use in the reader's clinical practice.

In the tables in Part Two the points highlighted in **bold** are those which I consider to be the most important, and which I find myself using most often. To avoid repetition, the points highlighted in the text are usually not included in the associated tables. By this means we hope to discourage readers from simply following a list of points, and instead rely more on their palpatory skills and knowledge of acupuncture to explore the best points to be used for any given patient. In addition, no mention is made of shunting or tonification because this is dependent on the overall deficiency or excess of yin and yang, the local deficiency or excess of yin and yang, and the presence of heat or cold. With these factors in mind, tonification or shunting is applied. Nevertheless, generally speaking, the yin meridians are tonified while the yang meridians are shunted.

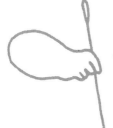

CHAPTER 14

NEUROMUSCULOSKELETAL DISEASES

THE SUBJECTS COVERED in this chapter include stiff shoulders, stiff neck, whiplash, trigeminal neuralgia, facial paralysis, shoulder pain and frozen shoulder, stroke, chest wall pain and herpes zoster, joint pain, lower back pain, sciatica, lower extremity problems, and trauma. These are all problems that are commonly seen in the clinic. In traditional thinking, these diseases are regarded as those that affect the body hair, blood vessels, sinews, and bones, and are therefore classified as outer or external (外 gai/wài) diseases. Hemiplegia is included in this chapter because, although it is the result of a circulatory disorder, it involves the brain and rehabilitative treatment is an important component of the disease. Herpes zoster is of course a skin complaint, but because of its strong connection with intercostal neuralgia, it is also included here.

Outer diseases are part of the meridian sinew system. Because of this, some people believe that they are not connected with the organ system. It is true that there are occasions when there are no symptoms associated with the yin or yang organs. However, all diseases occur as a result of deficiency of the essence of the yin organs, even if there are no symptoms of internal disharmony.

Pain, swelling, and/or paralysis are the main complaints in cases of outer diseases. These disorders are said to occur as a result of external pathogens such as wind, cold, or dampness. These external influences can only affect the body when there is a deficiency in the essence of the yin organs.

When the pain is caused by the wind pathogen, it will tend to move around, and the pulse will be floating and large. Wind can also cause paralysis. The type of pain induced by cold is characterized as stubborn and fixed, occurring spontaneously, and the associated pulse is tight. Dampness gives rise to numbness and swelling as the main complaint, and is associated with a sunken pulse.

Outer diseases can also occur as a result of other factors that include overwork, blood stasis, and internal phlegm and thin mucus (discussed further below). If the causative factor is overworking, while there will be pain, fatigue will be the main symptom, and the pulse will be big and floating. If there is blood stasis, the pain will be stubborn and fixed in location, often manifesting at night. The pulse will be sunken, rough, and excessive. When phlegm and thin mucus are the cause, numbness and swelling will be the main symptoms. The pulse will be sunken and slippery, or sunken and wiry.

Whatever the disease, if the pattern is clearly understood and the appropriate treatment is administered, the patient will recover. There are, however, cases where the root treatment by itself is not sufficient to affect a cure. In these cases, the points used in the root treatment and the tonification and shunting methods are modified slightly. Sometimes even this is not enough.

Take, for example, a case of Liver deficiency/yin deficiency/heat. The tonification of the fluids of the Kidneys and the Liver should result in a quenching of the deficiency heat and a corresponding disappearance of the symptoms. If, however, the deficiency heat has reached other organs and meridians, then the 'local' areas must be treated as well or the symptoms will not be resolved. The important thing is to determine which meridians the heat has entered. This can be learned by understanding the symptoms in detail as well as by discerning the six positions of the pulse in terms of their respective qualities. For example, the pulse at the Kidney and Liver positions of a patient with Liver deficiency/yin deficiency/heat is sunken and wiry. If this is indeed the case, and if the patient has a cough that is often worse at night, then the pulse in the upper positions should be investigated. The cough could well be a result of Lung heat, in which case the Lung pulse might be sunken, rough, and forceful. Also, the path of the meridians can be examined for hard and painful areas.

Note that when heat or cold enters a meridian, the points on that meridian often move and cannot be found in their normal location. It is also important to remember that reactive points used in the branch treatment will change according to the pattern. For example, with patterns of Spleen yin deficiency, the reactive points most likely will appear along the Stomach and Large Intestine meridians. It is with these factors in mind that the points used for branch treatment should be carefully determined.

14.1 STIFF SHOULDERS

Diagnosis

The term stiff shoulders (肩凝り *kata kori*) refers to stiffness in the areas of the neck, shoulders, and between the shoulder blades. Stiff shoulders manifests in many diseases, and if the disease is not dealt with, the stiffness will of course remain. Even if there is no apparent disease, body constitutional factors may be at play, reinforcing the need for determining the underlying pattern and treating the body as a whole.

In Edo period texts, stiff shoulders are referred to as 痃癖(*ken peki/xuán pǐ*). The character 痃 is taken to mean cramping, while 癖 means habitual, which is taken to mean chronic or long-standing. The two terms together then mean chronic cramping of the muscles. According to these premodern texts, causes for stiff shoulders include the following: phlegm, wind, cold, dampness, and deficiency overwork (虚労 *kyo rō/xū láo*). In addition, blood stasis (Liver excess) can also be connected with stiff shoulders.

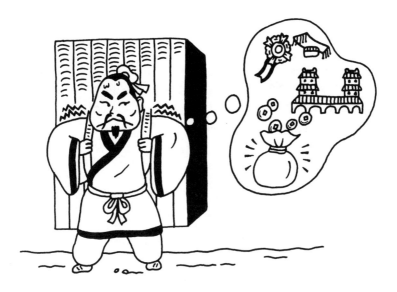

Carrying large loads leads to stiff shoulders

1. Phlegm is part of the category of secondary pathogens known more generally as phlegm and thin mucus (痰飲 *dan in/tán yǐn*), of which there are many types. According to Edo period texts, phlegm is produced when water collects internally and combines with heat. When heat is added to the water, it becomes sticky and ceases to flow freely. Because of this, the circulation of qi and blood is impaired, causing heat to collect and giving rise to stiff shoulders. Phlegm and thin mucus is often present in patients with weak digestive systems, and therefore the most common presenting pattern is Spleen deficiency. With stiff shoulders due to Spleen deficiency, the crest of the shoulders along the Large Intestine meridian is stiff but the muscles over the rest of the shoulders are reasonably pliant.

2. Wind, cold, and dampness are external pathogens that can also cause stiff shoulders. When this happens, the occurrence of pain in the shoulders, neck, and the area between the shoulder blades is preceded by a fever. Even if the shoulder pain occurs without any clear precipitant, an external pathogen is nevertheless involved, and the treatment should be extremely light or the condition will be made worse. These patients may present with any of the basic patterns.

3. Deficiency overwork refers to overuse of the arms (as is often seen, for example, with computer workers, chefs, and waiters) or doing too much work while seated, causing the shoulders to become stiff. The underlying pattern is often that of Spleen deficiency. If there is emotional fatigue and overall body fatigue, Liver deficiency is probably the culprit. With this deficiency pattern, the area from inside the shoulder blades to the neck becomes stiff and the muscles are prone to developing cramps.

4. In cases of blood stasis, the shoulders will be as hard as a rock, with the stiffness running from the medial shoulder blade area all the way up to the neck.

Patients that present with stiff shoulders as a main symptom do not normally have a life-threatening disease. However, high blood pressure is very common in these patients, and if the pulse is either sunken (with or without being tight as well), tight, or rapid, it would be wise to check the blood pressure. If the overall pulse is soft, there is no need for concern.

Treatment

The strategy outlined below is concerned with the branch treatment and so it is not always necessary, or even advisable, to use all the points outlined. Although there are often points that are thought to be especially effective for a given disease, as a general rule, I don't think this way. If the treatment is based on the correct pattern, the stiff shoulders will recover sooner or later regardless of the branch treatment; doing the correct branch treatment allows the shoulders to recover much more quickly. If, however, the treatment is not based on the correct basic pattern, while the shoulders may feel good immediately after treatment, they will soon revert to their old status.

With the branch treatment, it is very important to be able to locate and differentiate the following: areas of deficiency in the protective qi or nutritive qi, hard areas of blood stasis or excess, and hot or cold areas. Depending on the status of the local area, the treatment is weighted toward specific acupuncture and moxibustion techniques. For instance, for yang deficiency (protective qi deficiency), the needling would be very shallow. For yin excess, however, the needling must be more intense.

Generally speaking, it is not as good to needle deeply into the shoulders because deep needling can temporarily affect the flow of blood to the brain, leading to fainting. Preparing the area by rubbing and patting, and then using techniques that encourage the flow of qi and blood, are preferred. If there is a particularly hard area, shunting of the nutritive qi using scatter needling is appropriate. If the muscles are soft, the protective qi should be tonified using soft scatter needling. Often, contact needling of points such as GB-21, ST-12, SI-12, SI-13, SI-14, SI-15, TB-15, and BL-11 has a great effect. It is also good to needle the sides of the neck and the region around the sternocleidomastoid muscle using scatter needling.

There are some cases where strong stimulation is necessary. For instance, I had a patient who was a very heavy drinker with high blood pressure who began to feel stiff and uncomfortable in his shoulder and neck area. He decided to take things into his own hands and nicked his shoulders with a razor to let out some blood. Afterward, he felt much better. It is interesting that this treatment method is mentioned in the late eighteenth-century book *Secret Selections of Acupuncture and Moxibustion*. The text discusses using bloodletting on GB-21, LI-12, and LU-5 for an individual who was in a life-threatening state. Today, this approach is thought to be applicable for patients who have very high blood pressure that leads to stiff shoulders.

When a patient complains of spontaneous pain in the shoulders, only tonification of the protective qi (using contact needling) should be done. The shoulders should not be pressed or massaged in any way. There are also instances where the patients feel stiffness in the shoulder as well as pain on pressure at various points on the chest; nowadays this phenomenon is known in Japan as 痃癖 (*ken peki/xuán pǐ*), a term which used to simply mean chronic cramping of the muscles. In these cases, contact needling is the best method for treating the chest. If heat is present, heat perception moxibustion should also be applied. To treat any chest pain, retain the needles at LU-1 and LU-7 and at stiff areas on the abdomen; this should be followed by heat perception moxibustion.

If the abdomen appears to be weak overall, contact needling (to tonify the protective qi) is administered in this area. If, on the other hand, there is evidence of blood stasis around the sides of the navel, moxa head needling should be done.

On the back, select the hard points from the posterior Kidney meridian[1] and the Bladder meridian in the area from BL-10 to BL-17. Needles are retained in these hard points, followed by the application of moxibustion. This is very effective in removing stiffness throughout the shoulder region. For stiffness of the neck, treat the hard areas between the shoulder blades. However, for stubborn hard knots up around BL-10 and GB-20, it may be necessary to needle directly into these points and to perform Do In massage. Another option is to needle BL-54 and GB-35.

Finally, it is important to needle the back-associated points that are deficient in nutritive qi, which are found by firmly pressing the points. Those that are deficient in nutritive qi will reveal a small hole with the diameter of a loading tube. Needles are inserted and retained at these points.

....

[1] In China, these points are referred to as Hua Tuo's paravertebral points (*Huá Tuō jiá jǐ*) and are located 0.5 to 1.0 units lateral to the depressions below the spinous processes of the thoracic and lumbar vertebrae. As a group, they are also referred to as M-BW-35. In Japan, at least as far back as Sawada Ken (1877-1938), these points are viewed as constituting a posterior Kidney meridian (and will be referred to as such in the text).

Many of the important points in the branch treatment for stiff shoulders are shown in TABLE 14-1.

Table 14-1	Branch Treatment Points for Stiff Shoulders
Location	Points
ARMS AND LEGS	Lesser yang meridian: **GB-21**, GB-36, **GB-39 to GB-40**, LR-5 Greater yang meridian: SI-2, **SI-3**, **BL-54**, **BL-66**, BL-66 Yang brightness meridian: **LI-4**, **LI-10**, **ST-36**
CHEST	**LU-1**, ST-13, KI-27, PC-1
HEAD	**BL-10**, GB-12, **GB-20**, GV-16, GV-18
ABDOMEN	**ST-19**, KI-18, GB-29, **LR-14**, **CV-4**, **CV-12**
BACK AND SHOULDER	**SI-14**, BL-12, BL-22, **BL-37**, **BL-38**, BL-40, **GB-21**, GV-1, GV-11, GV-14

Case History

PATIENT: 59-year-old woman

CHIEF COMPLAINT: A month earlier this patient had contracted a cold, after which pain had begun to spread from her right shoulder down to and including her whole upper arm. The pain was spontaneous in nature and was sufficient to cause insomnia. She could not raise her right arm because of the pain.

HISTORY: This revealed nothing special except that the subject had a number of cups of coffee with something sweet every day.

VISUAL: The subject was of medium to slender build, and her complexion lacked luster, perhaps due to fatigue. Her tongue was moist with a thin coating, which indicated a lack of excess heat.

ABDOMEN: The area on both sides of the abdomen from ST-19 to ST-21 was found to offer resistance upon palpation.

PULSE: The overall pulse was found to be rapid and tight. Both the left distal and middle position pulses were sunken, tight, and excessive. The left proximal pulse was deficient on both light and firm pressure. The right distal position pulse was sunken and rough. The right middle position pulse was deficient on light pressure. The right proximal pulse was sunken, wiry, and deficient.

TREATMENT: In this case, the yin and yang of the Kidneys were both thought to be deficient; Liver excess and Heart heat were also present. Also, perhaps as a result of the excessive intake of coffee, the Stomach was deficient, with water collecting below the Heart.

The root treatment consisted of needling only KI-7 bilaterally. This was followed by the application of heat perception moxibustion at CV-12. The patient was then made to lie down on her left side. Needles were then inserted and retained at LI-15, LI-16, and TB-14. After 20 minutes the needles were removed and contact needling was applied to areas of the upper arm where the protective qi was found to be deficient. Points such as LI-11, TB-14, SI-9, and SI-11 were used. After the treatment, the shoulder pain had completely disappeared. The following day, a small amount of pain remained, and so the same treatment was repeated, which resulted in a complete cure.

14.2 STIFF NECK

Diagnosis

If the shoulder is persistently stiff and the individual becomes exhausted as a result, the person may wake up one morning unable to move the neck at all. (This is sometimes called torticollis or wry neck.) In severe cases, the sufferers are in such pain that they literally do not know what to do with their own heads. There is no position in which they can be comfortable, including lying face down, face up, or on their side. Even when there is no other complicating disease factor, the sufferers may complain of dizziness and nausea. The causative factors of this condition are similar to those listed for stiff shoulders, the most important of which being overuse of the arms and getting chilled. However, all the basic patterns can potentially lead to this condition.

The painful cramping areas include those near the top of the neck, the area around BL-10 and GB-20 down to BL-11, and on the shoulders from SI-14, SI-15, and TB-15 over to GB-21. Alternatively, there may be stiffness and cramping in the areas between GV-14 and SI-15 or lower down between the shoulder blades around the area of BL-43. These are all regarded as variations of the same problem. All the basic patterns discussed in Part One can be seen in these patients.

Another ailment that is closely related to stiff shoulders and stiff neck is occipital neuralgia where the back of the head throbs with pain. This pain is not always a result of neuralgia; rather, it can also be considered an extension of the symptoms associated with stiff shoulders. In this case, arteriosclerosis and high blood pressure are important in the etiology of the condition, but the treatment is the same as for stiff shoulders and stiff neck. The most common pattern in these cases is Liver deficiency/yin deficiency/heat.

Treatment

If possible, the patient should slowly recline in a supine position and light scatter needling should first be performed on the abdomen to allow the patient to relax. Next, the root treatment is performed followed by scatter needling around the sternocleidomastoid muscle on the affected side. When this is performed, if there is pain referring down to the chest, scatter needling is done on the chest around LU-1. Subsequently, the patient turns face down and needles are retained from the back of the head down to the back. If lying face down is impossible, the patient can lie on the side, with the needles retained on alternate sides. When doing this, it is important that the head cushion be raised to avoid straining the neck.

Finally, to finish the treatment, the exact area of pain is found. Strong needling or massage should not suddenly be applied to the neck as this will adversely affect the area, even resulting in muscle spasms. Instead, light contact needling is applied. Alternatively, ask the patient to move the head until the patient finds one or more positions where movement is difficult or painful. While the patient maintains one of these positions, tender points are located and light needling or heat perception moxibustion is applied. If the patient is in a seated position, it is important that the stimulation not be strong, as this could cause fainting.

Again, it must be stressed that all types of massage should be avoided. Often a patient will come in after receiving a massage from a friend or acquaintance with the result that the painful neck has become so bad that the patient cannot move the head. This type of patient will take about six treatments to recover, whereas normally (without the friendly massage beforehand), it would take only three treatments.

The types of points to be used are more or less the same as for stiff shoulders. The points GV-14, BL-10, GB-20, GB-21, and SI-15 are essential. Also, the use of the points TB-10, SI-1, SI-3, BL-40, and GV-1 can often result in quick recovery. These points should be used with the basic pattern in mind.

The same basic treatment is given to those with occipital neuralgia. However, in these cases, there should also be needles retained at sites of pain on the occiput. Fukaya mentioned that direct scarring moxibustion to GV-17 is particularly effective for occipital neuralgia. At the same time, he also stated that while GV-15 is very good for pain in the frontal region of the head, it is not effective for pain in the occiput.

14.3 WHIPLASH

Diagnosis

In Japan, patients suffering from whiplash normally arrive at an acupuncturist's doorstep after first receiving medical attention at a hospital. The reason they go to the hospital first is often due to insurance concerns rather than the effectiveness of the treatment. Two of the main causes of whiplash are, of course, traffic accidents as well as any incident that places mechanical pressure on the neck. The assault often causes greater damage to the soft tissue than is at first thought. The sudden shock associated with this kind of trauma usually results in blood and yang deficiency, which is what leads to the stiffening and cramping of the muscles. If there is significant internal bleeding associated with the trauma, blood stasis will ensue. Thus, the patient will often have either Liver deficiency/yang deficiency/cold (i.e., deficiency of both blood and yang) or Spleen deficiency/Liver excess/blood stasis.

Common symptoms include pain and stiffness of the neck and shoulders, inability to move the neck, numbness in the hands and fingers, feelings of nausea, dizziness, headaches, and lower back pain. The pulse is commonly found to be sunken, rough, and fine. If the pulse is also deficient, the diagnosis is usually blood deficiency; if the pulse is excessive, the diagnosis is often blood stasis.

Treatment

The treatment consists of scatter needling on the abdomen, the root treatment, and the retention of needles on the back. Last of all, the neck and upper back are finished with a little bit of light needling. It is important that strong stimulation be avoided at this time. If too much emphasis is placed on the neck, upper back, and shoulders, the patient may feel sick. There should be an inverse relation between the onset of the trauma and the severity of the symptoms and the intensity of the treatment: the more acute and strong the muscular pain and neuralgia, the lighter the treatment should be, with the use of contact needling.

It is also important to treat points on the hands and feet as well as the lower back (TABLE 14-2). Important points for loosening neck stiffness are BL-17 and BL-27 with the goal being to bring the qi down to BL-40, and eventually to BL-60.

By contrast, if there is no spontaneous pain and a number of days have passed since the problem began, then hard, stiff, and painful areas may be selected for shunting needling. This is achieved by retaining the needles at the reactive areas, and if this proves to be insufficient, then use Do In massage, blood letting, and slightly deeper needling with thicker Chinese needle at, for example, BL-10 and GB-20.

Case Study

PATIENT: 30-year-old single man

CHIEF COMPLAINT: The patient recovered well from a life-threatening traffic accident but was suffering from neck pain and stiffness that centered around the left BL-10, and from headaches. The action of chewing food caused the pain to travel from the back of the neck to the head.

VISUAL: The patient's frame was small, thin, and wiry.

SYMPTOMS: None of significance except for the chief complaint.

PULSE: The pulse was sunken, tight, and thin overall. The pulse at the left distal and right middle positions was deficient.

Table 14-2	Branch Treatment Points for Whiplash
Location	**Points**
ARMS AND LEGS	**LI-11**, **ST-36**, SP-6, **SI-4**, SI-7, **BL-40**, BL-60, TB-5, **GB-41**
CHEST	**LU-1**, LU-2, ST-12, ST-13
HEAD	**BL-10**, BL-17, **GB-12**, **GB-20**, GV-16, **GV-17**
ABDOMEN	**ST-19**, **ST-25**, **LR-14**, **CV-4**, CV-14
BACK AND SHOULDER	SI-9, **SI-14**, **SI-15**, **BL-17**, BL-22, **BL-23**, BL-24, BL-25, **BL-27**, BL-41, BL-42, **BL-43**, **GV-8**, GV-9, GV-11

TREATMENT: A root treatment for Spleen deficiency/Liver excess/blood stasis was performed using PC-7 and SP-3. SI-4 was used at the same time, as the Small Intestine is part of the greater yang system (related to the neck pain) and is also related to the digestive system. In addition, needles were retained at the rock-like tissue surrounding the left BL-10 and also at whichever deficient back-associated points were found by visual inspection and palpation. Several similar treatments were performed, but without much improvement in the patient's condition. On one occasion, the tight area was pressed firmly, but this only resulted in the patient feeling dizzy and nauseous. However, on one occasion, ST-36 was needled, and the patient soon recovered. The tightness at BL-10 completely disappeared, and with it, the pain and headaches. This case illustrates that there are some cases where stronger stimulation is required. Of course, it is not always necessary to cause dizziness to achieve a good result!

14.4 TRIGEMINAL NEURALGIA

Diagnosis

The cause of trigeminal neuralgia is often unknown, but factors such as overworking, fever, sinusitis, and dental caries are often involved. However, if the trigeminal neuralgia does not recover after an operation on an affected sinus or tooth, it is the trigeminal nerve itself that is the problem. Sometimes the pain attributed to trigeminal neuralgia may in fact be caused by a brain tumor. It is therefore important to monitor the pain with consecutive treatments. If a number of treatments result in no change in pain, then the patient should be referred to a medical physician for the appropriate tests.

According to modern medical theory, the pain can be located to one of the three branches of the trigeminal nerve. In traditional Oriental medicine, we think in terms of meridians. Thus, the first branch of the trigeminal nerve is associated with the greater yang and yang brightness meridians. The second branch is associated with the yang brightness and lesser yang meridians, and the third branch with the yang brightness meridians. Pain is said to occur when these yang meridians receive heat or cold, which ultimately is derived from a deficiency of essential qi in one of the five yin organs (see the Introduction). Once the pattern has been determined, a root treatment is administered and the local yang meridians are tonified and shunted appropriately. If this is done properly, the problem will resolve itself. There are cases that are simple to cure with the above methods, but unfortunately, there are others that do not respond and may actually get worse, particularly if the treatment method is wrong!

The two most common patterns are Kidney deficiency/yang deficiency/cold and Lung deficiency/Liver excess/blood stasis.

1. With Kidney deficiency/yang deficiency/cold, the yang qi of the yang meridians of the face is depleted. This leads to pain, poor facial color, and a generally tired look. Another possibility is that the complexion is red as a result of the last remaining yang qi being pushed up to the surface by the ever-increasing yin qi (true-cold, false-heat). The pulse is sunken, thin, and weak, but if there is severe pain, the pulse will be rough and tight. The pain from trigeminal neuralgia is often constant, so patients often require the use of pain killers. Because of this, their digestive function is often adversely affected, which interferes with the production of yang qi, and thereby worsens the condition.

2. With Lung deficiency/Liver excess/blood stasis, the deficiency heat from the Kidneys enters the yang meridians of the face and causes pain. At the same time, because of the blood stasis in the lower burner, the lower part of the body is cold while the upper part is hot and flushed. This results in a red face or at least a good complexion. The pulse is a little floating, big, and strong. When there is pain, the pulse will be tight or sunken, wiry, and excessive. Also, the left or right pulse may be flooding. The pain may be constant, but usually it occurs in waves. In the interim period, there is absolutely no problem at all, and so those with this pattern usually have a good appetite and no significant change in their stool and urine.

Treatment

Treatment of the face itself can be very difficult. Here is a selection of the points used for branch treatment by some famous senior practitioners.

- Bunshi Shirota used LI-10, LI-20, ST-3, ST-4, ST-5, ST-7, SI-18, BL-2, BL-11, BL-18, GB-1, GB-2, GB-3, GB-5, GB-12, TB-9, TB-22, and GV-12.

- Sodo Okabe believed that retaining the needles was necessary for the optimum relief of trigeminal neuralgia. The needles were retained at points in painful and stiff areas located on the sides of the neck, shoulders, and upper back until the symptoms subsided. For the branch treatment, LI-15, LI-18, LI-20, ST-1, ST-6, ST-7, ST-9, SI-18, BL-2, BL-10, BL-11, BL-12, BL-43, GB-3, GB-20, GB-21, GV-14, and CV-24 were often used.

- Soyo Kato included LI-3, LI-4, LI-11, ST-45, TB-1, and TB-2 in his point selection.

- Fukaya Isaburo, the famous twentieth-century practitioner of moxibustion, on the other hand, thought that applying heat perception moxibustion or needling the painful area for trigeminal neuralgia would make matters worse. He proposed applying scarring moxibustion to sites at a distance from the affected area. The points he used included SI-14, BL-10, BL-11, BL-12, BL-13, BL-15, BL-42, BL-43, GB-21, GV-10, and GV-11. Points on the shoulders and arms, such as LI-15 and TB-11, and a point on the center of the middle finger at the same level as PC-9, which is sometimes called middle PC-9 (中央中衝 *chū ō chū shō/zhōng yáng zhōng chōng*), were also mentioned. We will call this point simply the middle finger point.

I myself use two different approaches, depending on the effect of needling the painful area. In the first method, I treat for the overall pattern and retain needles at the painful sites. In the second method, I avoid retaining the needles at the painful sites. In general, when the pain is acute, it will probably make matters worse by retaining needles at the painful sites. When the pain is not so marked, then the approach of Okabe, that is, retaining the needles until the pain is diminished, is effective.

Basically, it is not constructive to touch the painful area; indeed, the painful area itself does not want to be touched. However, if the tonifying hand approach (that is, a warm, soft hand full of qi) is used, then the area may be touched and contact needling may be applied at BL-2, GB-14, ST-1, ST-2, ST-3, ST-4, ST-7, ST-5, SI-19, ST-6, ST-8, TB-17, GV-20, and M-HN-3 (印堂 *in-dō/yìn táng*), resulting in a reduction in pain.

When it is impossible to touch the painful area, points on the back, abdomen, arm, and leg should then be used. A successful example of this would include moxibustion at points such as LI-15, TB-11, and the middle finger point. In some cases, the points selected by Kato Soyo, that is, TB-1 and TB-2, are successful, and in other cases, selecting points on the yang brightness meridian, for example, LI-3, LI-4, and LI-11, is better. Also, the choice of points can be approached from an extraordinary meridian perspective, and thus using PC-6, SP-4, TB-5, GB-41, GB-40, or BL-62 can bring good results.

In addition to the points listed above, it is always good to needle and moxa the hard areas of the back. Direct scarring moxibustion (10 half-rice-grain sized cones) to the hollow just above GV-14 can bring good results, and applying moxibustion at LI-15, TB-11, and the middle finger point can bring better results. For LI-15 and TB-11, 7 to 10 half-rice-grain sized cones should be burned, but if the patient does not feel the heat, burning over 20 cones is acceptable. For the middle finger point, the number of cones should be less: three half-rice-grain sized cones is good. Shunting needling should be used on the hard areas on the back while the areas deficient in nutritive qi are tonified by retaining the needles (TABLE 14-3).

Table 14-3	Branch Treatment Points for Trigeminal Neuralgia
Location	**Points**
ARMS AND LEGS	LI-3, LI-4, **LI-11**, **LI-15**, ST-36, ST-45, SP-6, TB-1, TB-2, **TB-11**
ABDOMEN	ST-19, ST-25, CV-4, CV-12, CV-14
BACK AND HEAD	**BL-10**, BL-13, BL-15, BL-17, BL-19, BL-22, BL-23, **BL-42**, **BL-43**, **TB-17**, **GB-20**, **GB-21**, GV-10, GV-11

Case History

PATIENT: 70-year-old unmarried woman

CHIEF COMPLAINT: One year earlier, this patient developed trigeminal neuralgia, the pain extending from the right side of the nose up to and including the eye. There was also pain from the right TB-20 and from above the right eye to the top of the head. The pain came in waves every ten minutes, with each attack lasting around a minute. She also experienced pain when she washed her face, ate, or talked.

VISUAL: Overall the face was red with a little too much luster. There were no significant changes in the tongue. The patient looked much younger than her stated age.

SYMPTOMS: She had retired from a career in teaching and was living alone. Two years ago she had herpes zoster around the left part of her chest. After recovering, her face began to ache. One year ago she was prescribed some pain killers for her face. The side effects from this caused her skin to erupt all over her body to the extent that she had to be hospitalized. Her medical physician recommended surgery for her trigeminal neuralgia.

During the painful episodes, the application of either cold air or hot water to the face often served to dampen the pain. She also applied garlic to her face, or pressed the area of pain. Because the patient lived alone, she was inclined to overdo things, making all her food from scratch and being meticulously thorough about her housework. Because of this, her body was stiff and fatigued; she was completely unaware of these feelings. There were no significant changes in her urine or stool, and she did not complain of cold lower extremities.

PULSE: The overall pulse was sunken and tight, but not thin. The left distal pulse was flooding. The left middle pulse was floating and forceful, but was deficient on firm pressure. The left proximal pulse was deficient on firm pressure. The right distal pulse was wiry and forceful on firm pressure, and the right middle and proximal pulses were both slippery and forceful on pressure.

ABDOMEN: Increased muscle resistance to palpation was noted below both the left and right sides of the rib cage, as well as below the right side of the navel. Furthermore, there was an increase in resistance to palpation around the area of the appendix.

PALPATION: Pain on pressure was noted on the Stomach, Spleen, Lung, and Gallbladder meridians.

TREATMENT: The basic pattern was Liver deficiency/yin deficiency with deficiency heat radiating to the Stomach and Gallbladder meridians. It was also thought that stagnant heat was responsible for the response of the Lung meridian to pressure. The standard treatment of tonifying KI-10 and LR-8 and heat perception moxibustion at LU-6 was performed. The patient remarked that she could hardly feel the heat from the moxibustion. Finally, as a way of finishing the treatment, the upper back was needled very lightly with tonifying scatter needling.

The next day the patient complained that the pain was worse than ever despite her not touching her face. It was thought that this was caused by the deficiency heat entering the yang brightness meridians. The left LI-10, right LI-11, and left and right ST-36 were shunted.

On the following day the patient complained that the pain had worsened. Moxa head needling was performed at the left and right SP-6, and scarring moxibustion (seven half-rice-grain sized cones) was administered on the left and right LI-11 and the left and right ST-36. The root treatment consisted of a standard Liver deficiency/yin deficiency root treatment with shunting applied to the lesser yang meridian at GB-39. The hard areas (which were difficult to find) on the upper back were treated with heat perception moxibustion.

The next day the patient reported that while the treatment given on the previous day initially led to a reduction in pain, the pain had returned by the following morning. Again, the treatment was aimed at rectifying a Liver deficiency/yin deficiency pattern by tonifying KI-10 and LR-8. Needles were also retained at ST-1, ST-2, and GV-23. As on the previous day, half-rice-grain sized moxibustion was performed at LI-11 and ST-36, and heat perception moxibustion was applied to the right SI-11 and to BL-13, BL-43, and BL-44 bilaterally. Ten half-rice-grain sized moxa cones were also applied at BL-58 bilaterally. The above treatment was administered for three consecutive days, during which the patient complained that the pain was worse than ever.

At this point, the pulse was once again examined with considerable care. The right-side pulse was found to have settled down completely, while the left distal pulse was the same overflowing pulse. Also, while the Kidney deficiency was still evident, the Liver and Gallbladder pulses appeared to have become excessive. The first diagnosis of Liver deficiency may have been mistaken: the Liver was probably normal at the beginning. The patient's condition probably became worse because of the Liver excess, and this was corroborated by the indications of blood stasis in the abdomen. Her being single for such a long time probably contributed to the Liver excess condition. For women, blood and sex are intimately related. A woman's secretions during intercourse are derived from blood. Lack of sex causes a buildup of blood, leading to Liver excess. On the other hand, too much sex leads to blood deficiency in the form of Liver yang deficiency.

When she returned to the clinic three days later, a new diagnosis of Lung deficiency/Liver excess/blood stasis was adopted. KI-7 and KI-10 were tonified, and GB-38, GB-41, and LR-2 were shunted. While the standard Liver meridian point used for shunting is LR-8, because there was more heat and relatively less blood stasis here, LR-2 was more useful. As before, direct scarring moxibustion was applied at LI-11 and ST-36. Added to this, three half-rice-grain sized moxa cones were applied to SI-14, BL-42, BL-43, BL-13, BL-14, and BL-15. At this stage, the hard areas on the back became much more evident.

Even after all this, there was still no change, and so the midnight-midday relationship (based on the traditional clock) was investigated in connection with the Liver excess. From this, the Small Intestine meridian was palpated for reactive sites. The right SI-7 as well as SI-14 were found to be hard, and three half-rice-grain sized moxa cones were applied to these and the points used on the previous day. The root treatment was for Lung deficiency/Liver excess. In addition, needle head moxibustion was applied at the left and right SP-6.

Many different methods with good and not-so-good results were tried until at last her situation began to improve. The patient's face was no longer so red or shiny. Also, she was coming to the clinic by bicycle, riding for 20 minutes, seemingly unaware of the breeze striking her face. I was a bit concerned by this, so I advised her to try and cover her face as much as possible while riding her bike.

When she returned to the clinic four days later, the root treatment was again for Lung deficiency/Liver excess with tonification of KI-7 and KI-2. To shunt the Liver excess, a needle was retained at LR-2. Needle head moxibustion was performed at SP-6, and direct moxibustion was performed at ST-36, right SI-7, TB-11, BL-42, BL-13, GV-12, GV-11, right BL-43, BL-14, and right BL-15. A treatment was performed almost every day, but the patient insisted that her condition was gradually getting worse. Having said this, she was nevertheless sleeping at night with no pain, and was able to lie face down now without any pain while being treated. The pulse also showed that the right side was completely normal. In addition, she was now aware enough to recognize that her feet were cold.

Four days later the patient reported that for the previous 24 hours she had begun to feel stiffness around the inside of her right shoulder blade. The root treatment consisted of tonifying KI-7 and KI-2 and shunting retention of needles at LR-2 and ST-36. Abdominal needling consisted of CV-12, ST-25, CV-4, and ST-19. After that the patient was asked to lie on her left side. In this position, direct moxibustion was applied to the right LI-15, right TB-11, and right middle finger point. Three cones of moxa were applied to the middle finger point while the other two points had moxa applied until the heat was felt. LI-15 took 10 cones before the heat was felt, while TB-11 took 20 cones. On the upper back, needles were retained at hard and stiff areas such as BL-41, BL-42, BL-43, BL-13, and BL-15. Needles were also retained at sites where the nutritive qi was deficient, and at BL-60 and BL-62. After this treatment, the patient was able to turn over in bed without the usual pain in her face that she had previously experienced. Furthermore, the overall level of pain had diminished.

She came the next two days, and the same treatment was applied. This resulted in a further reduction of pain in the face. The patient reported that she had begun to be aware of shoulder stiffness that appeared to be alleviated by walking. She also mentioned that she completely forgot about the facial pain when she walked, but that she did not know what to do with her hands. After some thought, it was realized that she had always carried something while walking and that all her walks consisted of hurried strides to and from work. Walking for the sake of exercise had never been a part of her life.

At last this patient began to recover from this particularly severe case of trigeminal neuralgia. Her particular character and lifestyle made the recovery all the more difficult. For instance, she did not seem to feel that her shoulders were stiff, which meant that she was always prone to overdoing things. Also, the fact that she was single meant that she did everything herself, and her being particularly conscientious meant that she overdid things. The last follow-up visit was approximately two months later, when all that remained was a very slight pain around her nose.

14.5 FACIAL PARALYSIS

In the past, facial paralysis was known as deviation of the mouth and eyes (口眼歪斜 *kō gan ge sha/kǒu yǎn wāi xié*), which referred to the characteristic sagging expression of the facial muscles around the mouth and eyes. The cause of the problem is described at least as far back as the *Essentials from the Golden Cabinet* as wind afflicting the blood vessels, leading to sagging of the mouth and face. This means that the fluids within the blood vessels become deficient, giving rise to heat.

In actual practice, it has often been noted that a number of people who have ridden buses with their heads sticking out in the wind developed facial paralysis. More recently, the overuse of air conditioning has also led to cases of facial paralysis. Another causative factor is exhaustion from overworking or moving one's belongings; either of these can cause the shoulders to become extremely stiff. Afflicted individuals were also probably subject to the adverse affects of wind and drafts during the course of their labors.

Facial paralysis is regarded as an instance of the traditional disease category of wind-stroke (中風病 *chū fū byō/zhōng fēng bìng*). Various problems that cause hemiplegia also fall under this traditional rubric. If a patient is being treated for facial paralysis but is found to have extremely high blood pressure plus irregularities in the pulse quality, it is wise to refer that patient to a medical physician for tests. After saying this, it is important to remember that both hemiplegia and, of course, facial paralysis respond very well to acupuncture and moxibustion treatment.

A week of daily treatments should result in a noticeable if gradual improvement in the facial paralysis. After 20 days of treatment, even the most stubborn cases usually respond. According to my experience, some cases are completely cured after three treatments. However, if the individual has both facial paralysis as well as diabetes and high blood pressure, progress can be difficult. Obviously, if the paralysis is of a long-standing nature, good results will also be relatively difficult to achieve.

Facial paralysis can be found in the areas supplied by the yang brightness and lesser yang meridians. It is important to note that the Liver meridian runs underneath the yang brightness Stomach meridian all around the inside of the lips and cheek. It is for this reason that the most common pattern causing facial paralysis is one of Liver deficiency/yin deficiency/heat. The paralysis is produced by one of two mechanisms. In the first, the heat from the Liver yin deficiency is received by the yang brightness and lesser yang meridians themselves, thereby leading to the paralysis. In the second, the areas supplied by these meridians receive the heat, thereby also leading to the paralysis. Facial paralysis was regarded as a type of wind-stroke because of the localized production of heat.

Usually, the muscles on the afflicted side are sagging, while the muscles on the normal side have a healthy tone. If it is still difficult to determine which side is affected by a visual examination, then the patient is asked to tightly close both eyes. The eyelids of the afflicted side will not be able to close completely. Another method is to ask the patient to whistle. The lips of the affected side will not be able to purse properly.

The overall pulse is floating, big, and forceful, or it is sunken, big, and forceful. Another possibility is that the pulse is sunken, slippery, and deficient. Since deficiency heat is being produced, the pulse will generally be forceful. Sometimes it will feel as if the fingers are being bounced off the wrist, but this should not be taken as an excess pulse.

Treatment

First of all, needles are inserted and retained at the site of the paralysis as well as in the abdomen, hands, and legs. The root treatment can be done when these needles are in place. Heat in the yang brightness meridians is treated by retaining needles in the meridians using a shunting method, or by applying direct moxibustion to the meridians.

Next, soft skin needling using a normal needle, not a needle for children, is applied to the face. The method is as follows. Hold the needle at the tip between the thumb and the index finger. The hand is then delicately vibrated with the tip of the needle making contact with the skin. The patient should not feel pain. If the practitioner does not have enough confidence to use this method, simply touching the skin with the needle is another option.

Table 14-4	Branch Treatment Points for Facial Paralysis
Location	**Points**
ARMS AND LEGS	LU-7, LI-2, LI-6, LI-7, LI-11, ST-42, ST-44, LR-2
HEAD	**ST-1**, ST-2, ST-3, **ST-4**, **ST-5**, ST-6, **ST-7**, **SI-18**, BL-2, BL-6, BL-7, **BL-10**, **TB-17**, GB-2, **GB-3**, **GB-12**, GB-14, **GB-20**, **GV-24**
ABDOMEN	ST-19, LR-14, CV-4, CV-12
BACK	SI-14, **BL-37**, **BL-38**, GV-12, GV-14, **area between BL-11 and BL-17 on posterior Kidney meridian**

Lastly, the back, shoulders, and neck are treated because, if these areas are stiff, it can take longer than necessary to recover from facial paralysis. TB-17 is a very important point for this condition and should always be included along with BL-10 and GB-20 (TABLE 14-4).

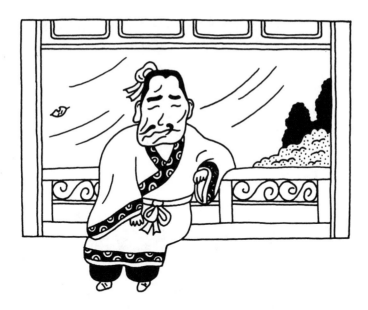

Paralysis is caused by being struck by wind

Case History

PATIENT: 66-year-old woman

CHIEF COMPLAINT: Facial paralysis of the right side

HISTORY: The patient was diabetic and had frequently been to the clinic for sciatica and lower back pain. One day, she awoke to find that the right side of her face was sagging. At the same time, the tips of her right hand and foot felt numb. She was sent to the local hospital for a thorough examination and tests. The results indicated that the problem was not that of the central nervous system; rather, it was caused by her diabetes. The blood sugar level of the patient was double that of normal, and she also had high blood pressure and high cholesterol. In addition, she suffered from a frozen right shoulder: she was only able to raise her arm halfway before it became painful.

VISUAL: The patient was overweight (being fond of sweets) and had a reasonable complexion. The tongue was red and cracked.

SYMPTOMS: Her eyesight had deteriorated to the point where she was seeing double after going up a flight of stairs. She suffered from a little constipation, had a tendency to become excited, whereupon she flushed easily, had a stronger than usual thirst, and tired easily.

PULSE: Overall, the pulse was sunken and slippery, and when it was pressed firmly, the left proximal pulse was found to be deficient. The deficiency at the left middle position was difficult to discern. The left distal pulse was sunken, slippery, and forceful.

ABDOMEN: Overall, the abdomen was rather distended and difficult to judge. However, it was clear that the area below the navel was lacking in normal resilience.

PALPATION: There were no areas of significant tenderness.

CONSIDERATIONS: From the pulse, the main pattern was that of Kidney yin deficiency, with a little Liver yin deficiency as well. The yin deficiency heat rose to the Heart, causing the high blood pressure, to the Spleen, causing the diabetes, and to the Small Intestine meridian, causing the frozen shoulder. When this heat attacked the yang brightness meridian, it caused the facial paralysis.

TREATMENT: KI-10 and LR-8 were tonified, and two rounds of moxa head needling were applied at ST-36 and SP-8. Five rice-grain sized moxa cones were applied bilaterally at the Spleen back-associated point, BL-20, as well as GV-6. Also five moxa cones were burned on the left LI-11. For the frozen shoulder on the right, two rounds of moxa head needling were applied on the right SI-9 and SI-11. For the face, needles were retained at right BL-2, ST-1, ST-2, ST-4, ST-7, GB-4, and GB-14. After this, the needles were removed and contact needling was applied to the skin.

This treatment was repeated two or three times a week for a period of a year, after which the paralysis completely disappeared. Not only this, but the eye problem and the frozen shoulder had also completely disappeared. Furthermore, her blood sugar level had dropped to normal and her blood pressure had also stabilized. Presently, the patient enjoys good health and is seen occasionally for treatment of relatively mild symptoms such as colds or overworking.

14.6   SHOULDER PAIN AND FROZEN SHOULDER

Diagnosis

Most shoulder pain cases seen in the acupuncture clinic are caused by a frozen shoulder. From a traditional standpoint, it usually belongs to one of the following three traditional Oriental disease categories: wind attack (中風 *chū fū/zhòng fēng*), painful wind (痛風 *tsū fū/tòng fēng*), or painful obstruction (痹 *hi/bì*).

1. Wind attack occurs when the Liver is deficient and wind pathogen invades the body. The contractile structures of the body that are controlled by the Liver, that is, the muscles, become numb and/or painful and begin to experience cramps. The wind pathogen has the effect of drying the fluids, which induces heat, and so this condition leads to Liver deficiency/yin deficiency.

2. In a frozen shoulder caused by wind attack, the muscles between the shoulder blades atrophy and frequently cramp up as well. Most of the pain occurs upon movement, with little spontaneous pain. In these cases, it is impossible to raise the arm because of the deficiency heat that spreads into the meridians of the hands, adversely affecting the circulation of qi and blood in these areas and thereby causing the local problems. It is important to find these so-called blocked meridians and treat them; otherwise, recovery will not be possible.

3. In painful wind disease, the Liver deficiency/yin deficiency results in extremely strong pain. In the *Pulse Method Handbook*, the pain is described as "extreme, like that of being bitten by a tiger. For this reason, it is called white tiger painful wind. At night, the symptoms always worsen because the blood enters the yin areas." In my own experience, there are patients with this type of frozen shoulder pain: no pain during the day, but severe pain at night.

4. Painful obstruction disease occurs when there is a combination of three external factors—wind, cold, and dampness—leading to the condition. The resulting diseases vary because of variability in the nature of the dominant factor. In a frozen shoulder caused by painful obstruction, the most common dominant factor is either cold or dampness. When cold is the dominant factor, the pain is fixed, and because the condition is brought about by an attack of cold, the pain is often worst in the morning when it is impossible to raise the arm. The most common pattern that is seen in patients with this type of shoulder problem is Liver deficiency/yang deficiency.

   When dampness is the dominant factor, the shoulder pain usually gets worse just before it rains. The arm, though painful, can be raised a bit. This helps to differentiate this condition from cold painful obstruction. Damp painful obstruction occurs when there is excess fluid collecting in the tissues controlled by the Spleen. This type of frozen shoulder is best treated as a Spleen deficiency/yin deficiency pattern. Interestingly, it is very common in people who have had surgical treatment of gastrointestinal ulcers.

When patients arrive for treatment, is it best to ask them to raise their arms in every direction. When this is done, the direction in which pain is experienced is examined. For instance, when the arm is raised to the front, the patient should be asked whether pain is experienced at the back of the shoulder, front, or side. The affected yang meridians can be deduced from the location of the pain, and the tight meridians and their paired yin meridians should be treated.

Occasionally, there will be cases of shoulder pain caused by traffic accidents or by overuse, such as that seen in laborers and caregivers of invalids. The pain in these cases often becomes worse after the individuals take a break, such as at Christmas or New Year. In these cases, cold is the real source of the problem.

Often, the pulse is found to be sunken and hard, which indicates that the fluids have dried out. This pulse, however, should not be mistaken for yang deficiency. In addition, the left middle and proximal pulses are deficient when firmly pressed. The pulse can also be used to determine the meridians that have been attacked by deficiency heat: the associated positions will have a stronger pulse. For instance, two different pulse patterns can be seen if the deficiency heat has spread to both the Lung and Large Intestine meridians. If the deficiency heat has spread only rather recently, the Large Intestine pulse will be floating and strong. But if the deficiency heat has been around for a long time, the Lung pulse will be sunken and strong.

Treatment

As far as the branch treatment is concerned, it is vital that the hard areas around the upper back, shoulders, and shoulder joints be relaxed. In order to achieve this, acupuncture, moxibustion, Do In massage, and other methods should be considered. Half of the problem is fixed by simply getting this area to relax. It is, however, important to understand that if there is spontaneous pain, the needling for the local treatment should be light.

Regardless of the type of shoulder pain, distal points on the hand should be treated as well (Table 14-5). For example, if the deficiency heat has entered the Lung meridian, tonify LU-10, shunt LU-6, and perform Do In massage between the heads of the biceps. If the deficiency heat has entered the Heart meridian, tonify KI-2, shunt HT-2, and perform Do In massage at HT-1. If deficiency heat has entered the Pericardium meridian, tonify PC-3 and treat the hard areas between PC-1 and PC-3 with acupuncture and Do In massage. If deficiency heat has entered the Large Intestine meridian, perform scarring moxibustion or needle head moxibustion at LI-15 and LI-14. LI-4, LI-10, and LI-11 can also be used. If deficiency heat has entered the Small Intestine meridian, perform scarring or needle head moxibustion at GB-21, SI-10, and SI-11. Shunting of SI-4, SI-6, or SI-8 is also effective. Finally, if deficiency heat has entered the Triple Burner meridian, perform needle head moxibustion at TB-13 and TB-14, and shunting at TB-2, TB-5, or TB-10. Scarring moxibustion can also be applied at TB-12.

Case History

PATIENT: 50-year-old rural woman

CHIEF COMPLAINT: Pain in the left shoulder that started two months previously. It had gradually become worse to the point where there was spontaneous pain that prevented her from getting a restful sleep.

Table 14-5	Branch Treatment Points for Shoulder Pain
Location	**Points**
ARMS AND LEGS	Lung meridian heat: LU-6, LU-10 Large Intestine meridian heat: LI-4, LI-10, LI-11, **LI-14**, **LI-15** Heart meridian heat: **HT-2**, KI-2 Small Intestine meridian heat: SI-4, SI-6, SI-8, SI-10, SI-11 Pericardium meridian heat: hard areas between PC-1 and PC-3 Triple Burner meridian heat: TB-2, TB-5, TB-10, TB-12, TB-13, TB-14
CHEST	LU-1, LU-2, PC-1
ABDOMEN	ST-25, CV-4, CV-12
BACK	SI-14, SI-15, BL-10, **BL-13 to BL-17**, **BL-42**, **BL-43**, GB-20, GB-21

VISUAL: Her face looked a bit fat, with a large number of freckles. The skin had a reasonable luster.

SYMPTOMS: There were no abnormalities in the stool or urine, but her appetite was diminished because of the persistent shoulder pain. She was unable to raise the shoulder at all. It was almost as if the shoulder joint and shoulder blade were totally fixed to the trunk.

PULSE: The overall pulse was sunken and tight, with a deficient left middle and proximal pulse.

CONSIDERATIONS: As noted above, the patient's severe, nocturnal, spontaneous pain is compared in the classical literature to being bitten by a tiger. The pulse was sunken and tight because of deficiency in the fluids of the Liver and Kidneys. The lack of fluids created the hard, tight pulse as well as the deficiency heat that spread to the meridians supplying the left shoulder, leading to the pain. Her lustrous complexion was probably due to the deficiency heat. The spontaneous pain coupled with the scarcity of internal symptoms meant that this case was, as far as the symptoms were concerned, focused in the yang meridians.

TREATMENT: The patient was treated for Liver deficiency/yin deficiency with tonification of KI-10, LR-8, LI-11, and ST-36. She was then asked to lie on her right side, and needles were retained at left LI-14, LI-15, TB-13, SI-9, and SI-14. After the treatment, the patient still had pain in the shoulder but was able to sleep that night. The following day, the same treatment was performed and the patient reported sweating afterward, with a feeling that unwanted heat had been discharged. On the third day, the pulse had changed; it now showed a Spleen deficiency pattern. However, the treatment regime was not changed; it was still directed at Liver deficiency because if the results are good, then the same root treatment should be performed even if the pulse has changed. By this point, the patient was able to do light housework and was able to raise her arm by 90 degrees. Raising the arm beyond this, however, still caused pain.

Similar treatments were carried out daily, and by the seventh day, the shoulder pain had completely disappeared, with the patient being able to resume her farm work. As there was no longer any spontaneous pain, Do In massage was performed on the hard areas around LI-15. After this, the patient felt as if something had been removed from her shoulder, leaving it freer to move. After two months, she was completely cured with no pain and a completely normal range of motion.

14.7 STROKE

Diagnosis

A person who has had a stroke is normally taken to the hospital for acute care. Patients suffering from the sequelae of stroke, such as hemiplegia or hemiparesis, usually go to see an acupuncturist after the acute condition has resolved. We will therefore deal mainly with rehabilitative treatment of hemiplegia from stroke.

While the focus of this discussion is on the sequelae of cerebrovascular accidents, the material presented here is also applicable to Parkinson's disease, brain infarction, or the after effects of brain surgery. Basically, we take a similar approach when treating any central nervous system disease or disorder where the hands and feet cannot move freely.

In the premodern texts, problems like cerebrovascular accidents were known as wind-stroke (see Section 14.5). Patients with this problem can be roughly divided into two patterns: Liver deficiency/yin deficiency/heat and Spleen deficiency/yang deficiency/cold.

1. The Liver deficiency/yin deficiency/heat pattern is the more common of the two. In this pattern, the deficiency heat from Liver yin deficiency spreads to various organs and meridians. The symptoms consist mainly of muscular cramps and paralysis. The face can be red and lustrous. However, if the face has no luster and the patient has speech difficulties and dementia, the prognosis is poor. If the facial complexion is overly lustrous or shiny, then there is a large amount of deficiency heat, which means that a cure is easier to obtain. It is also good to check the state of the hands and feet of post-stroke hemiplegic patients. Normally, the hands and feet are cool, but those patients that have hot, uncomfortable hands and feet have a large amount of deficiency heat.

The urination history should be checked. If the patient is incontinent, there is a severe Kidney deficiency and the prognosis is poor. Also, if there is nocturia, the person is affected by cold and is suffering from Kidney yang deficiency. Constipation is also very common because the large amount of deficiency heat can dry out the stools. Many people use laxatives on a daily basis. However, great care should be taken to avoid diarrhea because this leads to an even greater deficiency of fluids, resulting in even more severe constipation.

There are also many patients in this category who have a generous appetite. This too is due to the deficiency heat, and they should be advised to cut down on their food intake. When this is impossible, the prognosis is poor. There are also those that like to drink alcoholic beverages, which is acceptable in small quantities *if* the symptoms are stable. In addition, because the basic condition arose from Liver deficiency, many victims of stroke tend to be irritable and easily angered. They tend to reprimand their next of kin or some other person, which is again typical of deficiency heat. They should not become too agitated if possible, as this is obviously not good for their condition.

The pulse is floating, big, and forceful, which can be mistaken for an excess pulse. If the pulse is floating and slow, the recovery is easier; a rapid pulse indicates a more difficult recovery. When the pulse settles down during the treatment process, it will change from being big and floating to sunken and slippery or to sunken and wiry. The left and right distal pulses are sunken, wiry, and forceful, which indicates a large amount of heat in the upper burner.

2. The Spleen deficiency/yang deficiency/cold pattern occurs when there is insufficient yang qi, which causes the flesh to become slack and the hands, feet, and the rest of the body to become cold. Occasionally, the hands and feet become even colder, resulting in numbness and pain. There is no constipation, and often there is a loss of appetite. The facial complexion is pale and lifeless. When there is no color to the face, the prognosis is poor. The overall pulse is sunken, thin, and deficient. The right middle pulse is deficient, but sometimes the left proximal pulse is also deficient, which is indicative of a Spleen deficiency/Kidney deficiency/cold pattern.

Treatment

In order to speed up the recovery, it is best to begin treating stroke as soon as the patient's blood pressure has stabilized. Different masters have their own approaches to the treatment of stroke, among which are the following:

• The anonymous, late tenth-century work *Moxibustion Classic from the Yellow Emperor's Bright Hall* listed a set of points known as the seven internal wind points (中風七穴 *chū fū nana ketsu/zhòng fēng qī xué*). This set of points is often used to treat stroke and consists of GV-20, GB-7, LI-15, LI-11, GB-31, ST-36, and GB-39.

- In the Edo period book *An Anthology of Edified Learning*, Doha Manase mentioned that there are two types of strokes: "For those that affect the yang organs, GV-20, LI-15, LI-11, GB-31, ST-36, and GB-39 are good. For those that affect the yin organs [causing speech impairment], GV-20, GB-20, GV-14, GB-21, PC-5, LI-11, and ST-36 are good."

- In Bunkei Ono's late-1950s interpretation of the Edo period classic *A Collection of Acupuncture and Moxibustion Treasures*, he observed: "Acupuncture and moxibustion should be applied at CV-8, GB-20, GV-20, LI-11, TB-17, GB-31, GB-30 and LI-15 to disperse the wind. ... In whatever type of wind-stroke disease, if there are hard masses to be found in the abdomen, these should also be needled." The dispersion of wind probably refers to the dispersion of deficiency heat, while the hard masses in the abdomen refers to the five accumulations described in Chapter 56 of the *Classic of Difficulties*.

- In the *Principles of Acupuncture and Moxibustion*, the eighteenth-century writer Shukei Suganuma stated that CV-12, CV-15, and ST-36 should be needled, GV-20, GV-14, GV-20, GB-31, and ST-36 should be given scarring moxibustion, and BL-40 and LI-4 should be bled.

- In *Secret Selections of Acupuncture and Moxibustion*, Kimura Chuta stated that a point one unit lateral and two units superior to GB-31, and a point two units lateral to ST-36, should be needled.

- In the Edo period text *Ripples from the Way of Acupuncture*, the acupuncturist Ashiwara Kenko explained that to treat stroke: "First, the arms and legs [should be] needled all over using a round sharp needle. Then the area around 痞根 (hi kon/pǐ gēn)[2] and LR-13 as well as the shoulders and upper back are lightly needled over and over, without too much regard for point locations. Excess conditions are treated by bleeding lightly the area around GV-20 and in between the fingers and toes using a three-edged needle; deficiency conditions are treated by administering a large amount of scarring moxibustion to the hands and feet. If the treatment is carried out early, recovery is assured."

We can see from the selections above that the following points are common to most: LI-11, LI-15, ST-36, GB-29, GB-30, GB-31, GB-39, and GV-20. All of these points can be treated using scarring moxibustion, as detailed above. Alternatively, depending on the condition, GV-20 can be bled while the other points can receive moxa head needling. However, if the pattern is that of Spleen deficiency/yang deficiency, the stimulation should be as light as possible, even if the needles are retained. In this case, contact needling is often a better choice.

The prognosis is poor if the stroke patient has impaired speech. However, Fukaya stated that in this case moxibustion should be performed below the second and fifth cervical bones.

....

[2] This point is now called M-BW-16 and is located 0.5 units lateral to BL-51.

An additional area to treat is determined by measuring up from the navel the length of the patient's little finger, which is taken as the apex of a downward-facing equilateral triangle. The sides of the equilateral triangle are also the length of the little finger. Approximately 20 rice-grain sized cones of scarring moxibustion should be burned at each of the corners of the triangle. Finally, moxibustion at GV-15 is a well-known treatment for impaired speech.

Fukaya also recommended scarring moxibustion for paralysis on the distal phalanges of the fingers on the flesh above the bed of the nails. One to two cones are normally enough, but if no heat is felt, the number can be increased. Also, scarring moxibustion at SP-1 and KI-1 can also be effective.

Do In massage on the paralyzed areas is also important, and sometimes just this is enough to facilitate a cure. For best results, the massage should be applied along the flow of the yin meridians and against the flow of the yang meridians, as this would allow the yin to be tonified and the yang to be shunted. This is done when treating a patient with a yin deficiency pattern, which is the most common pattern. For yang deficiency, massage is contraindicated and contact needling or very gentle moxibustion is used instead. The skin at paralyzed areas is often felt to be dried out and lacking in moisture. In this case, massage should be continued until a natural moisturized texture begins to return to the skin. Conversely, if the skin is found to be overly moist, massage should be continued until it dries out a little and becomes normal.

Table 14-6	Branch Treatment Points for Stroke
Location	**Points**
ARMS AND LEGS	LI-4, LI-10, **LI-11**, **LI-15**, **ST-31**, **ST-36**, ST-41, TB-5, **GB-29 to GB-31**, GB-34, **GB-39**
HEAD	GV-14, **GV-20**
ABDOMEN	**LR-13**, CV-12, CV-15
BACK	BL-18, BL-23, **BL-45**, **M-BW-16**

Case History

PATIENT: 63-year-old man

CHIEF COMPLAINT: Numbness and paralysis reported from the left lower back down to the left leg. Also, the left arm was slightly paralyzed.

HISTORY: The paralysis began after an operation three months prior to remove a brain tumor.

VISUAL: He came to the clinic in a wheelchair, but he nevertheless had a strong constitution. His facial features gave a slight hint of dementia, and his speech was unclear. Because of his lack of mobility, he would often get angry with his wife. He was further irritated when he was unable to make himself understood properly.

SYMPTOMS: At night the patient would get up to urinate every two hours. Because he was constipated, an enema was used to evacuate his bowels. His sleep was normal. His left leg felt cold.

PULSE: The overall pulse was big and slightly sunken, with only a little force. When the left distal and proximal pulses were firmly pressed, they were found to be deficient, while the same amount of force produced an excessive pulse at the left middle position. The right middle pulse also proved to be deficient on firm pressure.

ABDOMEN: The hypochondria were a little tight. By contrast, the area below the navel was found to be lacking in resilience.

PALPATION: Overall, the left leg was cold to the touch, with pain on the inside of the knee upon bending and straightening.

TREATMENT: The pattern was that of Spleen deficiency, but in this case, the symptomatic treatment was even more important than the root treatment. Moxa head needling was applied at left LI-15, left and right ST-36, left GB-29, left SP-6, left LI-11, left BL-23, and left BL-25. Heat perception moxibustion was applied at the hard areas found on the inside of the shoulder blades, and Do In massage was given to the paralyzed area.

After this treatment the patient was able to lift his leg slightly and move his ankle. When he arrived for his second treatment, his face showed a return of health. After a few more treatments, the patient stopped using his wheelchair and began to walk with a slight dragging of his left foot. However, he was still a little unstable so his wife had to support him from behind.

14.8   CHEST WALL PAIN AND HERPES ZOSTER

Diagnosis

Intercostal neuralgia is a common cause of chest wall pain, but it is far from the only one. As there are other, and more serious, reasons for this problem, it is important to accurately diagnose the problem. Some of the more common organic reasons for chest wall pain are:

- Chest pain with fever may be indicative of pneumonia or pleurisy, in which case breathing symptoms should be checked.

- Chest pain, breathing difficulty, palpitations, and coughing in young men may be indicative of pneumothorax.

- Pain that is (usually) located in the center of the breast bone as well as numbness along the course of the Heart meridian can be indicative of cardiovascular disease such as either angina pectoris or even myocardial infarction. In the latter, the pain is so intense that breathing may stop (labored breathing).

Even this brief list shows that chest wall pain can be the manifestation of a very serious condition. For this reason, when there is even the slightest doubt as to the cause of the pain, patients should be referred to appropriate medical practitioners for a diagnostic workup.

Intercostal neuralgia often occurs as a sequela to problems such as stiff shoulders or the common cold. The most commonly seen basic patterns are Liver deficiency/yang deficiency or yin deficiency, Spleen deficiency/Liver excess/blood stasis, and Lung deficiency/Liver excess/blood stasis.

Areas with pain on pressure often include the medial and inferior edge of the scapula, the side of the chest, and areas close to the sternum. Often the patient complains of tight, gripping sensations in the chest that, if they are present on the left side, can be mistaken for angina pectoris. The overall pulse will be sunken, rough, and fine, indicating a poor flow of qi.

Intercostal neuralgia is often linked to herpes zoster, which occurs when the herpes virus enters a sheath of nerves, thereby causing inflammation. Usually it is the intercostal nerves that are attacked. However, in some elderly patients, it is the nerves of the buttocks that are attacked, and if the condition is treated incorrectly, the neuralgia will be resistant to further treatment.

Herpes zoster is a hot condition. It is often the result of deficiency heat from Spleen deficiency/yin deficiency spreading to the Lungs and giving rise to Lung heat. It is best if the practitioner is able to recognize herpes at first sight. In the beginning, it often looks like small insect bites, but instead of itchy areas, the lesions are red, filled with pustules, and painful.

Generally speaking, the pulse in patients with postherpetic neuralgia is often sunken, rough, and fine, with the left distal and right middle pulses being deficient. Although the overall pulse is weak, the right distal pulse feels somewhat stronger.

Costochondritis or fractures of the costal cartilage can also cause chest pain. Obviously, in this case, the pain is not life threatening and is usually caused by some sort of blow or collision. In old people these fractures can sometimes be caused by a belt buckle that presses against the ribs or cartilage while they are asleep. In other cases, the patient may experience seemingly inexplicable pain, or pain that appears after an extended bout of coughing. In these cases, the pain could be mistaken for intercostal neuralgia. However, the pain associated with costal cartilage fractures is confined to the rib cage, and so is easily distinguished from that of intercostal neuralgia.

Treatment

It is important to treat both intercostal neuralgia and an attack of herpes zoster as one would treat a cold and advise the patient to basically take it easy. Similarly, the patient should avoid drinking alcohol or taking baths as this may make it easier for the patient to catch cold. There are a variety of other ways to treat these conditions. For example, the moxibustion master Fukaya used scarring moxibustion on the tips of the fingers.

When the tissue close to the spine is palpated, hard areas will be found that run horizontally away from the spine. In addition, PC-1 and BL-42 often exhibit tightness. Needles should be inserted and retained in these areas. Other areas should also be palpated gently for pain and also treated with retained needles. Chief among these are the area running along the medial aspect of the scapula to its bottom angle, the armpit, and the epigastrium near the xiphoid process of the sternum.

To treat herpes zoster, one cone of scarring moxibustion should be placed on top of the herpes pustules. If there are a large number of pustules, only the larger ones should be selected for this purpose. Furthermore, needles should be retained next to the pustules. Usually, if this type of treatment is done early enough, the patient will recover within two to three days with no sequelae. For costal cartilage fractures, needles should be retained directly at the painful sites and a support bandage or plaster should be applied. The plaster or bandage is put on with the rib cage fully expanded. The patient can expect a full recovery in two weeks.

Table 14-7	Branch Treatment Points for Chest Wall Pain & Herpes Zoster
Location	**Points**
ARMS AND LEGS	**SI-4**, SI-8, TB-6, **PC-1, TB-10, GB-38**, GB-44
CHEST	**ST-14, ST-15**, SP-17, SP-18, **SP-21**, PC-1, **KI-25**
BACK	**BL-17, BL-44 to BL-46**, BL-47, BL-48, **along the medial edge of the scapula (including BL-42 and BL-43)**

Case History

PATIENT: 58-year-old man

CHIEF COMPLAINT: The patient reported bilateral shoulder pain, primarily around LI-15 and BL-42. However, inspection found that the pain spread below the right shoulder and around the chest to ST-15. Herpes pustules were found just below CV-22 and also on the right upper arm along the course of the Triple Burner meridian. The pain was such that the patient was unable to lie face up or face down for even 10 minutes.

VISUAL: The patient was overweight with a red face and had a white tongue coating.

SYMPTOMS: The stools were a little soft, and the patient reported slightly reduced urination. His appetite, however, was normal. He also reported shortness of breath. This patient was actually a heavy drinker with a fatty liver and diabetes. His fasting blood sugar often reached as high as 800mg/dL, and the fatty area on his liver was larger than the palm of the hand. Even when faced with these facts, the patient could not give up routinely drinking a third of a bottle of whisky every night; he insisted it relieved the pain. Approximately two months previously he had been admitted to a hospital with a myocardial infarction related to his diabetes, and it was after this that he began to experience pain on the medial aspects of the scapulae. Amazingly, the patient refused to stop his hobby of assembling plastic model planes, even though he was in great pain.

PULSE: The pulse was rapid and urgent to the point that it was difficult to discern any deficiency. The left proximal pulse was apparently deficient and both distal pulses were quite rapid, indicating heat in the Lungs and Heart.

TREATMENT: In this case there was heat in the Heart and Lungs. The treatment used the Kidney meridian fire point, KI-2, to clear heat from the Heart and the Lungs. As the taste of the fire phase is bitterness, these points are often used to remove heat. Similarly, LU-10 is used to clear the heat from the Lungs. KI-2 and LU-10 were tonified and scarring moxibustion was applied to the main herpes pustules. Needles were retained on the painful sites of the chest and shoulders. At first the patient could only lie face up for 10 minutes, but after a few treatments, he was able to do so for 30 minutes.

Needles were retained around BL-42 on the stiff points on the upper back. Then scarring moxibustion and intradermal needles were applied and kept in place at these same points. The above treatment was performed seven times, resulting in a drying out of the herpes and a reduction in pain.

Interestingly enough, from the end of 1994 through 1995, I suddenly began to see many patients with herpes zoster. I thought that this was a peculiarity of my clinic, and so I checked with the local skin dermatologist who reported the same phenomenon. It must have been due to the unusually hot summer of 1994.

14.9 JOINT PAIN

Diagnosis

One of the common ailments of the joints is pain. Pain that can affect all the joints of the body—usually caused by rheumatism—as well as pain of particular joints—the knee, elbow, wrist, finger, and temperomandibular joint—is looked at in this section, with a focus on pattern differentiation and treatment.

In *Essentials from the Golden Cabinet*, joint pain is classified as three types, all of which are related to external pathogens such as wind or cold: damp disease (湿病 *shitsu byō/shī bìng*), wind attack panarthralgia (中風歴節病 *chū fū reki setsu byō/zhòng fēng lì jié bìng*), and water qi disease (水気病 *sui ki byō/shuǐ qì bìng*).

1. Damp disease occurs when a person with a constitution that retains a large amount of water in the flesh is exposed to wind or cold. This results in a fever and swelling and pain of the joints. It is common for all the joints of the body to become swollen and painful. This overlaps with the modern medical disease of rheumatoid arthritis. The joint pain in patients with damp disease is a result of the following patterns:

    a. *Spleen deficiency/yang brightness meridian excess/heat.* This pattern can lead to joints that are swollen like a balloon, hot, and red, and that exhibit spontaneous pain. From the initial stages of the disease, there are fever and chills that differ from those associated with the average cold. After the fever has broken, the patient is left with a feeling of heat, pain, and some swelling. Urination is diminished, but the stool and appetite are normal. It is unusual for a patient to come in for treatment at this stage. After a few more days, as the disease becomes more entrenched, the pain, swelling, and feeling of heat in the joints become more extreme in the afternoons.

    b. *Spleen deficiency/yin deficiency/heat.* The pattern is based on a deficiency of the blood of the Spleen. The joint pain associated with the pattern can vary from spontaneous pain to only slight pain. If the pain is found in joints spread throughout the body, the patient will also have a feeling of heat, occasional redness, and so-called deficiency or pitting swelling, that is, swollen areas that, when pressed, retain their indentation. Occasionally, there may be a feeling of heat in the joints without any redness or pain, even on movement. If there is pain, it is often worse in the morning when the patient first moves the affected joints.

    c. *Spleen deficiency/yang deficiency or Spleen deficiency/Kidney deficiency/cold.* These patterns can result in an intense feeling of heat in the joints, but no local redness. The swelling is of a deficient nature and joint deformities are common. When you press on a swelling from deficiency there is a mild, almost pleasant, pain and a small dent is left in the tissues. Swellings from excess do not pit and pressure leads to intense pain. In many cases, the pain is spontaneous. However, it is also worse in the morning or whenever the joints are cold. This type of joint pain is commonly seen throughout the body and is known as polyarticular arthritis or rheumatoid arthritis. In this type of arthritis, joint deformities are common. These patients are often treated with steroids. Patients who are taking these drugs should not be induced to stop using them precipitously. Finally, other symptoms common to these patterns include reduced urination, constipation or diarrhea, sweating, palpitations, and shortness of breath.

2. Wind attack panarthralgia occurs when the fluids become deficient as a result of the wear and tear of overuse or of other causes, giving rise to deficiency heat. If the person is then exposed at this stage to wind, the fluid deficiency will worsen and there will be a corresponding increase in heat and pain in the joints. The pain is more pronounced at night, and because it is due mainly to deficiency heat, the pain will be severe, but there will be little swelling. However, there may be cases where the body is thin but an affected knee is huge in comparison, giving the appearance of a chicken's leg and knee. The joint pain in patients with wind attack panarthralgia is a result of the following pattern:.

   a. *Liver deficiency/yin deficiency/heat.* This is panarthralgia from *Essentials from the Golden Cabinet* and is often seen with the symptoms occurring mainly in the knees. In the early stages the patient may complain of heat and pain but little swelling. It is common for there to be both spontaneous pain and pain upon movement inside the knee joint. As the condition proceeds, the joint will become larger, but again with little swelling, and the pain will worsen at night. Small blood vessels soon appear in the affected area, and the joints are often deformed.

3. Water qi disease occurs when there is a large amount of water present in the skin and hair at the surface. Under these circumstances, the presence of wind adversely affects the ability of the yang qi to radiate out of the body, resulting in painful joints. This condition is seen in obese individuals who have large amounts of retained fluid and painful knees. However, while there is a large amount of stagnant water, there is little pain. The joint pain in patients with water qi disease is a result of the following pattern:

   a. *Kidney deficiency/yin deficiency/heat.* With this type of joint pain, the little bit of swelling is of a deficient nature. In addition, there is little redness, and the pain is mainly experienced on movement.

Treatment

As a general rule, needles should be retained in any joint that is swollen and painful, with the needles located around the swollen area. In addition, either heat perception moxibustion or direct scarring moxibustion in the form of five half-rice-grain sized moxa cones should be applied to hard and hot areas. In the paragraphs below, the treatment is set forth for various common joint pain.

KNEE PAIN

When treating the knee joint, retained needles are placed in two groups of points. The first group surrounds the patella itself and includes two points that are known as the eyes of the knees (膝眼 *shitsu gan/xī yǎn*),[3] M-LE-27 (鶴頂 *kaku chō/hè dǐng*),[4] two points to the left and right of M-LE-27 on the medial and lateral aspects of the rectus femoris muscle, and two other points located on the medial and lateral aspects of the patella itself. The second group consists of ST-36, SP-9, LR-7, LR-8, GB-33, GB-34, SP-10, and ST-34 with moxa head needling often applied at GB-33. The area between the first and second group of points should be palpated, since swelling is often found in between these points.

Normally, the patella has a little play and can be moved some, but when the knee has been injured, the patella cannot be moved. One clinical pearl regarding the treatment of knee pain is that if the treatment results in the patella regaining its normal range of motion, then the pain will significantly improve. In order to this, Do In massage should be applied to the points found in group one.

The eyes of the knee points (M-LE-16 and ST-35) are located in what look like two small dimples or depressions on the sides of the patella in a normal knee. When there is knee pain, these points sometimes develop fatty-like hard lumps. Finger pressure should be applied to them to help them return to their original state. Just doing this can be enough to cure some knee pain.

As is true for other joint problems, it is important to return the joint to its anatomically correct position, and Do In massage is the quickest method for accomplishing this. This can also be achieved through the use of moxibustion, but care must be taken when dealing with a cold pattern because too much moxibustion can cause dispersion, which then leads to a further cooling of the area.

Other points used to treat knee problems and rheumatic pain elsewhere in the body are listed in TABLE 14-8. Note that the relevant patterns should be kept in mind when choosing

....

[3] The alphanumeric appellation of this pair of points is M-LE-16, and they are located in the depressions on either side of the patella with the lateral point being ST-35.

[4] This point is located in the depression of the midpoint of the superior patellar border.

among these points. Thus, for example, BL-40 or BL-60 can be used to treat joint pain associated with Bladder meridian heat or cold; SI-4, SI-6, or SI-8 can be used to treat joint pain associated with Small Intestine meridian heat or cold; LI-2 or LI-3 can be used to treat joint pain associated with Large Intestine meridian heat or cold; and TB-3 or TB-10 can be used to treat joint pain associated with Triple Burner meridian heat or cold.

Table 14-8	Branch Treatment Points for Joint Pain
Location	**Points**
ARMS AND LEGS	Large Intestine meridian heat or cold: **LI-2**, LI-3
	Stomach meridian heat or cold: **ST-40**, ST-36
	Small Intestine meridian heat or cold: **SI-4**, **SI-6**, SI-8
	Bladder meridian heat or cold: **BL-40**, BL-60
	Triple Burner meridian heat or cold: TB-3, **TB-10**
	Gallbladder meridian heat or cold: **GB-38**, **GB-40**
	Other points: ST-31, ST-32, ST-35, **BL-58**, BL-64, GB-29, **GB-30**, GB-31, **a point 3 finger widths above BL-40, a hard point 1 unit above GB-30**
ABDOMEN	ST-19, ST-25, right SP-25, LR-14, CV-4 to CV-7, CV-9, CV-12
BACK	BL-20 to BL-23, **BL-28**, **BL-30**

ELBOW PAIN

Elbow pain is usually caused by some sports-related activity, the most common of which are tennis elbow and baseball elbow. First, needles are retained at the painful areas, after which it is helpful to perform Do In massage and heat perception moxibustion. In addition, taping the area can be surprisingly effective. The main treatment points include BL-41, LI-13, TB-10, LU-5, SI-8, HT-3, LI-12, LI-11, LI-10, TB-1, SI-4, and any hard areas near TB-11.

WRIST PAIN

The pain is usually a result of tendonitis from overuse of the wrist and arm. Again, needles are retained at the painful areas after which it is helpful to perform Do In massage and heat perception moxibustion. If the area feels warm, a cooling pad like the one used for sports injuries can be useful. However, it is best to apply heat perception moxibustion to points on the wrist such as LI-6; the heat perception moxibustion can discharge the heat effectively without overcooling the area. Alternatively, have the patient grasp a suitably sized natural crystal with the affected hand. This has the effect of cooling the wrist and leads to a cure.

Writer's Cramp

As the name suggests, attempting to write causes the individual's hand to shake or cramp up. Since this condition has an emotional component, a total body treatment is important. In most cases, it is best to treat for Liver deficiency/yin deficiency with special attention paid to clearing hard spots on the Governing and Bladder meridians of the upper back. Applying moxibustion to the fingertips is also useful.

Finger Pain

There are patients who suffer from finger joint pain just before retiring to bed, probably as a result of blood deficiency. The pattern is therefore either one of Liver deficiency/yang deficiency or Liver deficiency/yin deficiency. It is therefore essential to treat the overall body because otherwise there is no real chance of recovery. According to Fukaya, applying one to two rice-grain sized moxa cones to the knuckles is effective. The patient should also refrain from overusing the fingers by, for example, typing on a computer keypad for any extended period.

Other patients may suffer from so-called trigger finger where the offending digit can be bent normally, but trying to straighten the digit results in a feeling of constriction. Straightening the digit cannot be done smoothly; rather, it extends in an abrupt fashion. Treatment of this condition should include needle retention and moxibustion to any hard areas on the upper back between the shoulder blades, and also at BL-17. At the same time, the meridians that run through the clicking digit should be examined at the forearm and upper arm, and once again, needles should be retained or moxa applied at any hard areas.

Temporomandibular Joint Pain

Pain when opening the mouth in a certain way may not be life-threatening, but it can cause great discomfort. Basically, the problem can more easily resolve itself when the shoulders are relaxed and the hard areas on the upper back, including the Governing meridian, are treated.

Case History

PATIENT: 50-year-old housewife

CHIEF COMPLAINT: Treatment was sought for the swelling and pain of her right knee.

VISUAL: The wrist and ankle joints were also slightly swollen, with some evidence of joint deformation, but they exhibited no pain. She was suffering from rheumatism affecting many of the joints throughout her body, but she had not seen a medical physician for treatment of this condition.

SYMPTOMS: The patient felt spontaneous pain and a sensation of heat in her joints. She said that the rheumatism had begun after giving birth twenty-five years earlier and that later her husband had suffered a stroke, leaving her with a large amount of work (rice seller) to be done. She felt cold overall, her stools were normal, and her urine was decreased. She also had a reduced appetite and stiff shoulders.

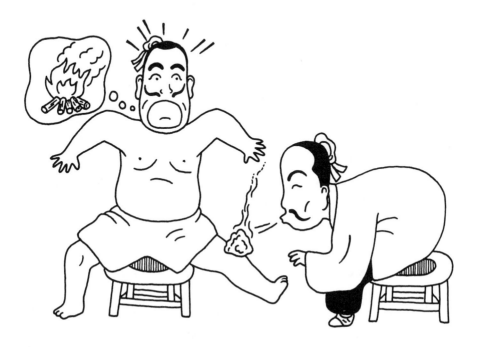

Heat perception moxibustion for joint pain

PULSE: Her overall pulse was sunken, weak, and rapid, and the left distal and right middle pulses were deficient.

ABDOMEN: The right ST-19 showed a slight resistance to pressure but the rest of the abdomen was weak with evident accumulation of water. In addition, the Stomach meridian below the navel was tight.

TREATMENT: The root treatment was for a pattern of Spleen deficiency/yang deficiency/cold and consisted of tonifying PC-7, SP-3, ST-42, SI-3, and GB-41. Needles were retained on the back at points including BL-29, BL-30, BL-23, and BL-20. Contact needling was applied to the rest of the back.

The next day the spontaneous pain had disappeared, and on the following day, the swelling around the knee had decreased. After that, it was a case of two steps forward followed by one step back. However, after about 20 treatments, the swelling of the right knee had completely disappeared and the treatment was discontinued.

14.10　LOWER BACK PAIN

Diagnosis

Lower back pain is the most common neuromusculoskeletal complaint seen in acupuncture clinics and is also one that can be effectively treated by acupuncture and moxibustion. This is true even in cases of a herniated disc in which surgery has been recommended. However, lower back pain that is caused by cancer does not respond completely to acupuncture and moxibustion, although the pain can usually be reduced considerably even in these cases. What is needed in those cases is the consent of the patient, the family, and whenever possible, the physician in charge.

The overall state of the patient and the type of pain is important and should be observed closely. For instance, if the pain is constant, not even allowing the patient a moment's sleep, or if the onset of the pain coincides with a sudden loss in weight, then the patient should also consult a medical physician for tests.

The pulse is also a very important barometer of the patient's condition. It is not within the scope of this book to include every detail, but if the pulse quality is found to be the opposite of what one would expect based on the patient's constitution, one should be careful. Also, generally speaking, a sunken, tight, and rapid pulse in a patient with lower back pain is not a good sign. In addition, if the pulse and abdominal diagnoses seem to indicate that the problem is not neuromusculoskeletal in nature, the patient should be referred to a medical physician for tests. Finally, if the pain does not respond to five or six treatments, or becomes worse after these treatments, the patient should be referred to a medical physician.

There are many types of lower back pain, all of which should be treated using the appropriate pattern-based treatment. I will now give an approximate guide on how to differentiate the various patterns. The most common type of lower back pain is acute lower back pain, which results from lifting a heavy object and thereby causing damage, primarily to the lower back muscles. There are even cases where a sneeze or simply getting up from a chair has triggered this type of pain.

Acute lower back pain is often seen in individuals with Liver or Kidney deficiency, and in these cases, areas of the Gallbladder meridian will always exhibit pain on pressure. In addition, individuals with this type of acute lower back pain can often move very carefully without significant pain, but once they strain their back in any way, the muscles spasm and cause intense pain. This is a sure sign that the Gallbladder meridian needs treatment.

Chronic lower back pain is most evident in the morning when the stiffness is such that it feels as if a board has been attached to one's back. Also, the intensity of the pain can result in emotional paralysis. These symptoms indicate that the treatment should focus on Kidney deficiency.

The type of lower back pain where there is no pain on movement but the lower back feels sluggish, heavy, and tired is caused by dampness. This type normally gets worse on days when it rains and is best dealt with by treating it as Spleen deficiency. Finally, lower back pain can occur together with a fever, in which case it is due to either Lung deficiency or Spleen deficiency.

An important point to assess is whether overwork or exhaustion lies at the heart of the lower back pain. Other contributory factors might include overindulgence in sex, walking excessive distances, standing for excessive lengths of time, or cold that enters the body via the legs and collects in the lower back. Of course, blood stasis and diseases of an internal organ, say, the intestines, may lead to lower back pain. All of these possible causes have to be pondered in the light of the information gained from the pulse and symptoms, and treatment is carried out according to the appropriate pattern. This is, of course, applicable to all treatment strategies.

Treatment

Chapter 1 of the *Divine Pivot* can be interpreted as saying that the affected area should be needled, and that delicate needling should be used to regulate the meridians to effect a cure. Both of these methods should be used, with the affected area being tonified or dispersed according to the deficient, excessive, hot, or cold state of the area. This is the branch treatment. The regulation of the meridians that are connected with the affected area is known as the root treatment.

However, for extremely strong symptoms, it is best to treat by needling well away from the affected area. It is good to start, for instance, from the leg meridians; the lower back proper should only be treated directly after the pain has diminished to some extent. In some cases, just the root treatment is enough to obtain relief.

In addition to providing treatment, it is important to advise the patient concerning the following factors:

- Do not receive a massage from untrained, though well-meaning, people as this will aggravate the condition. Therefore, at home, it is important to just relax and not strain oneself. Even acupuncturists should not suddenly attempt to treat extremely painful lower back pain by working on the back directly, and this is truer still for massage work.

- Do not take hot baths. While the pain may decrease temporarily during the bath, it will actually get worse after the lower back cools down.

- Do not use ice packs on the affected area.

- Do warm the area, but do not induce sweating as this will increase the pain.

- Do not consume alcohol, as this will lead to an increase in pain.

- Do not sleep on surfaces that are either too hard or too soft.

- Do light stretches for the lower back. In addition, after the acute phase is over, strengthening exercises should be done regularly.

- Do not allow the feet to get cold.

- Do not overindulge in sex.

TREATMENT OF ACUTE LOWER BACK PAIN

Since patients with acute lower back pain find it difficult to move, they should assume the most comfortable position they can for acupuncture. Then needles can be retained in the most painful areas in cases of yin deficiency, or contact needling can be performed in cases of yang deficiency. Generally speaking, the pain and level of stimulation should have an inverse relation: the more acute and painful the problem, the lighter the stimulus. The next step is to apply heat perception moxibustion.

In the clinic, the following presentations are commonly seen:

- In some cases, the pain is so severe that movement of any kind is impossible. In these cases, the most painful area is selected for contact needling. At this time, the left hand is used to fix the needle in place firmly, and this position is held for a number of breath cycles until the muscular tightness is felt to release beneath the left hand. When this release happens, the lower back pain is resolved.

- There are cases where any sort of movement leads to cramping of the muscles and an increase in the pain to such an extent that the patients find it difficult to breathe. The treatment for this type of lower back pain should always include Do In massage along the entire length of the Gallbladder meridian, or needle retention on the painful areas.

- In other instances, the patient can somehow manage to walk and is able to lie face up or down on the treatment table. For these cases, needles should be retained at the muscular areas that exhibit the greatest muscular tension. Thereafter, the most painful, hard, tense areas are found and needled so that the tip of the needle reaches just down to the hard tissue. After insertion, the needle is held firmly in place with the left hand and a few deep breaths are taken. At the same time, the tension and hardness of the muscular tissues are monitored. When they relax, the lower back pain will be resolved. It is also permissible to perform direct moxibustion to the hard areas; around five half-rice-grain sized moxa cones are usually sufficient.

It is not easy to perform Do In massage on individuals with acute lower back pain without risking negative effects, but if the practitioner is qualified, it can be done. The thumb is pressed flat onto the tense muscles and a firm, continuous pressure is applied until the muscles are felt to relax under the belly of the thumb. When this relaxation response occurs, the lower back pain will be cured.

Treatment of Chronic Lower Back Pain

In the clinic, the following presentations are commonly seen:

- In some cases, the posterior Kidney meridian will contain a hard line approximately 1cm long and 5cm wide. This will often be noted on the inside of BL-25, extending vertically above and below the point. Moxa head needling should be applied to this line. If the line is present in a case of acute lower back pain, contact needling should first be applied, after which moxa head needling can be administered. Women with lower back pain caused by blood stasis will also exhibit this characteristic line of hardness. If moxa head needling is applied, the menstrual period will commence and the lower back pain will disappear.

- In these cases, there are small hard spots about the size of the tip of the little finger distributed from around BL-25 to the iliac crest. These areas of hardness continue around the iliac crest to the front up to the top of the inguinal folds. It feels like an almost continuous thin rubber band wrapping itself around the loins. If this band is not softened, the lower back pain will not improve. The branch treatment involves moxa head needling along the hard areas and at points such as GB-26 to GB-31 and GB-34. This type of lower back pain is often seen in athletes.

- These cases are characterized by overall stiffness of the lower back, especially around BL-23. Retain needles and apply heat perception moxibustion all over the lower back. Since the area surrounding BL-23 is tense, moxa head needling should be applied to BL-23. This condition is commonly seen in women who present with what appears to be hard areas of fat from BL-27 to the inside of BL-29, and in such cases it is best treated by scarring moxibustion or moxa head needling. Depending on the degree of stiffness of the area, thicker Chinese needling is perhaps also warranted.

- These patients complain of lower back pain, but when the area is inspected, there is no sign of abnormal muscle tension. This type of back pain results from Spleen deficiency that leads to exhaustion of the flesh and is treated by simply retaining needles and applying heat perception moxibustion. Scarring moxibustion can also be applied to the Spleen back-associated point BL-20 and the Triple Burner back-associated point BL-22.

Do In massage can be effective in treating chronic lower back pain. Apply downward pressure in the direction of the feet to the extra point M-BW-24 (腰眼 *yo gan/yāo yǎn*). When the natural dimples of the buttock return and are plainly visible, the lower back pain will be gone.

OTHER THOUGHTS ON TREATING LOWER BACK PAIN

Other senior practitioners had this to say about the treatment of lower back pain:

- For back pain caused by lengthy sitting, Okabe used TB-5, and for acute lower back pain, he used LR-4. For lower back pain caused by lengthy standing and walking, he recommended GB-31, GB-34, and GB-38.

- In *Secret Selections of Acupuncture and Moxibustion*, Kimura Chuta recommends needling of BL-28 and BL-40 and scarring moxibustion of BL-31 through BL-34.

- Many classical texts, for example, Chapter 26 of the *Divine Pivot*, advise the use of blood letting at BL-40 as an effective treatment for lower back pain.

- In *Principles of Acupuncture and Moxibustion*, Shukei Suganuma recommends needling of M-BW-24, ST-36, and GB-34, plus any point that exhibits tenderness, scarring moxibustion on BL-23 and SP-9, and blood letting at BL-40.

- For acute lower back pain, Fukaya advocated applying scarring moxibustion at BL-60 and LR-4 as well as midline flow moxibustion (中条流の灸 *chū jō ryū no kyū).*[5] He also recommended applying moxibustion to a point just on the outside of BL-39, on the line between BL-39 and LR-8.

In my experience, LR-4 and GB-38 are good for acute lower back pain, and BL-40 and BL-57 are particularly good for chronic lower back pain. Especially when the right distal pulse is strong, LR-4 is very effective. For any type of lower back pain, BL-60 is good. The inguinal areas should be checked for tender points, and needles should be retained there. An additional point that is quite useful is M-BW-25, located just below the spinous process of the fifth lumbar vertebra (this point is known in Japanese as 'above the sacrum' 上仙 *jo sen,* and in Chinese as 'below the 17th vertebra' 十七椎下 *shí qī zhuí xià).* Also, if there are hardness and pain around the navel, indicating blood stasis, needle head moxibustion should be performed at these points (TABLE 14-9).

---

[5] Midline flow moxibustion is performed on two specific points on the lower abdomen and is most often used for treating infertility in women. The points are found by measuring the width of the lips and taking this length to form an equilateral triangle. The apex of the triangle is placed at the navel. Direct scarring moxibustion using rice-grain sized cones is normally performed on the lower two corners. In China, the method for locating points for moxibustion is known as three-cornered moxibustion (三角灸 *sān jiāo jiǔ*), and the most common English alphanumeric appellation for the points is M-CA-23.

Table 14-9	Branch Treatment Points for Lower Back Pain
Location	**Points**
ARMS AND LEGS	ST-33, **ST-36** SP-8, **BL-40**, BL-57, **BL-60**, BL-62, **GB-38**, **LR-4**, LR-5, LR-9, a tender point within 1 unit of GB-31
ABDOMEN	**ST-25, ST-27, ST-28**, ST-29, **SP-13**, **GB-27 to GB-30**, LR-14, CV-3, CV-4, CV-7, CV-12
BACK	BL-18, **BL-23**, **BL-28**, **BL-30**, BL-32, BL-53, BL-54, GB-26, GV-1, GV-2, GV-4, M-BW-25

Case History No. 1

PATIENT: 28-year-old mother of two

CHIEF COMPLAINT: Sought treatment for an uneasy feeling in her stomach and for lower back pain.

VISUAL: There was nothing significant to be noted in either her face or tongue. She had a good constitution.

SYMPTOMS: The patient had been suffering for two days from vomiting and diarrhea, and although these symptoms had stopped, at the time she came for treatment her stomach nevertheless still felt uneasy, her lower back was painful, and she had constipation and no appetite.

PULSE: The pulse was sunken and slightly big as well as a little rapid and wiry. On firm pressure, the left distal pulse was found to be deficient while the left middle pulse was excessive. The left proximal, right distal, and right proximal pulses were slightly deficient. The right middle pulse was deficient.

ABDOMEN: Palpation revealed an increase in muscular resistance and tenderness in the epigastric area.

CONSIDERATIONS: The pulse was thought to indicate that the patient was in the process of changing from Lung deficiency to Spleen deficiency. At the same time, there was some Liver excess as the rapid, wiry pulse was thought to be due to heat remaining in the Liver meridian, which was causing the symptoms in the lower back and stomach. The patient reported that she did not have an elevated temperature when she experienced the diarrhea and vomiting.

TREATMENT: The root treatment was for Spleen deficiency/yang deficiency/cold pattern and consisted of tonifying PC-7, SP-3, and ST-42. As this was proceeding, the patient remarked that she felt very good, especially when ST-42 was tonified. The next part of the root treatment was to shunt GB-41, which was found to be painful on pressure.

The painful areas of the lower back were located around the iliac crest. These structures are related to the Girdle vessel and problems here often occur because of Liver excess. Needles were retained at BL-17, BL-19 to BL-23, BL-25, and BL-27. Afterward, heat perception moxibustion was applied at these points. The pain in the lower back was eased, but the patient now complained of pain along the inguinal areas. This was regarded as a problem with the Girdle vessel. Although this vessel is said to encircle the waist at the height of the navel, in practice I find that it encircles the lower body following the iliac crest and the inguinal fold. The tender areas along the inguinal fold were needled superficially (just breaking the skin), after which the pain subsided. The patient's stomach also felt much better and she began to feel hungry.

The patient was pain-free for two days but returned to the clinic when the pain reappeared. The same treatment was performed, resulting in easing of the pain. However, a few days later the pain returned yet again. I examined the pulse and found it to be sunken and wiry, displaying a Spleen deficiency/Liver excess pattern, and the pain was still evident along the iliac crest and inguinal fold. It was obvious that the heat was still stuck in the Liver meridian, and palpation of the Liver and Gallbladder meridians revealed them to be extremely tender, further confirming this hypothesis.

Treatment consisted of tonifying PC-7 and SP-3 followed by shunting of LR-2, GB-40, and LR-14. After this, the tenderness along the Liver and Gallbladder meridians disappeared. However, there was still an uncomfortable feeling left in the lower back, and so I applied Do In massage to M-BW-24, after which she was completely cured and did not report another relapse.

Case History No. 2

PATIENT: 49-year-old male industrial worker

CHIEF COMPLAINT: Three days prior, the patient had hurt his right lower back while working and had taken time off work to recover. The pain was so severe that he took some over-the-counter pain medication, including a suppository, but to no avail. The night before his visit to the clinic, he asked his wife to massage him, resulting in an increase in pain. On his first visit, he was only able to lie face up.

VISUAL: Due to the severity of pain in his lower back, he was unable to shave. His face was slightly red. His constitution was normal, with a slight tendency to being overweight.

SYMPTOMS: The pain was only present when he moved. He had a history of lower back pain that he managed by massaging himself and getting moxibustion on the painful areas. His lower back was full of moxibustion scars. He was fond of drinking. There were no other significant symptoms.

PULSE: The left radial artery was displaced, and thus could not be used in the diagnosis. The right distal pulse was sunken, wiry, big, and forceful. The right middle pulse was sunken, rough, and forceful. The right proximal pulse was rough.

ABDOMEN: The epigastric area had a feeling of fullness and hardness with resistance and tenderness under both sides of the costal margin, which was probably related to his drinking; it had no immediate connection to this back problem.

BACK: The muscles of the back from BL-17 to BL-19 were bulging, probably as a result of the alcohol consumption.

CONSIDERATIONS: It is likely that this patient usually had a Spleen deficiency/Liver excess/heat pattern and had gotten his lower back chilled or something similar, causing his present lower back pain. Presently, his right middle and distal pulses showed no deficiency. Because this ruled out deficiency of the Lungs, Spleen, or Kidneys, it indicated that he was developing Liver deficiency.

TREATMENT: LR-4 and KI-7 were tonified. Shortly thereafter, his leg was bent and BL-60 was tonified, after which he was able to turn over with reasonable comfort. Needles were retained at BL-25 for 20 minutes, and heat perception moxibustion was applied to hard points from BL-23 downward.

After this treatment, the patient felt better and was able to walk home normally. However, in this type of lower back pain, it is common for it to return the following morning. I cautioned the patient about this and asked him to return the following day. The next day he was a little stiff first thing in the morning, but then quickly loosened up. After three similar treatments he had completely recovered.

14.11 SCIATICA

Diagnosis

After stiff shoulders and lower back pain, sciatica is one of the most common complaints in patients seeking acupuncture and moxibustion treatment. It is the most common of the various types of neuralgia. In this section, pain and numbness of the lower back and buttocks down to and encompassing the thigh and lower leg are included under the term sciatica.

Most patients who complain of sciatica have some history of lower back pain, and neuralgia is quite common after a number of these episodes. If the patient presents with sciatica but has no history of lower back pain, then, depending on the pulse and disease pattern, it may be advisable to refer the patient for a basic medical workup. The reason for this is that the cause of the neuralgia may be some serious disease, including a tumor in the pelvic cavity, tuberculosis of the spine, diabetes, or syphilis. Providing that there is no associated serious organic disease, sciatica usually improves very quickly after several treatments. However, if the muscles of the affected leg have atrophied, full recovery usually requires several months of treatment.

The intensity and location of the pain can vary. For instance, some will have pain that starts in the lower back then disappears only to resurface in the buttocks and along the Bladder meridian of the thigh and lower leg. Other cases can involve lower back pain as well as pain along the entire length of the Bladder meridian. Still others will complain of pain located along the Bladder meridian in the buttocks, but in the leg, the pain resides along the Gallbladder, Stomach meridian, or Triple Burner meridian of the leg (see Chapter 4 for a description of this meridian). It is also common for pain to be present from the ankle downward along the Gallbladder, Bladder, and Stomach meridians, and occasionally along the Spleen meridian. It is unusual to see someone with bilateral pain, and even in such a case, one side will be crucial as far as the treatment is concerned.

The intensity and type of pain will vary greatly. Some people feel numbness rather than pain, while others have such severe pain that they cannot sleep at night. Most sciatica is made worse by cold and tends to improve with warmth. Therefore, it is common for patients to enjoy long baths and drinking alcohol. Unfortunately, the body will become cold afterward and the pain will increase, and so it is best to advise the patient to take short baths and abstain from alcohol and intense exercise.

The most common pattern is Liver deficiency/yin deficiency, in which case just retaining the needles on the tender sites will greatly relieve the pain. However, there are times when the use of retained needling and moxa head needling will actually make the condition worse, especially when the condition is caused by a Liver deficiency/yang deficiency pattern in which sweating occurs easily. Therein lies the problem: any attempt at warming the body results in sweating, which immediately cools the body and makes things worse —a vicious cycle. Therefore, warming the body has to be done in a different way, and deep needling must be avoided.

Treatment

If possible, the patient should lie face down and needles should be retained at the tight areas and points that are found to be tender on pressure from the buttocks down to the lower legs. If lying face down is too painful, the procedure can be administered with the patient lying on the more comfortable side, with needling applied to the most painful and hard areas of the buttocks.

The practitioner must understand when to use retained needling and when to use moxa head needling. Moxa head needling is appropriate when the pain is particularly strong or the site of the pain is deep. If both of these methods make the condition worse, it is probably due to yang deficiency. In that case, direct scarring moxibustion with five half-rice-grain sized moxa cones per point should be used. Keep an eye out for any sweating while doing this since patients with Liver yang deficiency tend to sweat easily. If while performing the moxibustion the sweat dries out, the pain will disappear. Another method for achieving this is to substitute contact needling. If the pain is still present, Do In massage may be used to good effect, but the results tend to be temporary.

The points listed in Table 14-10 are usually effective. However, it should be emphasized that points must be chosen from stiff or tender areas, or from an area where the muscles are contracted. If points are needled purely on their textbook topographical locations, the therapeutic effect will be reduced, if not completely lost. The main thing is to let your fingers become sensitive so that you can locate the correct points. For areas suffering from atrophy, select stiff, tender areas for direct scarring moxibustion of half-rice-grain sized moxa cones. This is performed until the heat is felt.

Table 14-10	Branch Treatment Points for Sciatica
Location	**Points**
LOWER BACK	**BL-23, BL-25,** BL-26, BL-27, **BL-52, M-BW-16**
BUTTOCKS	BL-28, BL-30, **BL-53, Bl-54,** GB-30, GV-3, **point lateral to BL-53, point above BL-53, point lateral to Bl-54**
THIGH	**BL-37,** BL-40, **BL-56, GB-31, points above and below BL-40**
LOWER LEG	**ST-36,** ST-42, BL-56, BL-57, **BL-58, BL-60,** BL-65, GB-34, GB-36, **GB-38, GB-39, point lateral to BL-58**

Case History

PATIENT: 60-year-old woman

CHIEF COMPLAINT: The patient reported sciatica of the right leg with pain in the Bladder meridian at the thigh and the Triple Burner meridian of the leg.

VISUAL: There were no remarkable visual findings.

HISTORY: While working as a teacher, the patient had suffered from lower back pain on numerous occasions. After she retired, she reaggravated her lower back while helping her child move. At first she appeared to make light of her pain and persisted in taking long car trips to go mountain hiking and to visit hot springs, despite my advice to the contrary. Because of this, her pain became worse, and she said that the acupuncture she was receiving at my clinic was not working. It was shortly after this that she stopped coming to the clinic. Two months later, however, she returned saying that she had been receiving other forms of treatment that helped reduce the pain somewhat. However, an examination of the right leg showed considerable atrophy: the pain had been exchanged for numbness, as neuralgia set in.

PULSE: The overall pulse was sunken, thin, and deficient with the left middle and proximal pulses being especially deficient. The right middle pulse was thin and rough but did not become deficient even after applying pressure.

SYMPTOMS: She sweated very easily, for example, entering even a mildly warm room induced sweating.

TREATMENT: Treatment was administered for a Liver deficiency/yang deficiency pattern. KI-3, LR-3, and SP-1 were tonified, and then direct scarring moxibustion was done using seven half-rice-grain sized moxa cones, which were placed on each of the following tender points: BL-23, BL-53, a point two finger widths above BL-53, another point two finger widths lateral to BL-53, GB-30, BL-54, and another point three finger widths lateral to BL-54. Interestingly enough, from about the fifth day after treatment commenced, the patient developed insensitivity to moxibustion at BL-23, and so the number of cones was increased, reaching up to 60 cones before heat was felt. Direct scarring moxibustion was also performed at the following points on the lower leg: ST-36, GB-39, SP-6, and a point just lateral to BL-58. All of these points, except ST-36, received seven half-rice-grain sized moxa cones. ST-36 had around 50 cones burned on it before any heat sensation was felt. After this, contact needling was applied to the painful areas of the lower leg.

After the second treatment she felt that her leg had warmed up, even at night, and after one month the atrophied leg began to become more fleshed out. After three months, the leg reached its normal thickness, she was able to walk two kilometers without any problem, and she had no pain at night. At around this time, she also began to feel the heat from the moxibustion, and so it was continued only at BL-23 and ST-36 for five more treatments.

14.12 LOWER EXTREMITY PROBLEMS

Weak Legs

There are some patients who have weak legs and are prone to falling over even though they do not have a history of hemiplegia or Parkinson's disease. There are also patients who have intermittent limping, which is sometimes characterized by pain in the legs and is often the result of walking long distances. These patients are thought to have a

Kidney deficiency pattern; treatment should include needle head moxa at BL-23 and a large number of cones of direct scarring moxibustion at ST-36. Other points that are also suitable for moxibustion are LR-7, BL-40, ST-33, GB-30, and GB-31. ST-35 and GB-34 are good points when there is pain below the knee.

During the summertime, a patient complaining of fatigue in the legs should be treated using ST-36 and ST-40. Interestingly enough, shunting at PC-4 is also said to be effective. Those complaining of leg fatigue often sleep with their legs out from under the covers, and so a light blanket wrapped around the legs at night will often relieve the problem.

In the past, leg qi disorder (脚気 *kakke/jiǎo qì*), a problem related to beriberi, was also a problem. Fukaya recommended applying three cones of direct scarring moxibustion to SI-3 on both sides. The primary Edo period texts recommend leg qi eight point moxibustion, which consists of direct scarring moxibustion at GB-31, ST-32, ST-35, M-LE-16, ST-36, ST-37, and GB-39.

Heel and Achilles Tendon Pain

The underlying problem is always cold caused by a Kidney deficiency pattern, and the treatment consists of needle head moxibustion at BL-23 and retained needling at BL-59 and BL-60.

Heat perception moxibustion can be performed on the bottom of the heel as well as on the

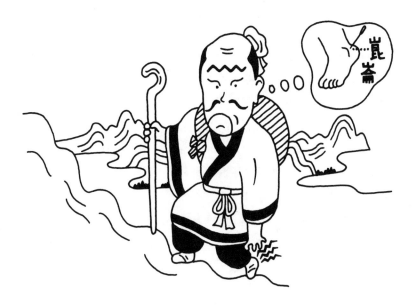

BL-60 (the Kunlun Mountains point) is for pain of the Achilles tendon

area where the Achilles tendon inserts into the heel. Direct scarring moxibustion can also be performed at KI-7 and BL-59.

Calf Muscle Cramps

In Edo period texts, there is mention of twisted sinews (転筋 *ten kin/zhuǎn jīn*); twisted refers to cramping. This condition can be caused by cold, walking too much, congestion of the veins of the lower limbs during pregnancy, thrombophlebitis, varicose veins, diabetes, and alcohol-induced hepatitis.

Some cases are severe enough to warrant calling an ambulance, but in most cases, this condition responds quickly to acupuncture and moxibustion treatment. It is usually a result of a Kidney deficiency pattern, but those patients that complain of dull achy legs in the summer that later develop into muscle cramps are often best treated as if they have a Spleen deficiency pattern. Needles are retained at BL-56 to BL-59, and at a tender point that is lateral to BL-58. Pricking SP-1 to let out a few drops of blood can also be effective. Finally, the patient should be advised to stretch the Achilles tendon during any episodes of muscle cramps.

14.13 TRAUMA

Diagnosis

In Japan these problems are generally the domain of bone setters, but they often end up appearing in acupuncture clinics. When dealing with contusions, sprains, and possible bone fractures, it is important to determine the initial and subsequent history of the injury. In any case when a fracture is a possibility, a qualified practitioner should evaluate the patient quickly. In any event, if the pain increases rather than decreases in a 24-hour period, an x-ray should be done to check for a possible bone fracture.

If an elderly person falls over and is unable to walk because of the resulting pain, it is likely that the individual's hip was fractured. In these cases, it is important to refer the patient to an orthopedist. I have twice found hip fractures that were misdiagnosed as something else by internal medicine physicians.

Any fracture requires that the area be put in a cast for a lengthy period of time, resulting in immobile and stiff muscles. After the plaster is removed, acupuncture, moxibustion, and Do In massage are very effective in promoting a speedy recovery.

Treatment

From a modern medical perspective, contusions and sprains are usually dealt with by icing, but in traditional medicine they are warmed. This may sound strange, but the goal of warming is to discharge heat by localized sweating, leaving the injured area cooler as a result. Accordingly, for contusions and sprains, moxa head needling of the injured area is followed immediately by heat perception moxibustion. Needling of the area using quick insertion and withdrawal is then performed, followed by Do In massage. When doing the massage, apply enough pressure to cause the blood vessels to rise to the surface. Finally, the area is bound in place. It is not normal practice to cool the area, but if it is very hot, a cooling pad can be used.

Moxa head needling is used to bring to the surface any bruising that occurs deeper in the tissues. Sometimes this causes a temporary increase in pain. Next, local heat is dispersed by the use of heat perception moxibustion, followed by quick insertion and withdrawal to remove the heat. Another method is to apply a large amount of heat to the affected areas using thread-size direct scarring moxibustion until the area feels hot to the patient. Pricking to let out a few drops of blood is also useful when there is a lot of heat and pain and the site of injury has very clear swollen blood vessels.

For the aftereffects of fractures, it is good to apply moxa head needling to points within the stiff muscular areas. This should be followed by quick insertion and withdrawal needling, and finally Do In massage.

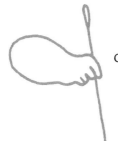

CHAPTER 15

RESPIRATORY DISEASES

IN TRADITIONAL MEDICINE, bodily areas are defined by words such as exterior (表 *hyō/biǎo*), interior (裏 *ri/lǐ*), outer (外 *gai/wài*), and inner (內 *nai/nèi*). The exterior includes the areas where the yang meridians flow while the interior represents the areas where the yin meridians flow and the organs are located. The areas where the meridians flow represent the outer aspect of the body, which also includes the hair, blood vessels, flesh, muscles, tendons, and bone. Inner indicates the aspect where the organs are found.

Because the yang organs are in the outermost part of the inner region, they are adjacent to the yin meridians and heat and cold can easily spread between them; that is, a yang organ can receive heat or cold from a yin meridian and a yin meridian can receive heat or cold from a yang organ. The exterior, interior, and yang organs are all under the control of the yin organs. It is for this reason that disease occurs when there is a deficiency of essential qi in a yin organ.

Most of the diseases in this chapter occur as a result of a deficiency of essential qi in the Lungs. With this deficiency, areas that are under the control of the Lungs, as well as possibly the Lungs themselves, will manifest disease. This basic deficiency will manifest in such symptoms as acute fever, cough, and sore throat. The names given by modern medicine for diseases of the Lungs include, for example, rhinitis, sinusitis, wheezing, asthma, pneumonia, pleurisy, pulmonary emphysema, pulmonary edema, lung cancer, pulmonary tuberculosis, or lymphadenitis. Not all of these conditions are suitable for treatment with acupuncture and moxibustion, but some of them are.

Febrile diseases cover a very wide range of illnesses, but the approach used by traditional medicine provides us with a framework for dealing with all of them. Still, the actual number of patients that come to our clinics presenting with serious febrile conditions is actually quite small, and the treatment can be difficult. Therefore, the type of fevers that are considered here are those that are relatively common, that is, those associated with colds and influenza. The coughs and sore throats that are discussed here are mainly those that linger on after the patient has more or less recovered from the original infection.

Nasal symptoms, of course, occur with a cold, but the types of rhinitis and sinusitis that we will look at here are those that are not accompanied by an elevated temperature. While some may consider even this to be the domain of the otolaryngologist, it is included under the traditional rubric of Lung disease and will be considered in this chapter.

Night sweats and profuse sweating are also covered. I include sweating here under respiratory disorders because, in traditional medical thinking, the Lungs are connected with the skin. Therefore, changes in sweating are usually related to Lung pathology.

The final section in this chapter deals with pulmonary diseases that are not covered in the earlier sections. Acupuncturists today do not often see patients with these illnesses. However, they are sometimes found in the history of many of the patients, and it is important to be familiar with their diagnosis and treatment. It is also important to know when to refer the patients for medical tests or for medical treatment.

15.1 ACUTE FEBRILE DISEASE

Diagnosis

It is common for a disease to begin with chills and/or fever. In traditional terms, this would be a disease that started in the exterior part of the body and would include influenza and colds. There are also cases that are less common where the fever is the product of an internal visceral disease, including pneumonia, pleurisy, hepatitis, enteritis, and pyelitis. From my perspective, what traditional medicine calls external pathogens are actually bywords for the effects of internal deficiencies. Thus, the external pathogen 'wind' refers to a drying effect that is often a sign of a Liver yin deficiency pattern. Any external pathogen can exacerbate the problem, but the pathogen is not considered the source of the disease. Fevers associated with rheumatic and other connective tissue diseases are also considered in a similar light.

As previously mentioned in Chapter 2, while traditional medicine has methods for treating any febrile disease, in practice, the treatment can be very difficult. Also, there are some cases where the patients will recover better under the care of medical practitioners. It is important, therefore, to question the patient, check the pulse carefully, and determine the pattern of deficiency. Based on this, choose whether or not it would be better to refer the patient to someone else for treatment.

In traditional medicine, chills and fever-related conditions are known as cold damage (傷寒 *shō kan/shāng hán*). There are also specific types, including wind attack (中風 *chū fū/zhòng fēng*), warm disease (温病 *un byō/wēn bìng*), summerheat disease (暑病 *shō byō/shǔ bìng*), malarial disease (瘧病 *gyaku byō/nuè bìng*), and sudden turmoil (霍乱

kaku ran/huò luàn). Each of these has its own pathology and is treated accordingly. The basics for understanding and treating these diseases are all contained in the *Discussion of Cold Damage*. With just this one book, you have the potential to treat any febrile disease. However, most of the treatments involve herbal formulas, and the contents can be difficult to understand at first. Therefore, I will summarize some of the main points. To avoid unnecessary repetition, I will focus on the diagnosis of febrile diseases. The treatments are discussed under the various basic patterns in Part One. For example, Chapters 1 and 2 deal with greater yang and yang brightness diseases, Chapter 4 deals with lesser yin diseases, and Chapter 8 deals with lesser yang diseases.

HOT AND COLD PATTERNS

Acute febrile diseases usually originate from Lung deficiency, and therefore the first symptom will typically be chills (literally, aversion to cold), followed by fever. Lung deficiency/yang excess/heat and Lung deficiency/yang deficiency/heat are examples of patterns where events proceed in the normal sequence. However, there are cases in which the chills are not followed by a subjective feeling of feverishness, even in the presence of an objective elevation in temperature. This is termed a yang deficiency cold pattern regardless of which yin organ is found to be deficient (see Chapter 3). Also, there are cases where chills are absent from the very start; in these cases, fever is predominant throughout. These are known as warm diseases and are thought by those in the tradition of the *Discussion of Cold Damage* to be due primarily to exhaustion setting in during the winter months. With the arrival of spring, the exhaustion prevents the yang qi from being released and discharged from the body as it should be; instead, it remains stuck in the exterior of the body. In these cases, the fever can be treated as a Lung deficiency/yang brightness meridian excess/heat pattern.

The three types of febrile disease just discussed can, through mistaken treatment or through natural causes, lead to heat or cold in other parts of the organ-meridian system. It is important to correctly diagnose and treat these cases, which can be rather confusing. Accordingly, there have been a number of books written on this subject, including two that were written during the Edo period by Kitetsu Naito, *Selections from the Discussion of Cold Damage* and *Solutions to Medical Puzzles*. These books examine the *Discussion of Cold Damage* with cross reference to the *Divine Pivot*, *Basic Questions*, and the *Classic of Difficulties* and are therefore useful for acupuncture and moxibustion therapy as well. In the text that follows, I will outline a few points mentioned in these books that are particularly relevant.

EXTERIOR AND INTERIOR DISEASES

As noted above, diseases that begin with chills and fever are thought to pertain to either a

Lung deficiency/yang excess/heat or Lung deficiency/yang deficiency/heat pattern. There is, however, one stipulation: there cannot be *any* symptoms of an interior deficiency pattern, for if there are such accompanying symptoms, then even a fever cannot be considered a sign of yang excess. It must be stressed that, in this case, interior includes the yin meridians as well as the yang organs, and deficiency refers to either yang deficiency cold or yin deficiency heat. Also remember that interior deficiency can be induced by mistaken treatment. For example, when a patient with Lung deficiency is treated with deep needling or with needles that are retained too long, there is a strong likelihood that interior deficiency will result. This is actually not uncommon. When in doubt, always go for more superficial insertions and shorter retention than you would normally do. In the discussion that follows, the deficiencies are divided into those of the upper, middle, and lower burners.

Yang deficiency of the upper burner: In this state, the chills and fever resemble those found in the Lung deficiency/yang excess/heat pattern. However, if the symptoms include a sore throat, copious saliva, chills, nasal discharge, and a productive cough with thin sputum, then yang deficiency of the upper burner may also be present. The relevant pattern in this situation is either Lung deficiency/yang deficiency/cold or Lung deficiency/Lung cold.

Yin deficiency of the upper burner: Chills and fever that are accompanied by dryness and discomfort of the throat, dry mouth, coughing and wheezing with sticky sputum, chest pain, palpitations, and shortness of breath may indicate yin deficiency of the upper burner. The relevant pattern in this situation is Liver deficiency/yin deficiency, which produces heat and thereby dries out the fluids of the Lungs.

Yang deficiency of the middle burner: Chills and fever that are accompanied by vomiting and diarrhea followed by fatigue, lack of thirst and appetite, and either copious or scanty urination are indicative of cold and phlegm in the Stomach and Intestines. These symptoms are best resolved by a treatment aimed at a pattern of Spleen deficiency/yang deficiency/cold. This pattern is seen in instances of sudden turmoil disease (霍亂 *kaku ran/huò luàn*), which is characterized by headache, vomiting, diarrhea, and fever. Alternatively, there will be chills, fever, vomiting, diarrhea, dry mouth, and palpitations, in which case the relevant pattern is Liver deficiency/yang deficiency/cold.

Yin deficiency of the middle burner: Here, the mild chills and fever are accompanied by general lassitude, stomachache, either constipation or diarrhea, variable appetite, dry mouth, and copious or scanty urination, all of which suggest the presence of heat or heat with phlegm in the Stomach and Intestines. These symptoms are best resolved by a treatment aimed at Spleen deficiency/yin deficiency/heat. This pattern is found in instances of sudden turmoil disease.

Yang deficiency of the lower burner: Chills and fever that are accompanied by cold legs, frequent and pale urination, lack of vigor, and diarrhea without subsequent abdominal pain are indicative of deficiency of the yang qi of the Kidneys. These symptoms are best resolved by a treatment aimed at a pattern of Kidney deficiency/yang deficiency.

Yin deficiency of the lower burner: Chills that are accompanied by a feeling of exhaustion and lassitude, palpitations, shortness of breath, dry mouth, and copious or scanty urination are best treated as a pattern of Kidney deficiency/yin deficiency.

Transmission through the Meridians

The first stage of acute febrile diseases begins with excess or deficiency heat in the greater yang meridian. If this is left untreated, the heat can make its way or be transmitted to other meridians. The heat moves into the yang brightness meridian next and can be dealt with at this stage by a treatment aimed at Lung deficiency.

If the heat proceeds as far as the lesser yang meridian, it should be treated as a pattern of Spleen deficiency/Liver excess/heat. Malarial conditions are examples of this pattern and typically exhibit chills followed by fever that is broken by sweating. This process then repeats itself once or twice a day.

After proceeding to the lesser yang meridian, the heat can enter the yin meridians. When this happens, the heat is transferred from the yin meridians to the neighboring yang organs and also to the Lungs. Clinically, the symptoms at this stage are thought to be the result of heat in the yang organs and are treated as a pattern of Spleen deficiency/yang excess/heat. If there is heat in the Lungs, it is treated as a pattern of Spleen deficiency/Lung excess/heat.

All of these patterns are discussed in detail in Part One. It is suggested that the reader review the relevant chapters to gain more confidence in understanding and utilizing these concepts.

Treatment

Treatment methods are discussed in the first half of this book, and so I will not mention them at all here. However, I would like to make a few general remarks.

In the treatment of a febrile disease, irrespective of what name is given to the disease by Western medicine, if the diagnosis, point location, and treatment techniques are correct, the patient will recover. Having said this, there are times when it is best to refer the patient to a medical physician. I would suggest that you consider this course of action in the following instances:

• When you have no confidence in the outcome of the treatment.

- When the chills and fever become worse after the treatment.

- When there is internal pain with vomiting and diarrhea that does not respond to the treatment.

- When you believe that it is important that your patient receive a modern medical examination. Of course, the opinions and thoughts of the patient should always be respected.

In general, when there is a fever, it is best to use contact needling. However, when treating fever from constraint in the meridians, it is essential to use shunting or the treatment will be ineffective.

When there are chills and fever, direct moxibustion at GV-14 often breaks the fever. Approximately 20 half-rice-grain sized moxa cones are generally enough to accomplish this. Sometimes, however, when there is a great deal of stagnant heat, moxibustion can make the situation worse. In my experience, this type of moxibustion is best done when dealing with a Lung deficiency/yang excess/heat or Lung deficiency/yang deficiency/heat pattern.

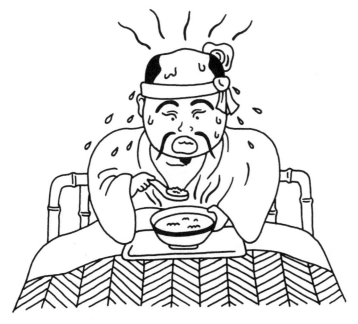

Fevers are cured by sweating

Case History

PATIENT: 32-year-old woman

CHIEF COMPLAINT: The patient complained of fever, chills, headache, sore throat, and exhaustion. The fever began just the night before, and the exhaustion was so severe that she was unable to open her eyes properly.

VISUAL: Even though the patient had a fever, her face showed no signs of redness. Her tongue had no coating, and her lips were somewhat dry and lacking in luster.

SYMPTOMS: She had a temperature of around 39°C (102°F). She had no appetite, but she had neither diarrhea nor constipation. To make matters worse, her father had suddenly passed away, and so she was unable to rest, being very busy with the funeral arrangements.

PULSE: The overall pulse was slightly floating and rapid, but also somewhat tight and thin.

CONSIDERATIONS: As there was no sweating and the pulse was a little tight, I thought at first that the patient may have a pattern of Lung deficiency/greater yang meridian excess/heat. However, I rejected this choice based on the accompanying symptoms: inability to keep her eyes open, exhaustion, lack of appetite, and lack of redness in the face. I eventually decided that the tightness in the pulse was not a result of heat stagnation, but was actually the result of a buildup of cold pathogen. Therefore, the yang qi of the patient had to be tonified, and this would be accomplished by tonifying the Spleen and building up the yang qi of the Stomach. If this was done successfully, then the yang qi of both the Lungs and the Bladder meridian would be strengthened, and together they would push out the cold pathogen.

TREATMENT: Although I chose to perform a Spleen deficiency pattern treatment, within this, I selected metal points—namely, PC-5 and SP-5—because they are related to the Lungs. These points were tonified using contact needling. I also gently burned three half-rice-grain sized moxa cones at KI-6. After this, scatter needling was performed on the back to tonify the protective qi.

Following this treatment, the patient felt a little better and her sore throat disappeared. That night she still had a fever, but it had disappeared by the following day, allowing her to perform all the tasks for her father's funeral.

15.2   COUGHING AND WHEEZING

Diagnosis

Patients may present with coughing only, coughing accompanied by wheezing, or simply wheezing, all of which can be associated with either colds or influenza. The types of coughing and wheezing that we will discuss here are those that occur after the onset of a fever.

In premodern texts, coughs and wheezing are referred to by three basic terms: 咳 (*gai/ké*), 嗽 (*so* or *soku/sòu*), and 喘 (*zen/chuǎn*). The term 咳 refers to a noisy, nonproductive cough, and 嗽 is a cough that is not so intense but is marked by copious sputum. If both the coughing and the production of sputum are significant, it is known as 咳嗽 (*gai so/ké sòu*). The word 喘 is used when wheezing is the main problem, although to some it simply means the presence of breathing difficulties.

These terms exist because they represent three different pathologies: 咳 is indicative of a Lung problem, 嗽 is marked by phlegm and is associated with the Spleen, and 喘 is connected to the upward rebellion of qi. In the text that follows, these will be divided into the various patterns and the idiosyncrasies of each pathology will be outlined. While some of the patterns that follow are not explicitly discussed in Part One, they are simply variants of the basic patterns discussed there. Depending on where the heat and cold generated by those patterns go, there are a multitude of possibilities. As long as one grasps the dynamic of the major patterns, these are easily understood and treated.

YANG DEFICIENCY COLD PATTERN

There are many types of yang deficiency patterns, including Lung deficiency/yang deficiency and Lung deficiency/Lung cold. There are also cases where yang deficiency from sources other than the Lungs cause the Lungs to become cold, resulting in coughing and wheezing.

There are many causes for this state, including any fever-associated illness. After the fever has broken, sometimes a cough lingers on stubbornly. Another cause is the overconsumption of cold beverages, which may cause coughing and wheezing in a person who has a constitutional tendency toward Lung cold. In these cases the yang deficiency has progressed until the Lungs themselves have become cold. In such cases, the cough is usually nonproductive. However, if there is phlegm derived from Spleen deficiency, the cough will be productive, and if this state persists, wheezing will result. In these cases, the patients have thin sputum and nasal discharge, and they sneeze easily. Early morning cold air will induce either coughing or wheezing, the hands and feet of these patients are cold, and there is frequent and copious clear urination. The area around BL-13 on the upper back feels cold to the touch. Finally, because the circulation of qi is strongly effected, the overall pulse is either sunken and thin or sunken, rough, thin, and deficient.

SPLEEN DEFICIENCY/LIVER EXCESS/HEAT PATTERN

Spleen deficiency can be accompanied by stagnant heat in the lesser yang meridian (by way of the terminal yin meridian). In such cases, the Lungs are steamed by this heat, leading to coughing and wheezing. The coughing often occurs during a fever or just after the fever has receded. Asthmatic children may have a constitutional tendency toward this pattern.

The combination of this pattern plus a cough and a fever may be indicative of pneumonia or pleurisy. The Lung pulse should be checked, and if it is stronger than usual, the patient should be referred to a medical physician unless the practitioner is very adept at shunting the Lung heat, as serious conditions can develop.

Even after a fever has broken as measured by a thermometer, there may still be heat in the interior marked by thirst, constipation, and loss of appetite. Sometimes this interior heat will also cause pain in the chest.

In chronic conditions, this pattern is characterized by darkly colored urine, a reduced and unbalanced appetite, and some moss on the tongue. In the case of children, they will often be restless. The overall pulse is sunken and wiry, while the left medial pulse is wiry and forceful. By definition, the left distal and the right medial pulses are deficient.

Spleen Deficiency/Lung Deficiency/Heat Pattern

Sometimes a cough will linger on even after a fever has receded, or the cough will appear in the absence of a fever. This occurs when the heat produced from Spleen deficiency/yin deficiency spreads to the Lungs. At the same time, because of the Spleen deficiency, there will be phlegm, which will mean the cough is productive. In such cases, wheezing tends to occur when there is a high degree of humidity.

Often, when the body temperature rises, the throat becomes sore and coughing begins, sometimes resulting in bloody sputum. The expectoration of the sticky sputum often results in a decrease in the symptoms. Additional symptoms include a feeling of fatigue and a tendency toward constipation; the appetite is not strongly affected.

This state can also occur during the course of a fever in which case there will be a slight fever and a persistent nasal discharge or obstruction. There may also be chest pain when coughing. If the fever is intense, the patient may have pneumonia.

The overall pulse is sunken and wiry. The left distal and right medial pulses are deficient while the right distal pulse is sunken, wiry, and forceful because there is heat in the Lungs. Another possibility is that only the right medial pulse is deficient and the right distal pulse is forceful. The important thing to understand is that the Lung pulse will be just a little stronger than the overall pulse, even when the overall pulse is strong. The stronger Lung pulse of course indicates there is a great amount of heat in the Lungs.

The presence of phlegm is reflected in a slippery pulse. Phlegm can block the movement of heat outward, causing the heat to lodge in the Lungs, which will dry out the fluids and cause coughing. Also, since phlegm is sticky, it hampers the free circulation of qi, making it even more difficult to remove the heat from the Lungs.

LIVER DEFICIENCY/LUNG HEAT PATTERN

This pattern is commonly seen in cases of chronic coughing and wheezing. It occurs when the fluids of the Liver and Kidneys are deficient, which gives rise to deficiency heat that causes the Lungs to dry out. This in turn leads to coughing, fever, and wheezing. Again, as in the previous pattern, the sputum is thick, and there is a sense of relief when it is expelled. These patients often have a red face, constipation, no loss of appetite, and high blood pressure. Many of them suffer from heart disease and diabetes.

The overall pulse is forceful; commonly, it is also sunken and wiry or sunken and slippery. By definition, the left medial and proximal pulses are deficient, and the right distal pulse is sunken, slippery, and forceful. As there is heat in the Lungs, the Lung (right distal) pulse is usually a bit stronger than the overall pulse. This is somewhat similar to the one listed in Chapter 11 for Liver deficiency/yin deficiency/heat. If this type of pulse is present in an elderly patient and there is a continuous low-grade fever, that individual probably has pneumonia or a chronic pulmonary disease.

SPLEEN DEFICIENCY/LUNG EXCESS/HEAT PATTERN

In the *Discussion of Cold Damage*, this pattern is referred to as knotted chest (結胸 *kek kyō*/*jié xiōng*) and is characterized by phlegm and heat clumping in the Lungs. The phlegm and heat build up, resulting in coughing and wheezing. The pathology seen in this pattern is similar to that in the Spleen deficiency/Lung deficiency/heat pattern. However, the symptoms, abdominal patterns, and pulse seen here reflect an excess heat condition.

The chief complaint is usually constant coughing or wheezing. Often, there is no loss of appetite, but there is a tendency toward constipation. The abdomen will be swollen, and the area beneath the ribs in the epigastric area will be firm to the touch. The patient will feel a sensation of blockage in the epigastric area, heat in the chest area, and stiffness in the neck. The overall pulse is strong with the right distal pulse being especially sunken and excessive. The dorsal pedis pulse (taken at ST-42) will be big and forceful. When this state becomes chronic, thick phlegm collects in the Lungs and breathing becomes difficult. This disease used to be called Lung abscess disease (肺癰病 *hai yō byō*/*fèi yōng bìng*).

SPLEEN DEFICIENCY/LIVER EXCESS/BLOOD STASIS PATTERN

Some patients always have the feeling that something is stuck in their throats and are constantly clearing their throats or coughing. With this pattern, the spreading and diffusing action of the yang qi of the Liver's blood is adversely affected, causing the qi stagnation (in particular, in the throat). The medial aspects of the shoulder blades are stiff in patients who have this pattern and who also wheeze.

In these patients the pulse is generally sunken, rough, and excessive, but it can be thin and slow. The left distal and right medial pulses are deficient when firmly pressed. The right distal (Lung) pulse is often a little stronger than usual, as it receives some heat from the Liver.

LUNG DEFICIENCY/LIVER EXCESS/BLOOD STASIS PATTERN

This pattern is characterized by Kidney deficiency and heat stagnation or blood stasis in the Liver as well as the buildup of heat in the Heart. The blood stasis is caused by a lack of Kidney fluids, which leads to a thickening or congestion of blood. This, in turn, changes over time into blood stasis. The buildup of heat in the Heart is caused by the Liver excess. At the same time, heat from the deficiency in the Kidneys makes the situation worse. All of these factors contribute to the swelling of heat in the chest, which leads to the wheezing. This pattern is commonly seen in chronic asthma sufferers.

Even though this condition presents a pattern of Lung deficiency/Liver excess/blood stasis, the Lung pulse is actually not deficient. This is because the Lungs receive heat from the Heart. Depending on the amount of heat, the Lung pulse is often quite strong. However, the left proximal pulse is floating and deficient.

KIDNEY DEFICIENCY/YIN DEFICIENCY PATTERN

In this pattern, Kidney deficiency causes the fluids on the outside of the body to increase. At the same time, the ability of the Lungs to circulate qi becomes impaired, causing pathogenic water to encroach on the Lungs. This leads to coughing and wheezing. There are many obese people that suffer from this pattern; these individuals often sweat a great deal and develop edema of the legs after standing for a long period. When they lie supine, their coughing and breathing difficulties worsen and their chests become painful. While their urination is scanty, they are not constipated. Because of the preponderance of water and obesity in these patients, the pulse is sunken.

Treatment

Here is a selection of points used by several famous senior practitioners for the branch treatment of respiratory complaints:

• For bronchitis, Fukaya recommended direct scarring moxibustion at many points, including a point one finger width above LI-11, GV-15, a point located on the inside of the crease formed when the big toe is bent at the first digit (very close to SP-2), CV-22, BL-13, BL-17, and PC-1. Presumably, Fukaya used these points when dealing with deficiency heat in the Lungs. For treating coughing and wheezing, Fukaya recommended the use of many points, including GV-12, GV-11, GV-10, BL-13, the asthma point (located by measuring 0.2 units lateral and 1 unit superior to BL-17), GV-9, BL-43, BL-12, BL-41, BL-42, BL-15, GB-21, SI-14, SI-15, BL-23, and BL-25.

- The Edo period text *A Collection of Acupuncture and Moxibustion Treasures* recommends direct scarring moxibustion at BL-13, GB-21, LU-11, KI-2, BL-18, LR-14, LR-2 and CV-23, and acupuncture at various points, including ST-19 and ST-21. This protocol was probably used to treat coughing as part of a Spleen deficiency/Liver excess/heat pattern. The text also sets forth more specific treatments, for example, using LU-9 for Lung coughs, SP-3 for Spleen coughs, KI-3 for Kidney coughs, ST-36 for excessive sleeping, TB-6 for coughs from heat with a red face, and scarring moxibustion at LU-1 to LU-3, CV-20, and BL-13 plus acupuncture at CV-12, LR-14, LR-13, and BL-13 for wheezing.

- For both coughing and wheezing, Okabe preferred scatter needling to the trunk and upper part of the body (except the head). Points he commonly used included BL-13, BL-10, GB-21, BL-43, BL-18, LU-1, LU-5, LU-9, CV-12, ST-21, ST-25, CV-6, and SP-5.

- For coughing and wheezing, *Rules for Acupuncture and Moxibustion* suggests acupuncture at LU-1, KI-21, CV-13, CV-14, PC-3, CV-12, and KI-19 and direct scarring moxibustion at BL-13, GB-21, ST-36, and CV-22.

- For coughing, *Selected Secrets of Acupuncture and Moxibustion* recommends the use of SI-2, PC-3, and BL-43, and for wheezing, KI-1 and PC-8.

Coughing can be difficult to stop, but moxibustion on the upper back leads to success in many cases. If cold is affecting the Lungs, tonifying direct scarring moxibustion to BL-13 is best. This type of moxibustion should not feel hot; rather, it should be administered until the upper back starts to feel warm, which generally takes about five to seven half-rice-grain sized moxa cones.

If the patient has a pattern of Lung heat, select hard points on the upper back and apply scarring moxibustion to them. Typical points are listed in TABLE 15-1. I also needle points on the chest, but I have never done direct scarring moxibustion on this area. However, if the abdominal diagnosis shows that there is heat in the chest,[1] I apply heat perception moxibustion to points on the chest.

If the patient is wheezing, this symptom will often resolve itself with only the application of a root treatment if the diagnosis, choice, and location of points (which are determined by palpation) are correct. Listed below are the points used to treat various patterns. Note that these point combinations relate the root treatment to the symptoms and so are different from the standard root treatment point prescriptions:

- For a Lung deficiency/yang deficiency/cold pattern, tonify SP-5 and LU-7.

- For a Spleen deficiency/Liver excess/heat pattern, shunt GB-41.

[1] As noted in Chapter 10, in this case, the area around the underside of the right ribcage is hard to the touch.

- For a Spleen deficiency/Lung deficiency/heat pattern, tonify SP-5 and LU-10.

- For a Liver deficiency/yin deficiency/Lung heat pattern, tonify LR-4.

- For a Spleen deficiency/Lung excess/heat pattern, shunt SP-5.

- For a Lung deficiency/Liver excess/blood stasis pattern, tonify KI-7.

- For a Kidney deficiency/yin deficiency/heat pattern, tonify LU-5.

As noted above, Okabe emphasized treating the upper body. In addition, moxibustion to hard areas on the upper back can make the treatment even more effective. Taking this all together, treatments that loosen the neck, shoulders, and upper back can help halt breathing difficulty attacks and bouts of coughing.

Table 15-1	Branch Treatment Points for Coughing and Wheezing
Location	Points
ARMS AND LEGS	LU-10, LU-5, SP-5, KI-7, LR-4, PC-5, GB-41, ST-36, SP-6
CHEST	CV-22, LU-1, CV-17, LU-2, KI-27, KI-26, KI-25, CV-20
ABDOMEN	ST-25, CV-12, ST-19, LR-14, CV-4
BACK	BL-13, BL-14, BL-42, asthma point, BL-41, BL-15, BL-43, GV-12, GV-11, GV-10, LR-13, GB-21, SI-14, SI-15, BL-23, BL-45

Case History No. 1

PATIENT: 68-year-old woman

CHIEF COMPLAINT: During the course of a cold, the patient developed a fever, at which time she began coughing. The cough persisted for an entire month. The fever and chills were no longer present at the time of the consultation.

SYMPTOMS: There were no significant changes in her stool, urine, or appetite. The coughing was worse at night, with scanty sputum.

PULSE: The overall pulse was sunken, rough, thin, and deficient. The left distal and right medial pulses were deficient on firm pressure, but the right distal pulse was sunken, wiry, and forceful.

TREATMENT: To treat a Spleen deficiency pattern using metal points, I tonified PC-5 and SP-5 and applied direct scarring moxibustion to the tight areas on the upper back. The points on the back were BL-42 and BL-43 bilaterally, GV-9, and points just medial to right BL-13 and BL-15, just lateral to BL-42, and at the lower edge of the right scapula; five half-rice-grain sized moxa cones were used on each point. The first treatment resulted in a reduction in the symptoms. After five treatments, the patient had completely recovered.

If the fever-induced cough and the fever are both present, treating the fever will normally cure the cough. However, if only the cough remains, direct scarring moxibustion to the stiff areas on the upper back is the quickest way to cure it. These stiff areas must be carefully located because the treatments will otherwise be ineffective.

Case History No. 2

PATIENT: 75-year-old man

CHIEF COMPLAINT: Three years earlier, the patient developed a cough during the winter that never seemed to stop. At the time of the consultation, he suffered from both coughing and wheezing.

VISUAL: The patient had a ruddy complexion with a well-developed physique. He definitely looked much younger than his stated age. Tongue inspection revealed a yellow coating.

SYMPTOMS: His stools and urine were normal, and he had a strong appetite. He was prone to sweating from the upper body. Despite his ruddy complexion, he did not drink alcohol.

PULSE: The overall pulse was sunken, wiry, big, rapid, and forceful. The left distal pulse was forceful, the left medial pulse was a little deficient, and the left proximal pulse was deficient. The right distal pulse was sunken, rough, and forceful, the right medial pulse was normal, and the right proximal pulse was rough and forceful.

ABDOMEN: Overall, the abdomen was swollen and exhibited increased resistance. The chest was warm to the touch.

TREATMENT: At first I considered the possibility that the patient had a pattern of Kidney deficiency/yin deficiency with heat in the Heart and Lungs. However, treating for this pattern produced no change. I therefore switched my treatment protocol to a Lung deficiency/Liver excess pattern and tonified KI-7 followed by shunting of LR-2. These changes were made to fit the root treatment to the patient. KI-7 is a metal (Lung) point and can be used to clear heat from the Lungs. LR-2 is the fire (Heart) point and here was used to clear heat from the Heart. This also produced no change.

Because there was no change whatsoever, I checked the dorsal pedis pulse (taken at ST-42), which was especially big and forceful. This made it clear that I was dealing with a pattern of Spleen deficiency/yang excess, that is to say, Spleen deficiency with excess heat in the Lungs. The heat in the chest must have been caused by the Lung heat, which I believed must be the source of the yellow tongue coating on the tongue. The six position pulse gave contradictory information. The Spleen pulse was not so deficient. If anything, it showed that the patient was Kidney deficient.

At this point, I concluded that the Kidney deficiency was normal for someone of his age and should not necessarily be the focus of treatment, but could be considered part of the background. I decided to treat this as a pattern of Spleen deficiency/Lung excess/heat, but keep the Kidney deficiency in mind. As there was a great deal of heat, I tonified SP-9, a water (Kidney) point, and shunted BL-40 to tonify the Kidneys. I also shunted ST-36 in a downward direction to clear the Stomach heat that is produced by Spleen deficiency, while also using this point to increase Kidney fluids. Heat perception moxibustion was then performed at LU-6 to shunt heat from the Lungs.

Following this treatment, the patient experienced diarrhea twice that night, after which his chest felt emptied and his breathing became easier. After two months of this treatment, the patient recovered completely. Additions to the basic treatment were heat perception moxibustion to the chest and retained needling with heat perception moxibustion at stiff points on the upper back.

15.3 SORE THROAT

Diagnosis

Throat diseases include pharyngitis, laryngitis, tonsillitis, vocal chord polyps, cancer of the larynx, and tuberculosis of the larynx. Symptoms usually include swelling of the throat, pain, hoarseness, and the feeling of something being stuck in the throat. There are also times when there actually may be a fish bone stuck in the throat.[2]

---

[2] *Translator's note.* I remember reading older texts where they mention what to do if a bone is stuck in the throat. I thought that it was something that happened a great deal in olden times but not in this day and age where the preparation and consumption of food is more precise. Of course, I was wrong! While attending a study session at Ikeda Sensei's place on the island of Shikoku, where they have the best fish in Japan, I gorged myself on some excellent fish while holding a conversation with three different people at the same time. All of a sudden, I felt a tearing sensation in my throat followed by the feeling that something was stuck in my throat that would not go away no matter how I coughed or swallowed. Needless to say, an excellent meal was ruined, although I did provide some entertainment for the other guests and a case study to see if acupuncture and moxibustion really worked. Direct scarring moxa, about 11 cones, to KI-6 helped to reduce the sensation to a reasonable level. That night I again could feel the pain and blocked sensation, making it difficult to sleep, and so another round of moxa was performed at KI-6, with good results. As I still felt a slight blocked sensation in my throat, I decided to go the local otolaryngologist for a checkup. "What a way to spend a Saturday night," I thought as we made our way to the hospital. Examination showed a small tear on the right side of my throat, which was irritating; but it was not a fish bone, which had evidently been there, but had long since disappeared. That night another round of moxa helped me fall asleep. In two days, I had completely recovered.

Whatever the name of the disease, it is important to identify the affected meridians and determine whether heat or cold is involved. The affected meridians are then treated accordingly. Note that throat pain is caused by local congestion of qi and heat. There are no throat problems caused solely by cold. Even if the overall pattern is that of yang deficiency cold, at a local level, the problem is caused by heat. In the case of a cold pattern, the heat collects as there is not enough yang qi to discharge or radiate it outward. Sore throats due to heat patterns have a similar mechanism: more heat is accumulating locally than can be discharged.

The tonsillitis, which often follows on the heels of chills followed by a fever, can range from mild discomfort when swallowing to pain so severe that swallowing is impossible. In any case, the pulse must be examined. If it is floating, big, excessive, and rapid, the pattern is that of Lung deficiency/yang brightness meridian excess/heat. In the initial stages of a febrile disease, a greater yang meridian excess/heat pattern or a greater yang meridian deficiency/heat pattern is common. This stage is still too early for the appearance of sore, swollen throats, but when the pattern progresses to that of yang brightness meridian heat, pain and swelling of the throat can occur. Clinically speaking, however, if it is believed that some heat is still left in the greater yang meridian, the heat should be shunted.

When heat remains in the yang brightness meridian for a long time, it can cause greater yin meridian heat. When heat builds up in the greater yin meridian (Lungs), it can spread into the Heart and Pericardium meridians as their related organs are also located in the chest. If the disease progresses to this stage, the fever becomes more severe and the throat becomes swollen and almost unbearably painful. Additional symptoms include irritability, restlessness, and insomnia. This condition should be treated as a pattern of Spleen deficiency/Lung heat.

There are instances of febrile disease where the chills that accompany a sore throat are the main symptom. These cases are a result of either:

1. *A decrease in the yang qi at the greater yang meridian level.* The decrease in the yang qi at this level brings about a shift in the balance between the Kidney and Bladder meridians, resulting in a relative preponderance of yin qi, and thus chills.

2. *Cold permeating the lesser yin meridian.* In this case, cold in the legs enters the lesser yin meridian, which normally is full of yin qi and contains only a small amount of yang qi. However, the presence of the cold results in a relative increase in yin qi, forcing the little bit of yang qi in the meridian to move upward and be trapped there. In this state, therefore, although other areas of the body have an abundance of yin qi, and are consequently cold, there is yang qi trapped in the throat, and is consequently sore.

If this continues for a long time, the heat trapped in the throat increases. Thus, even when there are some slight chills, the patient will also have a fever at the same time. Over time, the fever becomes even more prevalent than the chills, and the sore throat worsens. By this time, the pattern is one of Spleen deficiency/Lung heat. Even when the fever begins to die down and swallowing does not produce pain, the throat still feels a little strange; this too is best treated as a Spleen deficiency/Lung heat pattern.

3. Finally, in other cases, the onset of the cold is marked by a sore throat but no chills or fever. Whether due to a decrease in the yang qi at the greater yang meridian level or cold permeating the lesser yin meridian, the pulse will be sunken, thin, and weak. All of these can be taken care of by tonifying the lesser yin meridian. However, if over time the sore throat is accompanied by a significant fever, this should be treated as a Spleen deficiency/Lung excess pattern.

Patients often come to the clinic complaining of a sensation of something clogging their throats, including women in menopause who often have this problem as their chief complaint. There are three basic patterns. The first is Spleen deficiency/yang deficiency with the collection of qi and phlegm; this pattern leads to qi stagnation. The second is either Lung deficiency/Liver excess or Spleen deficiency/Liver excess; in both patterns, the yang qi of the Liver's blood cannot diffuse outward, leading to blood stasis and the blocked feeling. The third type is a Kidney deficiency pattern in which there is a feeling of something pushing upward, often into the throat. Classically, this was referred to as running piglet qi (奔豚気 *honton ki/bēn tún qì*).

Hoarseness can occur during the course of a cold or as a result of overusing the voice. Hoarseness can be a result of Spleen deficiency/Lung heat—where the Spleen deficiency causes a lack of fluids, leading to heat in the Lungs—or of Kidney deficiency/yang deficiency.

Finally, some vocal cord polyps can be large enough to block the throat. The occurrence of polyps on the larynx is becoming more common due, it is thought, to the popularity of karaoke. These cases should be left to the care of medical physicians.

Treatment

For sore throats caused by Lung deficiency/yang brightness meridian excess/heat, tonify the Lung meridian and shunt points on the greater yang meridian, including SI-1 and SI-2. For sore throats caused by yang brightness meridian heat, points such as LI-1 and LI-2 are shunted. Additional points such as LI-4, LI-5, ST-45, and ST-39 are also useful.

For sore throats caused by Kidney deficiency/yang deficiency/cold, perform direct scarring moxibustion at KI-6. Needling is also acceptable, but moxibustion with three to five half-rice-grain sized moxa cones is very effective, especially for the present pattern. However, if the point location is even a little bit off, there will be no effect. HT-7 and KI-3 are effective when there is a great deal of cold, while KI-2 is used when there is a lot of heat.

When treatment directed at a sore throat caused by Kidney deficiency and/or Lung deficiency is ineffective, perhaps the diagnosis should be changed to that of Spleen deficiency/Lung heat, which is a common cause of sore throats. To treat this pattern, tonify PC-5, SP-5, and LU-10. This is usually enough to resolve the sore throat, but when there is a great deal of heat, the affected meridians must be shunted. If there is heat in the Lung meridian, LU-11 and LU-5 are shunted. If there is heat in the Pericardium meridian, PC-8 is shunted.

For a blocked throat that is caused by stagnant qi, points on the Governing vessel, including GV-12, GV-11, and GV-10, are often found to be reactive (TABLE 15-2). After the reactive points are treated, a root treatment for Spleen deficiency/yang deficiency is added to ensure the treatment's efficacy. For a blocked throat that is caused by Liver stagnation, treat according to the pattern. There is no need for any special points or methods, although care should be taken to treat stiff areas on the shoulders and upper back.

Table 15-2	Branch Treatment Points for Sore Throat
Location	**Points**
CHEST	**Points on or near the sternocleidomastoid muscle (ST-9, CV-22, SI-17, LI-17, LI-18, ST-11, ST-12, ST-10, KI-27), sensitive points on and around the sternum**
BACK	GV-12, GV-11, GV-10, BL-13, BL-14, BL-42, BL-43, BL-22, BL-23, GB-20, GV-14, sensitive points around GV-14

There are a few other useful points for treating sore throats. One is an extra point that is found one finger width above LI-11; if this point is tender, direct scarring moxibustion should be applied here. Another is either SP-1 or an extra point that is found on the medial edge of the crease formed when the big toe is folded at the first digit. This extra point can be thought of as a variation of SP-2, and one cone of direct scarring moxibustion is sufficient. Finally, there is another extra point (鬼当 *ki tō/guǐ dāng*) that is found on the lateral edge of the crease of the thumb when it is folded at the first digit (on the Lung meridian). This is also treated with one cone of direct moxa.

I remember that some time ago, a patient came to my clinic with a fish bone lodged in the throat. I recall saying that it would be best if the patient went to an otolaryngologist, but for some reason I ended up treating him. I used KI-3, and shortly after needling this point he reported that the pain had disappeared. From that time on, I have made use of the lesser yin meridians—Kidney and Heart—for sore throats, with good success.

Case History

PATIENT: 48-year-old woman

CHIEF COMPLAINT: The patient reported the recent onset of chills, fever, joint pain, and a sore throat.

VISUAL: The patient had a small frame and a red face. This redness was, however, not a healthy glow, but was felt to be caused more by yang qi floating up to the face. The tongue body was slightly pale. The throat was red and swollen.

SYMPTOMS: There were no significant changes in her stool or appetite, but there was a reduction in her urination.

PULSE: The overall pulse was sunken, thin, rough, and rapid.

CONSIDERATIONS: Even though there was a fever, the pulse was not floating. Rather, it was sunken, which meant that the red face was due to false-heat, true-cold. The fever was also misleading because it was also a case of false-heat, true-cold. Because of all this, I told myself to be careful in this case.

TREATMENT: Direct scarring moxibustion was applied to KI-6, and contact needling was performed on the upper back. After this, the fever broke and the sore throat disappeared. However, a few days later after overdoing it, the patient's symptoms returned, but the sore throat was even worse than before, preventing the patient from sleeping for four or five nights. At this point, intense heat had gathered in the throat, which led to chills elsewhere.

This time, extensive shunting would be important if a favorable result was to be achieved. Direct scarring moxibustion at KI-6 and heat perception moxibustion at ST-9 were applied. After this, HT-7 and KI-3 were tonified and contact needling was applied to the upper back. Finally, Do In massage was slowly applied to BL-10, GB-20, and GB-12. By "slowly," I mean applying a gentle, even pressure while breathing in and out slowly. I also slowly transferred my hand from one point to another to achieve the best effect. The Do In massage allowed the trapped heat in the upper body to be recirculated; it is especially effective for severe sore throats. Thirty minutes following this treatment, the fever broke, the patient's appetite was restored, and she was able to eat some noodles without any problem. The next day her temperature had returned to normal.

15.4   NASAL DISORDERS

Diagnosis

The most common nasal problem in recent times is allergic rhinitis, which is characterized by sneezing, nasal discharge, nasal obstruction, and itchy red eyes. In Japan, the most common forms of allergic rhinitis are said to be due to cedar tree pollen and cypress tree pollen. The only problem with this theory is that these trees have been around for ages, but it is only recently that allergic rhinitis has become so common. Maybe the problem is caused by adverse changes in the quality of the air, water, and food. Another factor is that many more people lead lives in sealed, fully heated and cooled air-conditioned dwellings, which subjects the body to what is referred to from a traditional perspective as pathogenic wind.

The nasal discharge seen in cases of rhinitis is caused by heat raising the fluids in the Stomach to the nose. Heat has a tendency to move up and outward, and normally this heat is appropriately discharged from the body. However, when there is deficiency of yang qi, the heat cannot be properly discharged; instead, it begins to collect in the upper burner from where it moves the fluids and causes the nasal discharge. The sneezing, nasal obstruction, and itchy eyes are also all due to the trapped heat in the upper burner.

Rhinitis occurs mostly in the spring and is a result of overusing one's energy during the previous winter, primarily by being too soft and indolent, which leads to a weakened body. This means that in the spring, the body does not have the ability to create sufficient yang qi. Also during the winter, because of the increased reliance on heaters, the body is constantly being exposed to heat, which acts as a pathogenic wind, creating heat during the winter. Exposure to the yang qi of spring then leads to the buildup of heat because the body does not have the capacity to discharge it. The external heat and the heat trapped in the upper burner then combine to cause rhinitis.

Based on this, it is clear that, in order to prevent an attack of rhinitis, a reasonable amount of exercise should be undertaken, not molly coddling ourselves while sitting next to the heater day and night! On the other hand, the body should not be allowed to get cold and the Stomach and Intestines should be treated properly. When the Stomach and Intestines are in good condition, there will be ample amounts of yang qi for the spring.

Blocked nasal passages, sneezing, and nasal discharge during the course of a cold all share the same pathology—a large amount of heat trapped in the nose. There are cases where people recover from a fever only to find that they have lost their sense of smell. This too is from the large amount of heat trapped in the nose. I now see the problem of blocked nasal passages less frequently than before, perhaps because people are going to their doctors first and receiving a treatment there. However, I do see people that come to me after having received an unsuccessful operation for the same problem.

Nasal polyps, which are quite uncommon, are caused by heat in the yang brightness meridian. So too are the red noses seen on some patients; in these cases, overeating and overdrinking are also factors. Sometimes, however, the redness may be due to blood stasis, in which case, pricking prominent dark-colored and small blood vessels on the nose and upper back to let out a few drops of blood is an effective treatment.

The nose is governed by the Lungs, but the yang brightness meridian also runs through this area. The yang brightness meridian is, in turn, governed by the Spleen and Stomach. Finally, one part of the nose is also connected with the greater yang meridian.

Nose problems start with heat in the Lungs, but then the heat gets trapped in the yang brightness meridian and the symptoms begin to appear. There are cases where the disease ends at this stage. Some of the nasal problems are connected to the greater yang meridian, which are easy to cure. Most of the time, the disease in the yang brightness meridian progresses, resulting in Spleen deficiency and various heat-related symptoms such as fever, joint pain, and itching. If the disease progresses further, the heat will migrate to the greater yin Lung meridian; in these cases, the heat always enters the Governing vessel as well.

The above pathology can be seen both during the course of acute febrile disease as well as in nonfebrile chronic nasal problems. Allergic rhinitis, for example, is often due to Lung deficiency with heat in the yang brightness meridian. However, there has been a shift in people's general health such that even children are now found to have patterns of Spleen deficiency rather than Lung deficiency, which used to be more prevalent in the past. This means that there is more strain being put on the digestive system than before.

The branch treatment for nasal problems is actually quite straightforward, as long as you bear one thing in mind: regardless of the pulse, nasal symptoms can always be attributed to heat in the yang brightness meridian and the Governing vessel. The Governing vessel is an extra meridian and receives the overflow of heat when the ordinary meridians have too much of it and cannot deal with it by themselves. Chapter 27 of the *Classic of Difficulties* states that once the heat has gone into the extra meridians, it cannot return to the ordinary meridians. Stubborn nasal symptoms are therefore due to yang brightness meridian heat overflowing and becoming stuck in the Governing vessel.

In premodern texts, nosebleeds were regarded as nasal diseases. There are various types of nosebleeds. Instead of menstruating, young women often suffer from nosebleeds. Young children who have a weak constitution and are exhausted get nosebleeds. In men, nosebleeds are basically a result of stiff shoulders; hot-headed men with high blood pressure are particularly susceptible to this problem. Each of these has a different cause, but the actual nosebleed is caused by heat in the yang brightness meridian.

Treatment

Points that have traditionally been used are GV-23, GV-22, GV-20, and BL-7 (see TABLE 15-3). *Classic of Nourishing Life with Acupuncture and Moxibustion* mentions the use of GV-24 to GV-27. For blocked nasal passages, Keiri Inoue—a famous master practitioner and my brother's teacher—would always use M-HN-3, GV-22, and GV-23.

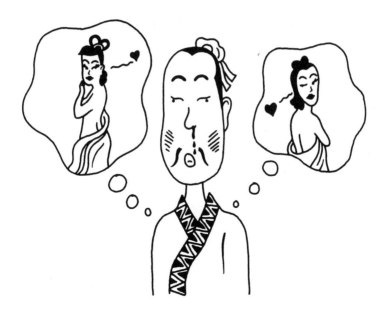

Blood rushing to the nose causes nosebleeds

Other points for the face include BL-2, ST-2, and LI-20. For the occipital area, use BL-10 and GB-20. There are cases where BL-2 is enough to clear a blocked nose. For blocked nasal passages with facial pain, good results can be obtained by using retained needles or heat perception moxibustion at sensitive points around ST-2. Another common symptom in these cases is a heavy feeling in the occipital area, in which case BL-10 and GB-20 are essential.

Table 15-3	Branch Treatment Points for Nasal Disorders
Location	Points
ARMS AND LEGS	ST-36, BL-67, LU-5, LI-4, LI-10, LU-6, LI-2, LI-3, SI-3, SI-2, BL-62
HEAD	GV-23, GV-22, GV-20, BL-7, GV-24, BL-2, ST-2, LI-20, **points around both sides of nostrils**
BACK	BL-10, GB-20, BL-13, BL-43, BL-42, BL-41

Some patients come in after a cold unable to smell anything. This type of problem responds well to retained needling or direct scarring moxibustion (about seven half-rice-grain sized moxa cones) applied to BL-10, GV-23, and GV-22.

When there is a nasal problem, the shoulders become stiff, which in turn makes the problem worse. In this case, hard, stiff areas should be treated by using retained needles or applying direct scarring moxibustion to reactive points such as BL-41 to BL-43 and BL-13.

Nasal problems can also be cured by using points on the arms and legs. The points that are used most often are found on the Large Intestine meridian, for example, hard points that resemble a grain of rice anywhere around LI-10 can be used. Direct scarring moxibustion is applied to these points, but the moxibustion should be applied in such a way that no heat sensation is felt. If this is the case, then rhinitis, itchy eyes, or blocked nasal passages are often resolved on the spot. Of course, when this treatment is combined with points on the head, the results will be even better. If the heat has penetrated deeply into the body, direct scarring moxibustion using half-rice-grain sized moxa cones is applied at LU-6 until the heat is felt.

Other points used for nasal problems include ST-36, BL-67, LI-2 to LI-4, SI-3, SI-2, and BL-62. The points are pressed thoroughly and painful stiff points are selected for treatment. If possible, it is best to discern the location of the heat. An examination of the pulse can reveal whether it has reached the yang brightness meridian, stopped at the greater yang meridian, or gone as far as the greater yin meridian.

15.5   SWEATING ISSUES

Diagnosis

Night sweats and oversweating can be considered as one. Patients may either have sweating as their chief complaint or suffer from this as a result of some other disease. The absence or presence of sweating can be important in discriminating between patterns, and I would therefore like to briefly outline the pathology of sweating.

In premodern texts, we find sweat-connected terms, including lack of [normal] sweating (無汗 *mu kan/wú hàn*), spontaneous sweating (自汗 *ji kan/zì hàn*), night sweats, or literally the 'sweat of thieves' (盗汗 *to kan/dào hàn*), white sweat (白汗 *haku kan/bái hàn*), yellow sweat (黄汗 *ō kan/huáng hàn*), and bloody sweat (血汗 *ketsu kan/xuè hàn*). All of these are briefly described below.

LACK OF SWEATING

This is defined as an absence of sweating when there should be some. In acute febrile disease, the lack of sweating indicates a Lung deficiency/yang excess pattern. However, we cannot make this diagnosis solely on this one piece of information. The patient must also present with fever, chills, and a floating, rapid, excessive pulse. If, on the contrary, the pulse is floating but weak, then the pattern is that of yang deficiency even in the absence of sweating. Also, when we speak of a fever, we are talking about the patient's subjective feeling of a fever and not a quantitative measurement on a thermometer. For instance, chills that are accompanied by a hot, red face can be called a fever.

On the other hand, even if there is a measurable fever, as long as the face and lips are pale, the urine is clear, and the patient has chills but no sweating, then the pattern is that of yang deficiency. It could be Lung deficiency/yang deficiency transforming into Kidney deficiency/yang deficiency, or perhaps into a Spleen deficiency/Kidney deficiency/cold pattern. Of course, the yang deficiency pulse would be sunken and weak.

In the midst of summer, there are some individuals that do not sweat a drop. This is not indicative of a febrile disease, but it does suggest that there is not enough yang qi to produce sweating. This condition is often treated as Spleen deficiency/yang deficiency or Kidney deficiency/yang deficiency.

Spontaneous Sweating and White Sweat

This is defined as sweating that occurs in the absence of a febrile disease or particular physical activity. In most cases of acute febrile disease, the patients present with chills, fever, and sweating; in these cases, the pattern is that of Lung deficiency/yang deficiency/heat. However, the presence of a great deal of sweating, strong chills, and aversion to drafts— but no fever—indicates that, although the pattern is still that of yang deficiency, it is nonetheless approaching that of yang deficiency cold.

Sweating can also occur even when the extreme state of yang deficiency cold is reached. This should really be called sweating from collapse, as it occurs when the yang qi is about to fade away completely, often in life-threatening situations. This type of sweating is known as white sweat because when it occurs it leaves the body cold and pale.

The other extreme is reached when internally trapped heat causes sweating; for example, heat that has entered the lesser yang meridian can sometimes induce whole body or upper body sweating. This is usually treated as a pattern of Spleen deficiency/Liver excess/heat, and if the heat penetrates as far as the yang organs, the sweating will continue unabated and the chills will disappear.

There are also those who suffer from chronic sweating, most of whom have yin deficiency heat. These individuals are thin in the initial stages. However, as the yin deficiency becomes chronic, many of them tend to become obese (although they still suffer from chronic sweating). There are also obese people that sweat profusely; these individuals are Kidney deficient. They are obese because the contractive power of their Kidneys is weak, and they sweat because of the outward movement of the deficiency heat. In these cases, the profuse sweating is also a result of water collecting near the surface of the skin, which is a consequence of poor circulation of Lung qi. Recall that both the Kidneys and Lungs are adversely affected in individuals with a Kidney deficiency pattern.

NIGHT SWEATS

This is defined as sweating that occurs during one's sleep and is a result of internal heat. At night, the yang qi migrates to the interior of the body. If heat is already present in the interior, the two contend with each other, leading to night sweats. As mentioned earlier, the internal heat can be due to yin deficiency or Liver excess, and if the night sweats continue for any length of time, Lung deficiency/Liver excess/heat can result, which is an acute version of Lung deficiency/Liver excess/blood stasis. In this pattern we have the circulation of the Lung weakened with deficient Kidney fluids, all combined with heat containing blood lodged in the Liver. The heat in the blood is responsible for the sweating, which, during the night, occurs in the upper body and face. In this pattern, the right distal and left proximal pulses are deficient. The left medial pulse will be sunken, rough, and excessive; sometimes this pulse is excessive in both the superficial and deep levels. The combination of this pulse pattern and night sweats is often seen in patients with tuberculosis or hepatitis.

Pulse diagnosis is used to discern the cause of the night sweats. If the pulse is floating, big, and forceful as well as deficient on pressure, then the patient has yin deficiency. Of course, an acute febrile disease must be ruled out before arriving at any decision. Another thing to check is the strength of the appetite, because a strong appetite would confirm the yin deficiency.

A sunken, rough, and excessive pulse or a sunken and slippery pulse means that heat can be found somewhere in the internal organs. In this case, it is good to check for other symptoms such as the extent of the appetite and fever. In cases of yin deficiency, there is normally a slight fever and the pulse will often be rapid.

There are patients who sweat from the palms of the hands and soles of the feet. This is a result of Kidney deficiency in which a lack of fluids leads to quite a bit of deficiency heat, causing the hands and feet to sweat. Everyone has had the experience of being nervous and sweating from the palms of the hands. This nervous tension is due to the fear of failure or of being laughed at; individuals who experience this often have a predisposition toward weak Kidneys. Therefore, the only way to cure sweaty hands and feet is to strengthen the Kidneys. Those who sweat from the ankles downward are also Kidney deficient.

YELLOW SWEAT AND BLOODY SWEAT

Both of these occur as a result of a great deal of internal heat; bloody sweat requires a higher level of heat. It is important to determine whether this heat is from yin deficiency, excess heat in the yang organs, or excess heat in the Liver. In both yellow and bloody sweat, the sweat is darker than normal and may stain the patient's clothing; bloody sweat is darker than yellow sweat.

Treatment

When it is accompanied by chills and fever, lack of sweating, spontaneous sweating, or white sweat should be treated according to the appropriate pattern, as discussed briefly in Chapter 5. Night sweats as well as yellow and bloody sweat can also be treated successfully if the root treatment is made the focus of the treatment. Premodern texts also describe a variety of ways of treating different conditions marked by abnormal sweating. I will introduce a few here.

• The Edo period text *A Collection of Acupuncture and Moxibustion Treasures* states that spontaneous sweat is caused by yang deficiency and recommends direct scarring moxibustion at BL-20 and BL-13. However, GV-14 is more effective than BL-13 when treating fever plus spontaneous sweating. If BL-13 is chosen, then the patient should barely feel the moxibustion.

  In my experience, however, using moxibustion to treat spontaneous sweating is risky. If the wrong points are chosen or the correct points are incorrectly located, some patients will begin to feel worse as their yang qi is further depleted. A safer, more effective option is to apply contact needling to points on the back, including BL-13, BL-14, BL-21, and BL-22, which will tonify the protective qi.

• In the Edo period text *Principles of Acupuncture and Moxibustion*, acupuncture at LU-7, LU-11, LR-1, and KI-1 is recommended for treating spontaneous sweating. *A Collection of Acupuncture and Moxibustion Treasures* advises direct scarring moxibustion at BL-23 for night sweats, while *Principles of Acupuncture and Moxibustion* recommends direct scarring moxibustion to CV-6 and BL-23. *Selected Secrets of Acupuncture and Moxibustion* states that KI-19 and PC-5 are to be used for night sweats above the waist, while ST-25 and GV-4 are to be used for night sweats below the waist.

15.6   PULMONARY DISEASES

Diagnosis

Pulmonary diseases not covered so far include tuberculosis, pneumonia, pleurisy, pulmonary emphysema, spontaneous pneumothorax, and pulmonary edema. Inflammation of the cervical lymph glands should be added to this list, as it would fall under the category of Lung diseases in traditional medicine and can also occur secondary to pulmonary tuberculosis. Other difficult diseases such as diffuse bronchiolitis and lung cancer can also be included here. Of course, it is rather unusual to come into contact with patients with these diseases, and they are also difficult to cure with acupuncture and moxibustion. Still, it is important to be aware of their existence and to refer patients to the appropriate specialists if their pulmonary symptoms do not respond to acupuncture fairly quickly.

It is unusual to see tuberculosis nowadays, but if the patient has a low-grade fever, coughing, and night sweats, it is advisable to recommend a medical checkup. The pulse will be that of a Lung deficiency/Liver excess heat pattern.

Pneumonia has already been discussed earlier in this chapter, but I will repeat the information again. If the patient presents with cough, pains in the chest, and fever, and if the right distal pulse is sunken, wiry, and excessive or sunken, rough and excessive, and the patient also presents with cough and pain in the chest, then great care must be taken when treating this disease. You should be ready to refer the patient to a biomedical physician if necessary.

Pleurisy often occurs as a secondary infection after pneumonia, and the symptoms include chest pain, a feeling of pressure in the chest, wheezing, cough, and fever. The pattern is often that of Spleen deficiency/Liver excess. Great caution should be exercised when treating this disease.

A cold that worsens and presents with a continuous cough can lead to pulmonary emphysema. If a patient with this history also has breathing difficulties, pulmonary emphysema should be considered a distinct possibility.

There are a few cases every year in Japan of pneumothorax supposedly caused by acupuncture. If deep needling to the thoracic area is avoided, there can be no possibility of this happening. There are also cases where pneumothorax occurs spontaneously. This phenomenon seems to be more common in young men with a Lung deficient constitution. It is characterized by chest pain, breathing difficulties, coughing, palpitations, and a general sense of unease.

Pulmonary edema occurs as a result of heart problems. If the patient presents with cough, difficulty breathing, and whole body edema, and the pulse is rapid, pulmonary edema should be considered a distinct possibility.

Inflammation of the cervical lymph glands was traditionally known as scrofula (瘰癧 *rui reki/luǒ lì*) and occurred as a result of tuberculosis. It is not seen so often nowadays, but the cervical lymph glands can swell up from other causes as well. Deficiency consumption (虚 劳 *kyo rō/xū láo*), a form of exhaustion, is one of the key causes of this disorder, but there are also times when the cervical lymph glands swell up as a result of the presence of cancer. Again the rule is, if in doubt, refer the patient to an appropriate medical physician.

Ancient texts such as the *Essentials from the Golden Cabinet* mention a variety of Lung disorders that often overlap with significant pulmonary diseases as understood by modern medicine. These include Lung atrophy (肺痿 *hai i/fèi wěi*), Lung abscess (肺癰 *hai yō/fèi yōng*), and consumptive disease (癆瘵 *rō sai/láo zhài*). The pathology of all of these different Lung diseases involves Spleen deficiency or Liver excess heat patterns that generate Lung heat. You may think that Lung disease implies Lung deficiency, but Lung deficiency leads to yang excess or yang deficiency states in which the Lungs themselves are not yet affected by heat.

Treatment

Of the Lung diseases discussed above, pulmonary emphysema and pneumothorax respond extremely well to acupuncture and moxibustion. Swollen cervical lymph glands, provided the swelling is not caused by a malignant cancer, also respond well. If you have confidence in your ability and experience, you can also treat pneumonia and pleurisy. Diseases such as tuberculosis, pulmonary edema, and lung cancer have been treated by acupuncture in Japan, primarily before 1945 when other options were limited and practitioners had experience with treating these diseases. However, at present, modern medicine is the preferred method for the vast majority of patients, and acupuncture is only given when the family and the overseeing physician agree.

When treating with acupuncture and moxibustion, the basic rule is to treat according to the existing pattern, and for the particular diseases listed here, make sure that heat is removed from the chest. One way to clear the heat is to apply heat perception moxibustion or retained needling to the chest. Another way is to apply direct scarring moxibustion and retained needling to hard, stiff points on the back.

For spontaneous pneumothorax, retained needling is applied to painful areas on the chest to relieve the pain. For swollen cervical lymph glands, use contact needling and retained needling at the swollen areas. In these cases, the shoulders are normally stiff, and these should be treated and made to relax, as this will result in a cure.

Scrofula can be treated by applying direct scarring moxibustion to a point on the tip of the lateral epicondyle (a variation of LI-12). Around seven half-rice-grain sized moxa cones are applied on the left for right-sided symptoms, and on right for left-sided symptoms. Another method is to put slices of garlic over the swollen areas and apply moxibustion on top of these.

In *Collection of Acupuncture and Moxibustion Treasures* it is noted that, for consumptive disease:

> The qi and the body are weak, the Heart and the Kidneys are damaged by exhaustion. The Heart is associated with blood and the Kidneys are associated with essence. Both the blood and the essence are dried out. Heat flares up, there is coughing, and coughing of blood, nocturnal emissions of sperm, night sweats, chills, fever, irritability, and heat in

the five hearts [palms of the hands, soles of the feet, and center of the chest], a reduction in appetite causing the patient to waste away, with symptoms worsening in the evenings. With this disease pattern, the body becomes so exhausted that it feels like there are worms infesting it and that they are eating away at the bones. This spreads from person to person, exterminating whole families and clans. This was known as spreading of corpses [伝尸 *den shi/chuán shī*]. ... Direct scarring moxibustion should be applied to the four flower disease gates [四華患門 *shi ka kan mon/sì huá huàn mén*, discussed below], and to BL-43, LR-13, CV-6, and ST-36.

This text is describing what we call tuberculosis in modern medicine. However, the treatment is not only applicable to this disease, but to all pulmonary diseases, including cancer.

Many in Japan are familiar with Four Flower Disease Gates moxibustion, which was first written about in the *Classified Classic* by the seventeenth-century physician Zhang Jie-Bin. However, because it is not well known outside Japan today, I will explain it here. This method consists of administering scarring moxibustion at six points. These consist of two 'disease gate' (患門 *kan mon/huàn mén*) points and, not surprisingly, four 'flower' points (四華 *shi ka/sì huá*).

The first step is to use a piece of string to measure the length from the tip of the patient's big toe along the bottom of the foot up along the back of the calf to BL-40. This length of string is then taken, and one end of it is held at the tip of the patient's nose and run along the middle of the forehead, the middle of the head and down the back along the Governing vessel, all the while hugging to the body. The point where the end of the string touches the Governing vessel is marked. After this, another piece of string is used to measure from the bridge of the nose to both edges of the mouth, forming a shape resembling the two sides of a shallow triangle. This length of string is then taken, and the middle of it is placed on the spot marked previously on the Governing vessel. The string is placed at right angles to the Governing vessel, and the points at the two ends of the string are taken as the two 'disease gate' points.

To find the four 'flower' points, another string is draped around the neck, and the two ends are made to meet at the point CV-15. The string is then cut to this length and again draped around the neck at throat level, but this time, the two edges meet at the back along the Governing vessel. This point is marked. Finally, another piece of string is used to measure the width of the mouth. This length of string is then taken and its middle is placed on the point just marked on the Governing vessel. Two points are marked at right angles to the Governing vessel (one point to the right and one to the left) and another two above and below (that is, on the Governing vessel). These four points are 'flower' points.

Recently, there have been a large number of cases of atopic eczema in Japan. Looking at these patients, it is clear that they have Lung deficient constitutions, and in the past, these people would have developed tuberculosis. Nowadays, instead of developing tuberculosis, they develop atopic eczema; that is, instead of a Lung problem, they now develop a problem in its related tissue, the skin, However, the same constitution is present. Therefore, I believe that the Four Flower Disease Gates moxibustion mentioned in the text above is valuable for treating atopic eczema as well.

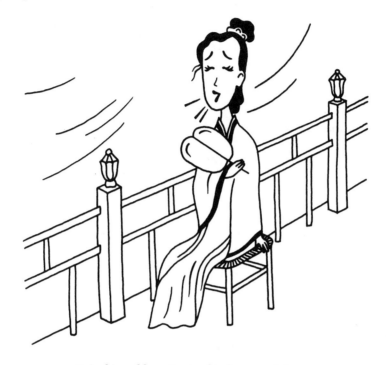

Fair skinned beauties tend to have weak Lungs

Case History No. 1

PATIENT: 88-year-old woman

CHIEF COMPLAINT: A member of the family consulted me concerning her grandmother who had suddenly lost all her vigor, appetite, and stopped talking altogether. She had already suffered from a brain infarction, leading to hemiplegia of the left side, and spent nearly all of her time lying in bed. However, despite this, she had an appetite and was reasonably vigorous. She suddenly took a turn for the worse the day before I was consulted.

SYMPTOMS: If her name was called, the patient replied but she would not open her eyes. She would easily fall asleep and her blood pressure was 180/100mmHg. I thought that maybe another brain infarction had occurred.

PULSE: The overall pulse was sunken, wiry, a little weak, and a little rapid. The right distal pulse (the Lung pulse) proved to be a little stronger than the rest. Because of her sudden loss of vigor, I thought that there could only be two possibilities: a second brain infarction or febrile pneumonia.

MANAGEMENT: Although the family was more relaxed after I saw her and said they would see how things went, I encouraged them to admit the grandmother into a hospital as soon as possible. I recommended the hospital of my acquaintance and accompanied them there. An x-ray was taken and sure enough, both Lungs were white, the diagnosis being febrile pneumonia. The patient received treatment in the hospital, and after three months, she was able to return home.

Case History No. 2

PATIENT: 75-year-old woman

CHIEF COMPLAINT: After suffering from a cold, she was left with a cough and a slight fever that would not go away. The patient was well known to me as I had been treating her regularly for some time.

SYMPTOMS: Her symptoms included lack of vigor, no appetite, and slightly soft stools. She had suffered from pneumonia once before and was therefore prone to getting it again. I observed her condition carefully.

PULSE: The overall pulse was sunken, rough, and weak. However, the Lung and the Large Intestine pulses were strong. This pulse pattern combined with the incessant coughing and slight fever made me suspect another bout of pneumonia.

MANAGEMENT: I contacted her doctor and asked for her to be tested, and sure enough, she was diagnosed with pneumonia. When the right distal pulse is sunken and strong, the patient then has either pneumonia, another serious pulmonary disease, a disease of the thyroid, or some hidden disease in the area above the chest. Also, even when a patient is thought to be over their illness, if their right distal pulse is still sunken and strong, they have not recovered fully. In such cases, using a root treatment for Liver deficiency/Lung heat or Spleen deficiency/Lung heat should bring good results.

Case History No. 3

PATIENT: 2-year-old girl

CHIEF COMPLAINT: For the past two weeks she had a slight fever and constant cough. She had a history of pneumonia.

SYMPTOMS: There were no changes in her stools or appetite.

PULSE: The overall pulse was sunken, wiry, and lacking in force; it was also a Spleen deficiency/Lung heat pulse.

CHEST: LU-1 and KI-27 were painful on pressure.

BACK: There were hard, stiff points found on the inside of the right scapula.

TREATMENT: For Spleen deficiency/Lung heat, PC-7, SP-3, and LU-10 were tonified and heat perception moxibustion was applied to the painful and hard points on the chest and back. This treatment was performed twice, resulting in a complete recovery.

Two years later she came to the clinic with the same symptoms after catching a cold. This time her overall pulse was fine and weak, and the right medial and distal pulses were deficient; in other words, a Lung deficiency/yang deficiency pattern. This meant that there was a pulmonary problem, but I was sure it was not pneumonia because the Lung pulse was not strong. Bearing in mind the overall weakness of the pulse, I began to suspect that she may have tuberculosis. I remembered the pulse pattern of tuberculosis patients that I had seen before, and it made alarm bells ring.

MANAGEMENT: Recently, because tuberculosis has become scarce, most young doctors have no experience with it. I therefore referred the patient directly to a pulmonary specialist I knew. In his hospital they had a tuberculosis ward, and so I was confident in his ability to diagnose this disease. The results indeed showed that the patient had tuberculosis, and she was then hospitalized for treatment.

Case History No. 4

PATIENT: 47-year-old woman

CHIEF COMPLAINTS: One year previously, she had an operation for cancer of the left breast. Three months later she had another operation for cancer of the uterus. At the time of the consultation, she had been diagnosed with lung cancer. Her main complaints were pain in the upper left back and around the Spleen associated points (BL-20). She did not have very high expectations for the treatment, but she also did not have many other choices.

SYMPTOMS: Even though she was in and out of the hospital, she still had time to run a small business (a small bar). Perhaps because of this, she had extremely sore and stiff shoulders. Her stools were slightly soft and she had lost her appetite.

ABDOMEN: There was resistance to pressure at the epigastrium and evident collection of water throughout the abdomen.

PULSE: The overall pulse was sunken and tight; it also had a dried-out feeling. The left distal and medial pulses seemed to be wiry and forceful, but overshadowing this was the dried-out feeling that gave the pulse its tight quality. The left proximal pulse was sunken, wiry, and deficient. The overall pulse on the right side was wiry with no deficiency discernable in the individual positions.

CONSIDERATIONS: The pulse felt like it was one step away from a terminal pulse. Cancer patients commonly exhibit a tight pulse. When there is no sign of deficiency in the pulse, it is considered a terminal pulse.

TREATMENT: The patient was treated for a Spleen deficiency/yin deficiency pattern. After a number of these treatments, the pulse became sunken, wiry, and rapid. The left distal pulse was deficient, and the left medial pulse was sunken and rough. The left proximal pulse was rough. The right distal pulse was wiry and forceful, while the right medial pulse was wiry and deficient.

The distal pedis pulse (taken at ST-42), which represents the Stomach qi, was hollow. This suggested that the postnatal qi was diminishing, which is not a good sign. It also confirmed the diagnosis of Spleen deficiency. The posterior tibialis pulse (taken at KI-3), which represents the lesser yin qi (and thereby the prenatal qi), showed a hidden pulse. This demonstrated that the postnatal qi was also beginning to weaken.

One month later, the overall pulse was rough, rapid, tight, and thin. The left distal and right medial pulses were deficient while the left medial pulse was rough and excessive. The right distal pulse was rough and excessive. The abdomen was tight in the epigastrium, and again, there was an evident collection of water. However, heat had begun to appear in the chest. Shortly after this, she was unable to continue the treatment and was admitted to a hospital where she passed away.

I have treated a number of patients with lung cancer and have found that acupuncture is very useful for dealing with pain that appears in various parts of the body. However, I was unable to affect the cancer itself. If the patient was not in a hospital, or if I had the permission of the attending physician and the family, I would like to have tried direct scarring moxibustion. I think that methods including the Four Flower Disease Gates moxibustion technique, described earlier in this section, would have been helpful.

Case History No. 5

PATIENT: 70-year-old man

CHIEF COMPLAINT: A week before consulting me the patient had a fever of 38°C (100°F) that abated, leaving him with a productive cough. The patient also suffered breathing difficulties, making it difficult for him to even walk. Six years before, he had been diagnosed with pulmonary emphysema and now he was suffering a relapse.

VISUAL: The patient had a red face, and it was clear that he had breathing difficulties. His physique was normal, and his tongue was dry.

SYMPTOMS: At the time of the consultation, the fever had dropped and there was no sore throat. He had diarrhea, but he still had an appetite. He also felt thirsty.

ABDOMEN: The epigastric area was swollen overall, with resistance to pressure at CV-12. Below the navel, there was a distinct lack of resilience on the Conception vessel and tightness on the Stomach meridians.

CHEST: The chest was hot to the touch on a line between the left and right LU-1.

BACK: Even though there was heat in the chest, the back was cold to the touch between the shoulder blades.

PULSE: The overall pulse was sunken, thin, fine, and rapid. The left distal pulse was a little strong, and the left medial and proximal pulses were sunken, thin, and fine. The right distal pulse was rough and forceful, the right medial pulse was rough and deficient, and the right proximal pulse was rough. The dorsal pedis pulse (taken at ST-42) was rough and thin, and the posterior tibialis pulse (taken at KI-3) was sunken and wiry.

CONSIDERATIONS: The abdominal diagnosis seemed to indicate Kidney deficiency with heat in the Stomach meridian. Another possibility was that the Kidney deficiency was to be expected of someone at his age, and the real pattern was Spleen deficiency.

The right medial pulse was deficient and the right distal pulse was forceful, appearing to confirm a Spleen deficiency/Lung heat pattern. Then again, I was still thinking about the possibility of there being a Kidney deficiency pattern as well. However, when I considered that the posterior tibialis (lesser yin) pulse was sunken and wiry, which is normal, I decided to use a Spleen deficiency/Lung heat pattern treatment.

TREATMENT: I retained needles at CV-12, ST-25, and CV-4 on the abdomen and LU-1 on the chest. After this, I applied heat perception moxibustion to the hot areas on the chest. The root treatment consisted of tonifying PC-5 and SP-4. These points are the metal (Lung) points of the Pericardium and Spleen meridians and are used to clear Lung heat while tonifying the Spleen. On the back, needles were retained at the deficient areas; there were no really stiff, tight points to be found.

The following day the heat in the chest had diminished and the overall pulse was bigger, more relaxed, and rapid. I repeated the same treatment as before. A week later the patient was able to breathe more easily, the diarrhea had stopped, and his pulse was relaxed and rapid. After another four treatments he was completely cured.

Of course, there is always a possibility that the symptoms of his emphysema will return, but other than the times when he catches a cold, the patient is now in extremely good health. I have treated a number of emphysema patients and have found that they respond surprisingly well to acupuncture and moxibustion.

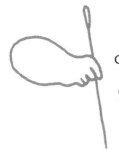

CHAPTER 16

CIRCULATORY DISEASES

CIRCULATORY DISEASES INCLUDE such problems as angina pectoris, arteriosclerosis, congenital and valvular heart disease, heart failure, high and low blood pressure, infectious endocarditis, myocarditis, myocardial infarction, pericarditis, phlebitis, Raynaud's disease, Takayasu's arteritis (also known as pulseless disease), and venous thrombosis. Congenital heart disease and valvular heart disease usually require surgery. Endocarditis, myocarditis, and pericarditis are often infectious in origin; therefore, they typically have a relatively acute onset and can be marked by fever, shortness of breath, chest pain, and palpitations. If these symptoms are present, the patient should be sent for a medical evaluation as soon as possible. While some of these problems do respond to acupuncture, it is prudent for the patients to have a medical workup first.

Other diseases listed above may also require the services of a medical physician, but diseases such as arteriosclerosis, high and low blood pressure, phlebitis, and Takayasu's arteritis may respond well to acupuncture and moxibustion. Symptoms such as arrhythmia, palpitations, and chest pain are also often effectively treated by acupuncture and moxibustion, especially when they are not caused by any specific disease. Most of the time, however, patients with these symptoms are not treated with only acupuncture and moxibustion. Rather, they are also receiving medication prescribed by a medical physician. Patients with these symptoms who are not under the supervision of such a physician should be referred to one at once. Many of these diseases can be life threatening, especially in the acute stages. Acupuncture and moxibustion are most effective when treating non-serious cardiac conditions, even if they have a large emotional component.

16.1   HIGH BLOOD PRESSURE

Diagnosis

The major types of high blood pressure are essential (or idiopathic) hypertension and secondary (primarily renovascular) hypertension. Regardless of the cause, the basic principle is to improve the flow of qi and blood, which will result in a stabilization of the blood pressure. Acupuncture is most useful in the treatment of essential hypertension. Renal hypertension is briefly touched on in the chapter on urogenital diseases, simply to say that often, once the Kidneys are working better, the blood pressure will take care of itself. From a traditional medical perspective, patients with high blood pressure can be classified into one of three patterns, discussed below.

KIDNEY DEFICIENCY/YIN DEFICIENCY PATTERN

Patients with this pattern normally have at least one parent who suffers from high blood pressure, and as a consequence, they have a body constitution that is susceptible to high blood pressure. Things would be all right if they followed a controlled diet, but they normally gravitate toward overindulgence in food, alcohol, and rich foods.

During their younger years, these individuals often have a pattern of Spleen deficiency/yang excess/heat. Because of the large amount of heat in the Stomach, they have a strong sexual appetite and are very active generally. Playing mahjong all night long is nothing for them. However, over time, the exhaustion, the overindulgence, and the drying out of the Kidney fluids by the Stomach heat causes these patients to develop a pattern of Kidney deficiency. Also, because they overeat, they become obese, which also contributes to the Kidney deficiency. At a certain age, heat derived from the Kidney deficiency spreads to the Lungs and Heart, resulting in fatigue, palpitations, an irregular heartbeat, shortness of breath, dizziness, high blood pressure, and a stiff neck. Additional symptoms can include nosebleeds, headaches, thirst, an uncomfortable feeling of heat in the legs, an inability to sleep properly, a decline in sexual performance, and a general feeling of unease. In addition, even slim individuals will start to become obese and develop a tendency toward, or actually have, high blood pressure.

The overall pulse for this Kidney deficient pattern is strong and hard (due to a lack of fluids); sunken, slippery, and floating; or big and slippery (due to the presence of a large amount of heat). Occasionally, a patient may have a sunken, thin, and hard pulse; if this evolves into a thin, tight, and rapid pulse, the patient may develop a problem such as stroke.

When those with high blood pressure have any of the overall pulse presentations, the left proximal pulse is deficient. However, sometimes the overall pulse is very strong, making it easy to miss this deficiency unless it is looked for carefully. Regardless of the associated pattern, the left and right distal pulses are strong. A stronger left distal pulse is indicative of heat in the Heart; the blood pressure in these individuals is difficult to control. By contrast, when the right distal pulse is stronger than the left, the high blood pressure is caused by overexcitement, which can be controlled rather easily.

In cases of Kidney deficiency, the area below the navel becomes weak and the chest starts to feel warm; both of these symptoms can greatly aid in the diagnosis of this pattern. In many cases, it is easier to detect the heat in the Heart or Lungs by palpating the chest than by feeling the pulse. Finally, heat in the chest in someone with Kidney deficiency can also be a prognostic indicator of developing high blood pressure.

LIVER DEFICIENCY/YIN DEFICIENCY/HEAT PATTERN

In these cases, the high blood pressure is a result of Liver deficiency heat spreading to the Heart and Lungs. In general, the heat generated in cases of Kidney deficiency/yin deficiency is more likely to travel to the Heart, while the heat generated in cases of Liver deficiency/yin deficiency is more likely to travel to the Lungs.

People with Liver deficiency are often easily irritated and tense, which leads to an increase in blood pressure. Once these individuals calm down again, their blood pressure will drop back to normal. Even if they get angry for no particular reason, their blood rushes, and even when they realize what is going on and try to calm themselves, they find it very difficult to do so. Once this pattern has become established, these people are often diagnosed by their physicians as having essential hypertension.

When they are young, patients with this pattern tend to be very thorough and systematic in everything they do. However, as they get older, they become Kidney deficient and begin to lose their vigor; they then find that they are unable to carry out their plans. Finally, since their Liver blood is affected, they become irritable as a result. When their irritability becomes ingrained, these patients are troubled by anything that others may do. When they were younger, they were able to handle this frustration, but after the age of fifty, Kidney deficiency begins to kick in and causes problems. In such cases, the deficiency heat from the Kidneys and Liver rises upward, causing the lower burner to become cold and the upper burner to become hot. When the heat moves into the Lungs and Heart, symptoms such as high blood pressure and palpitations become evident.

In young people, even if the blood rushes to the head, it is soon dispersed before the blood pressure is adversely affected. With the advancing years, however, while there may be enough deficiency heat to rise to the head, there is not enough yang qi to radiate the heat externally. The heat gets trapped in the head, resulting in a feeling of blood rushing to the head and a measurable increase in blood pressure. Worse yet, the Liver deficient patients will then become obsessed with trying to maintain a constant blood pressure level despite the fact that in healthy individuals the blood pressure varies according to the circumstances. While Liver deficient patients can understand this intellectually, they still worry about their change in blood pressure. To make matters worse, those with Liver deficient constitutions are very emotional, and thus their blood pressure tends to rise and fall more than the average person, leading to a sort of 'blood pressure neurosis.' When they come to the clinic, these patients always ask that their blood pressure be measured and expect to be told that it is a little high but stable. Therefore, it is good practice to tell them that it is a little lower than it actually is. This helps them to relax, and in a little while, their blood pressure will actually begin to fall.

The overall pulse is similar to that of Kidney deficiency in that it will be sunken and hard; sunken and slippery; or perhaps floating, big, and slippery. The left medial and proximal pulses are deficient, and the left and right distal pulses are strong. As noted above, if the left distal pulse is stronger, the condition is relatively serious, while if the right distal pulse is stronger, the high blood pressure is a result of a nervous condition. Regardless, the chest will be hot to the touch as a result of the rising deficiency heat. In addition, for a Liver deficiency pattern, the area of the abdomen below the navel will be lacking in resilience since both the Liver and the Kidney are deficient. At the same time, there will be resistance to pressure on the left side of the abdomen, and a pulsation can be felt to the left of the navel.

LUNG DEFICIENCY/LIVER EXCESS/BLOOD STASIS PATTERN

The symptoms are similar to those described above for both Kidney and Liver deficiency, but a characteristic of this pattern is depression. The pulse and abdominal findings have already been described in Chapter 10. This pattern occurs when both the circulation of Lung qi becomes poor, causing the Kidney fluids to become deficient, and heat and blood stasis increase in the Liver, causing heat to spread as far as the Heart. It is difficult to control the blood pressure in patients with this pattern.

In Ehima prefecture in the south of Japan where I have my clinic, there has always been a tradition of direct scarring moxibustion among the common folk (i.e., the nonprofessionals) that has generally been positive for a variety of complaints. This practice is slowly dying out, but those that still do it begin when they are children. People will generally apply direct moxibustion, using 100 to 200 cones, to the shoulders and upper back to points such as GV-12, BL-13, and SI-14. When some older people do this for their stiff shoulders, they find that they develop symptoms such as palpitations, headaches, and high blood pressure. This was described classically as fire pathogen; care should be taken not to apply a great deal of moxibustion to the upper body of older people. Those who develop high blood pressure from too much moxibustion can have any of the three patterns described here.

Arteriosclerosis occurs when plaque builds up on the inner walls of the blood vessels, leading to a reduction in their distensibility. Major risk factors include obesity, high blood pressure, diabetes, and smoking. Arteriosclerosis in turn can result in a higher risk of angina and myocardial infarction. From a traditional medical perspective, the problems of arteriosclerosis and high blood pressure are not really differentiated. The most common pattern seen in patients with arteriosclerosis is Kidney deficiency/yin deficiency/heat followed by Lung deficiency/Liver excess/blood stasis. The pulse will be hard and strong for both of them.

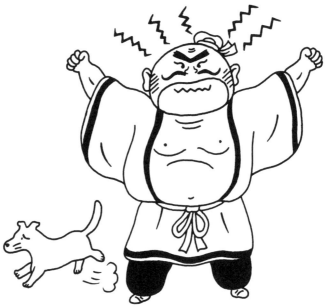

Anger raises the blood pressure

Treatment

It is good common sense to give some advice about diet to people with high blood pressure and arteriosclerosis. However, since it takes about five years for changes to appear, a little bit of perseverance is necessary. In my opinion, the first thing is to reduce the amount of salt, as too much of it makes the blood more viscous and raises the blood pressure. Traditionally, the salty flavor is said to have an effect on the Kidneys. It should be remembered that this effect is not in the form of tonifying the fluids and clearing the deficiency. The salty flavor actually prevents the excessive buildup of fluids in the Kidneys, thus preventing the body from becoming cold. However, too much of the salty flavor can injure the Kidneys; therefore, do not think that because high blood pressure is related to the Kidneys that salt is good for these patients.

It is not just salt that should be reduced, but also food items with a strong or rich flavor.

This can be quite difficult in practice because the people that make and consume the food in a household make the decisions concerning the level of salt and flavor in the food. While those in the household may think they have reduced their intake of salty, richly-flavored food, this is often not the case. It is important to really make an all-out effort to cut back on these prohibited foods because otherwise, there will be no change in the blood pressure.

Normally, alcohol is also thought to be bad for high blood pressure and heart disease. In actual fact, it is the flavor of the snacks consumed with the alcohol that is worse than the alcohol itself. Also, sweet things are not good. If a patient with high blood pressure or arteriosclerosis is not drinking alcohol, then it is often sweet foods that are the culprit. Of course, it goes without saying that smoking is also not recommended.

As far as treatment is concerned, we can start with retained needling in the abdomen, legs, and arms (TABLE 16-1). Just these steps are enough to stabilize some people's blood pressure. The next step is to perform a root treatment followed by retained needling in the back, neck, and legs. Finally, the shoulders are treated for stiffness. Many people with high blood pressure initially come for treatment of their stiff shoulders, but it is not good to treat the shoulders first because doing so may cause the qi to rise, making the blood pressure rise even higher.

Table 16-1	Branch Treatment Points for High Blood Pressure
Location	**Points**
ARMS AND LEGS	**LI-11**, ST-35, **ST-36**, **ST-42**, SI-10, **KI-1**, **KI-2**, GB-31, GB-39, **M-LE-16**
CHEST AND ABDOMEN	**LU-1**, ST-18, ST-19, **ST-25**, **KI-25**, LR-14, **CV-4**, CV-12, **CV-14**, **CV-15**
HEAD, SHOULDERS, AND BACK	**BL-10**, BL-17, BL-18, BL-22, **BL-23**, **BL-43**, BL-45, **BL-52**, TB-15, **GB-20**, **GB-21**, **GV-12**, **GV-20**

Case History

PATIENT: 64-year-old woman

CHIEF COMPLAINT: This patient suffered from high blood pressure and arteriosclerosis, for which she was taking medication. She wished to stop taking the medication.

VISUAL: She had a typical middle age spread, liver spots under her eyes, and a reasonable complexion. Her tongue was moist and unremarkable.

SYMPTOMS: Her highest systolic blood pressure was about 180mmHg. With the use of medication she had a systolic pressure of around 140mmHg. In addition, she had stiff shoulders, headaches, and constipation, although her appetite was normal. She felt cold easily, especially in her legs. She would wake during the night even though she did not need to go to the toilet. She was thirsty and sweated easily from the top half of her body.

PULSE: The left distal and medial pulses were wiry and forceful. The left proximal pulse was wiry and deficient. The right distal pulse was sunken, thin, and strong. The right medial pulse was sunken and thin. The right proximal pulse was sunken, thin, and deficient.

ABDOMEN: Overall, there was no resilience found in the lower abdomen, but there was resistance to pressure at areas around the navel and below the right ribs. The right ST-19 was tender, which is indicative of overeating. The chest was hot to the touch.

CONSIDERATIONS: Even though she had some signs of being cold, she nonetheless had a good appetite, suffered from constipation, and felt thirsty, signifying that although she had heat inside, the yang qi was unable to circulate to the periphery to warm her body. This state is characteristic of blood stasis (yin excess), and the diagnosis was confirmed by the resistance found around the navel and below the right ribs and by the excessive left medial pulse (the Liver).

The headaches, wakefulness at night, and upper body sweating were caused by heat in the chest. This symptom plus the forceful pulses at both distal positions are indicative of a great deal of heat collecting in the upper burner. This heat, which was a result of an underlying Kidney deficiency, was causing the high blood pressure.

TREATMENT: A treatment for Lung deficiency/Liver excess/blood stasis pattern was chosen. KI-2, KI-10, and LU-10 were tonified, and LR-8 and ST-36 were shunted. KI-2 is a fire (Heart/bitter) point which helps to generate the yin fluids of the Kidneys and clear heat from the Heart. KI-10 is a water (Kidney/salty) point and helps to restore the fluids and bring them to the Liver as a means of resolving blood stasis. LU-10 is a fire (Heart/bitter) point; tonifying it clears Lung heat. LR-8 is the water point of the Liver meridian and helps to restore fluids and resolve blood stasis. ST-36, an earth (Spleen/sweet) point, is used here to help move fluids from the Spleen to the Kidneys.

Needle head moxibustion was performed on the hard areas of the abdomen and at BL-23, and tonifying scatter needling was performed on areas with deficient nutritive qi. As a result of this treatment, her headaches, stiff shoulders, and constipation cleared, and the right distal pulse became weaker. The treatments were performed five to seven times per month, and after a year, her blood pressure stabilized, allowing her to be taken off her medication.

16.2 LOW BLOOD PRESSURE

Diagnosis

There are actually quite a few people that suffer from the effects of low blood pressure. Some of these people do not consider themselves un-well enough to do anything about it, and the remainder do not wish to take medication because of their side effects. The end result is that these people get on with their lives with symptoms such as difficulty in getting up in the morning and general lack of vitality. They also tire easily and may suffer from occasional dizziness, lack of appetite, a tendency toward diarrhea, stiff shoulders, cold hands and feet, palpitations, and tinnitus. The two most common body types associated with these symptoms are either thin people or obese women with water retention problems.

The symptoms mentioned above all fall into what traditional medicine calls a yang deficiency cold pattern. Low blood pressure is not so much a result of a disease but of a set of constitutional factors. There are various types of yang deficiency, and the ones that often manifest constitutionally are Spleen deficiency/yang deficiency and Liver deficiency/yang deficiency. Either of these patterns will result in a drop in blood pressure. In addition, during the course of an acute disease, low blood pressure often occurs with Lung deficiency/yang deficiency, Kidney deficiency/yang deficiency, and Spleen deficiency/Kidney deficiency patterns.

Symptoms such as profuse sweating, cold extremities, cramping of the hands and feet, palpitations, diarrhea, and frequent vomiting may occur after motor vehicle accidents and improperly aggressive treatments that lead to intense vomiting and/or diarrhea. In these cases, low blood pressure is usually also a factor. Of course, victims of motor vehicle accidents often experience a total loss of strength and an inability to move, that is, they are in shock. It is important that emergency steps be taken and that an ambulance be called. While waiting for help, and while minimizing the movement of the victim, the sweat should be toweled off and the body should be kept warm. If it is at all possible, at the same time, the Triple Burner channel of the legs (between the Bladder and Gallbladder meridians) should be tonified (see below).

Low blood pressure can also occur in less acute and less serious situations. People with constitutions that mimic either a Spleen deficiency/yang deficiency/cold pattern or a Liver deficiency/yang deficiency/cold pattern are likely to already have low blood pressure or are prone to sudden drops in their blood pressure. They are also prone to having some or all of the symptoms listed above. For Spleen deficiency/yang deficiency types, any diarrhea will be accompanied by fatigue and a lack of power in the arms and legs. Also, these individuals will have no appetite or a reduced appetite. Women with a Liver deficiency/yang deficiency constitution will have a tendency to develop diarrhea during menstruation. They also have no appetite but are able to finish a meal once they have started eating.

For Spleen deficiency/yang deficiency the pulse will be sunken, thin, and deficient, although there may be occasions where it is floating, big, and lacking in force. For Liver deficiency/yang deficiency, the sunken, thin, and rough qualities will be more noticeable. For Liver deficiency/yang deficiency, there will be times when the right medial pulse is found to be rough.

The abdomens of patients with a greater degree of yang deficiency (and consequently a greater degree of cold) will offer less resistance and feel less pain on palpation. The abdomens of these patients will feel quite mushy. However, proper treatment will improve the overall level of yang qi and the abdominal resiliency. For Spleen deficiency/yang deficiency patterns, the area around CV-12 will begin to become firmer. For Liver deficiency/yang deficiency patterns, the whole upper abdomen will start to become firmer.

Treatment

Diet is just as important for treating low blood pressure as it is for high blood pressure. People that only have a light breakfast, such as a piece of toast, are more likely to have low blood pressure. It is important that those with low blood pressure start each day with a solid breakfast. In Japan, we recommend that they always include rice in their breakfast, but as long as they have sufficient amounts of an easy-to-digest food item for breakfast, the type of grain is probably not that important. Generally, I recommend that people eat a large amount of grains and stay away from eating too much light food such as salads and fruit.

In yang deficiency patterns, there will be overall chilling of the body. Moreover, as the cold pushes the yang qi into ever smaller pockets, there may be areas of stiffness and soreness. Thus, individuals with either low or high blood pressure may have areas of stiffness and soreness, and these areas should be needled, for example, BL-10 and GB-20 should be needled if they are stiff and sore. Contact needling should be performed all over the upper back. Direct scarring moxibustion to LR-13 should be administered on those who do not respond well to treatments and who show a lack of vitality (see TABLE 16-2). Scarring moxibustion on BL-18 should be used to treat Liver deficiency/yang deficiency.

Modern emergency procedures are the treatment of choice for those in shock. If an ambulance is unavailable, the following points can be used: a point on the leg Triple Burner meridian just lateral to BL-58, PC-9, a point one unit proximal to TB-4, a point one unit proximal to PC-7, BL-17, LI-11, and points on the finger tips. Acupuncture, moxibustion, or simple finger pressure can be applied to these points.

Table 16-2	Branch Treatment Points for Low Blood Pressure
Location	**Points**
ARMS AND LEGS	**LU-4**, LI-10, **LI-11**, ST-36, SP-6, **TB-9**, **GB-31**
ABDOMEN	**CV-4 to CV-6**, CV-7, CV-12, **LR-13**
BACK	BL-13, BL-18, **BL-20 to BL-22**, BL-23, BL-43, GV-9, GV-10

Case History

PATIENT: 60-year-old woman

CHIEF COMPLAINT: This patient had bouts of low blood pressure, down to 80/60mmHg, and was lacking in vitality overall. When her blood pressure reached normal levels, she was full of vigor.

BACKGROUND: She had been suffering from low blood pressure for a long time. A few years ago, she fell over and bruised her lower back while trying to move her bowels.

SYMPTOMS: She was prone to headaches. She usually had a good appetite, but if she was feeling unwell, she would develop tightness around the epigastrium, sometimes even wanting to vomit. Her stools were either normal or slightly loose.

PULSE: The overall pulse was sunken, thin, and deficient. The left distal and right medial pulses were deficient; the right medial pulse was also slightly floating and rough.

ABDOMEN: This was lacking in resilience, with water collecting at the surface.

CONSIDERATIONS: The pulse pattern was clearly that of Spleen deficiency, and the sunken, thin qualities indicated that it was a pattern of Spleen deficiency/yang deficiency/cold. However, the headaches pointed to heat being stuck in the Stomach meridian, which was confirmed by the slightly floating, rough Stomach pulse.

TREATMENT: First, PC-7, SP-3, and ST-42 were tonified. Then the protective qi was lightly shunted at ST-44, in consequence of which the heat in the Stomach meridian was moved, curing the headaches. Direct scarring moxibustion (10 half-rice-grain sized moxa cones to each point) was performed on the back at BL-17, BL-21, and BL-22.

As a result of this treatment, the patient began to feel well. However, as she began to feel well, she had the unfortunate habit of ingesting too much fruit and fluids, which cooled her Stomach. This resulted in her blood pressure dropping, making her feel poorly again. This type of patient is very common and is often seen among those who have had stomach operations. It is important to give these patients guidance about their diet and to treat them regularly with acupuncture and moxibustion, which will definitely improve their condition. These facts should be explained to them, and a long-term relationship with such patients should be cultivated.

16.3   CARDIAC DISEASE

Diagnosis

It is unusual for patients to come to an acupuncture clinic with cardiac disease as their chief complaint. At my clinic, most patients with heart disease—including those with postcardiac infarction syndrome and postangina syndrome—are receiving treatment from cardiologists; they choose to combine it with acupuncture and moxibustion therapy. I remember having treated patients in the past with problems such as valvular heart disease and a ventricular septal defect. I also treat patients who have undergone heart surgery and are suffering from postoperative ailments. The operations were for valvular heart disease, ischemic heart disease, arrhythmia, palpitations, atrial fibrillation, atrial flutter, and myocardial enlargement.

These medical disease categories, of course, do not appear in premodern texts. However, in these texts we do see some cardiac-related problems, including the following:.

- Heart pain (心痛 *shin tsū/xīn tòng*). This can be further subdivided into collapsing Heart pain (厥心痛 *ketsu shin tsū/jué xīn bìng*) and true Heart pain (真心痛 *shin shin tsū/zhēn xīn tòng*). True Heart pain is characterized by the onset of cold extremities and a poor complexion, with death following within one to two years. This condition would be the result of what is called, in modern terms, cardiac infarction or aortic aneurysm. It would be unusual to see this type of patient in an average acupuncture clinic, and if they are seen, they should immediately be referred to the closest emergency facility. Collapsing Heart pain is characterized by cold invading the Pericardium meridian, giving rise to pain in the chest. It is not life threatening, but if there is habitual chest pain, a checkup by a medical physician is advised.

- Painful obstruction of the chest (胸痹 *kyō hi/xiōng bì*). This is a less serious form of Heart pain and is characterized by a feeling of something being blocked in the sternum. This can arise from a variety of problems such as cardiac disease, but it can also come about as a result of gastrointestinal disease or simple qi stagnation. In modern medical terms, it could be likened to the type of gripping chest pain seen in angina pectoris.

- Shortness of breath (短気 *tan ki/duǎn qì*). Shortness of breath, literally shortness of qi, occurs when there is shortness of breath or difficulty in breathing. While asthma can also cause shortness of breath, this symptom is especially serious if it occurs with heart pain or painful obstruction of the chest.

As noted above, it is unusual for patients to come in with these symptoms for treatment. If, however, they do come in with these problems, or a history of these problems, it is important to follow the golden rule: treat according to the pattern! In the average clinic, the practitioner will likely see symptoms that are closest to collapsing Heart pain. When the cardiac disease is caused by Heart cold, the overall pulse is sunken, slow, and irregular. The distal pulses may be sunken, thin, and deficient, while the proximal pulses may be wiry and deficient. If the overall pulse is sunken, thin, tight, and rapid, the prognosis is not good. This should be treated as a Spleen deficiency/yang deficiency/cold pattern. If the condition worsens, the pattern may have changed to one of Spleen deficiency/Kidney deficiency/cold.

As the condition becomes chronic, heat will become more prevalent, and this can cause circulatory problems and possibly blood stasis. The overall pulse for heat in the Heart is often sunken, wiry, and rapid. At the same time, the left proximal pulse is deficient while the left distal pulse becomes stronger. A pulse that also has a definite tight quality suggests a poor prognosis. If the chest is hot to the touch, the pattern is that of Kidney deficiency/yin deficiency/heat. If, however, the Liver pulse is rough and excessive, then there is blood stasis, and the patient should be treated for a pattern of Lung deficiency/Liver excess.

Treatment

Patients sometimes complain of a blocked feeling in the epigastrium and pain in the chest, which is characteristic of Spleen deficiency. Therefore, CV-12 and the area surrounding it should be treated in these cases, and patients should also be told to eat fewer and smaller meals. When there is borborygmus, relieving the tightness in the epigastrium will also help clear any chest pains.

For heat in the chest, heat perception moxibustion should be applied on and around CV-17 as well as at LU-1 and CV-15 (see Table 16-3). As heat in the chest is often caused by Kidney deficiency, CV-4 should be tonified. If there is a large amount of heat in the chest from the Kidney deficiency, KI-3, KI-1, and KI-2 should be tonified while PC-4 should be shunted.

For problems caused by Liver excess/blood stasis, LR-14 and ST-19 should be shunted. Often there are stiff areas on the inside of the shoulder blades that exhibit pain on pressure, including points such as BL-15 and BL-42 to BL-44. These should be treated with heat perception moxibustion, but retained needling and direct scarring moxibustion are also acceptable.

Table 16-3	Branch Treatment Points for Cardiac Disease
Location	Points
ARMS AND LEGS	LU-4, LI-11, SP-4, HT-7, **KI-1, KI-2, KI-3, PC-4**, PC-6, GB-41
CHEST AND ABDOMEN	**LU-1**, ST-19, LR-14, **CV-4**, CV-12 to CV-14, **CV-15, CV-17**
BACK	BL-15, BL-17, **BL-42, BL-43, BL-44**, GV-12

In the older texts, points such as LU-4, LI-10, LI-11, HT-7, BL-13, BL-17, KI-1, KI-3, PC-4, LR-2, and CV-10 to CV-12 were recommended to treat what in modern medicine are considered cardiac-related problems. Points within this range should be selected according to the presenting pattern. For instance, if the cardiac disease improves when the epigastric area is released, points such as BL-17, CV-10, and CV-11 should be used in subsequent treatments, and points like LU-4 and LI-11 should be used for heart disease caused by Lung heat moving into the Heart. Finally, in some premodern texts such as Kimura Chuta's *Secret Selections of Acupuncture and Moxibustion* and Fukuya's *Stories of Curing Disease with Moxibustion*, there is mention of direct scarring moxibustion to the plantar side of the base of the second toe in the middle of the crease for severe chest pains. Fukaya found that the third toe was useful for this problem as well.

Case History

PATIENT: 70-year-old male farmer

CHIEF COMPLAINT: This patient came to the clinic for atrial fibrillation

BACKGROUND: About 20 years before, he experienced occasional pain in the left side of his chest. At that time he did not know the cause of the problem. Over the last 10 years, he began to experience an irregular heartbeat. Two years prior, he was diagnosed with valvular heart disease and was operated on; an artificial valve was inserted. One year after the operation, his pulse would either be slow and irregular or too rapid. Regardless of whether the pulse was slow or rapid, he had difficulty breathing. His pulse measured 200 beats per minute.

VISUAL: His face was red overall, and his tongue was dry.

SYMPTOMS: His stools, urine, and appetite were normal. He suffered from insomnia and uncomfortably hot feet.

PULSE: The pulse was rapid overall, with a forceful, wiry left distal pulse. The left proximal pulse was wiry and deficient. The right distal and right medial pulses were rough and thin while the right proximal pulse was wiry.

ABDOMEN: There was a lack of resilience below the navel and the epigastric area along the left and right. The Stomach meridians were tight. Heat could be felt from the center of the chest to the right LU-1.

CONSIDERATIONS: Based on these findings, the pattern was thought to be Kidney deficiency with heat in the chest. The pulse—evidenced by the deficient left proximal pulse and forceful left distal pulse—and the lack of resilience below the navel were consistent with this diagnosis. The deficiency heat from the Kidneys was responsible for the tightness in the upper part of the Stomach meridian and the heat in the upper burner; the heat in the chest accounted for the insomnia, dry tongue, and red face. Furthermore, the uncomfortable feeling of heat in the feet was caused by Kidney yin deficiency.

TREATMENT: Heat perception moxibustion was applied to the right LU-1, ST-25, LR-14, CV-17, and CV-22. Needles were also retained at LR-14, CV-12, CV-4, and ST-25. Direct scarring moxibustion was administered at ST-36 using 20 half-rice-grain sized moxa cones, and 5 half-rice-grain sized moxa cones were burned at KI-7. LU-5 and KI-2 were tonified as the root treatment. (This is one of those cases where the root treatment is carried out after working on the tight areas on the abdomen and chest, as this makes things clearer and allows the root treatment to be more effective.) In addition, needles were retained on the back at BL-17, BL-19, BL-22, BL-23, BL-42, and BL-53. After this was done, the pulse dropped to 86 beats per minute, the heat in the chest was eliminated, and the patient felt much better. This treatment was performed three times a week for a month after which the patient came in every two or three weeks. There were only rare, mild recurrences.

16.4   PALPITATIONS AND IRREGULAR HEARTBEAT

Diagnosis

Palpitations and irregular heartbeat can be symptoms of heart disease. However, the patients discussed here have these symptoms but apparently do not have any organic cardiac disease.

Palpitations are usually felt as an uncomfortable beating of the heart; however, they may also be felt as an uncertain, vague feeling in the chest. In the older texts, palpitations were called 怔忡 (*sei chū/zhēng chōng*), which is literately translated as continuous palpitations or fearful throbbing. There are also those patients who are always easily startled and who are prone to palpitations. Most of these cases do not involve a problem of the heart itself, but if the palpitations are accompanied by shortness of breath, the patient should be referred to a physician for a medical evaluation.

In modern medicine, palpitations are often called cardiac neurosis. From a traditional medicine perspective, these problems are usually attributed to either a Kidney or Liver deficiency pattern. The former pattern is no surprise: whenever the Kidneys are deficient, palpitations are more likely to occur. Indeed, Kidney deficiency even plays a role in the Liver deficiency pattern.

The Kidneys and the Heart are constantly exchanging yin and yang energies, but when the yin of the Kidneys becomes deficient, the yang energy of the Heart increases abnormally, which causes palpitations. The term 'palpitations from being startled' (驚悸 *kyō ki/jīng jì*) can be found in premodern texts and is related to this concept, because when the Kidneys become deficient, the patient is easily startled and palpitations are more likely. Kidney deficiency leads to a feeling of being less settled than usual, and the state discussed here can be thought of as a pathological extension of this. In this state, the pulse is rapid and patients may experience a phenomenon known as running piglet qi (奔豚気 *hon ton ki/bēn tún qì*), which is referred to as a Kidney accumulation (腎積 *jin shaku/shèn jī*) in the *Classic of Difficulties*.

In running piglet qi, palpitations occur very suddenly, almost as quickly as having a seizure. The patient feels as if something solid is pushing up from their navel into their chest and throat, making it difficult to breathe and causing palpitations. At the same time, the heart rate goes up, and the patient feels like they will die at any moment. However, after a little while, the patient will settle down, sometimes being helped by a glass of cool water, and is normal again.

Trying to determine the cause of the attack is often difficult, but if the patient is thoroughly questioned, a consistent theme is a background of worry that comes to a head, that is, a type of worry that turns into fear. Unfortunately, when the patient feels the palpitations, they believe they are going to die at any moment, making the palpitations even worse. As noted above, the cause of running piglet qi is Kidney deficiency, which can be caused by events such as a miscarriage and abortions.

Neurosis or hysteria can also be the cause of this type of problem. For instance, someone with a domestic problem who is unable or unwilling to express it may develop running piglet qi. There are also cases where the person concerned is not even aware of holding things back and needing to express them. Whatever the contributing factors, running piglet qi is assumed to occur only when there is a Kidney deficiency. If this is not the case, then any neurosis or hysteria will manifest in other ways.

According to Zhang Zhong-Jing, running piglet qi is attributed to pathogenic fire that comes about from either mistaken moxibustion treatment, especially to the upper body, or extreme fear. The precondition for the former is again a Kidney deficiency where there is heat in the upper burner and a concurrent deficiency in the lower burner. In this state, the yin and yang balance of the body is disrupted, causing the qi to shoot up into the upper burner. At the same time, the exterior yang qi is lacking. As a consequence of all this, the patient may experience palpitations, feel irritable, and be unable to relax.

An occasional irregular heartbeat is almost always due to some premature contractions, which are usually of no significance and can be ignored without any harm coming to the patient. Irregular heartbeat also has Kidney deficiency as its root cause, where again the deficiency leads to a buildup of heat in the Heart. It can also occur as a result of Liver deficiency causing heat to build up in the Heart. In the latter case, it occurs when the person is angry, and is often accompanied by a rise in blood pressure.

The above symptoms can be very successfully treated with acupuncture and moxibustion, with near instantaneous results. However, if your treatments are unsuccessful, the fault may lie with your technique, or there may be a problem with the patient's heart. For this reason, treatment failures should be taken very seriously, and patients who do not respond to acupuncture and moxibustion should be sent for a medical evaluation.

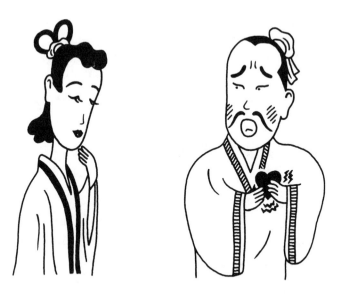

Meeting someone you fancy can also make your heart flutter

Treatment

Whatever you do, always treat KI-7, as this will usually reduce the speed of the pulse and eliminate the palpitations (see TABLE 16-4). If this proves to be unsuccessful, tonify BL-58 and LI-11. Tonification of LI-11 tonifies the Large Intestine meridian, taking heat from the

Lung meridian and thus cooling the Heart. If this still fails to bring relief, shunt LU-4. BL-58 is used to lead the heat in the chest down to the lower burner.

If the Heart heat is caused by Kidney deficiency and not by Lung heat, then, in addition to treating KI-7, HT-7 should be tonified and PC-4 should be shunted. As a last resort, if there is still no success, the Liver meridian should be tonified and GB-41 can be shunted. To find GB-41 correctly, it is always necessary to push deeply, pressing toward the fourth metatarsal from the lateral side.

Table 16-4	Branch Treatment Points for Palpitations
Location	Points
ARMS AND LEGS	LU-4, LI-11, HT-7, BL-58, KI-7, PC-4, GB-41
ABDOMEN	CV-4, CV-15, CV-17
BACK	BL-20, BL-23, BL-58

Case History

PATIENT: 60-year-old woman

CHIEF COMPLAINT: This patient felt discomfort in the epigastric area, as if something was blocked there. She also suffered from palpitations that at times felt as if they were rising up into her throat. During these episodes her pulse would speed up, causing her great discomfort.

VISUAL: She was obese with a large amount of fluids in her tissues; there were no significant changes in the tongue.

SYMPTOMS: She had heartburn and stomach pain but no loss of appetite. She was cold in general, had diarrhea and occasional hot flushes. She felt unsteady when she had her flushes. Her lower abdomen often felt bloated. She was also sexually frigid and had stiff shoulders and lower back pain.

PULSE: The overall pulse was sunken and wiry, with deficiency present at the left proximal and right distal positions.

ABDOMEN: Overall, the abdomen was soft and weak with resistance felt at and around CV-14. There was a distinct lack of resilience below the navel along the Conception vessel.

CONSIDERATIONS: All of the findings were indicative of Kidney deficiency. The hot flushes and diarrhea are known as rebellious qi with diarrhea. The bloated feeling in the lower abdomen was the result of cold in the lower burner. The flushes, with their attendant unsteadiness, and the palpitations were part of the running piglet qi phenomenon, which rises up from the lower burner to the epigastric region and to the chest, causing the various gastric problems and the palpitations. This case should not be mistaken for a Spleen deficiency pattern because the patient had a feeling of an object piercing upward from the lower abdomen to the chest.

TREATMENT: KI-7 was tonified first, which made the pulse slow down and relieved the palpitations. Then needle head moxibustion was applied at SP-6 and LU-5 was tonified. This was followed by retained needles at BL-23 and BL-30. After this treatment was performed, there were still occasional episodes of palpitations, which were eventually remedied by a course of similar treatments.

At the time of her first visit, this patient was unable to lie face up due to the severe chest pain. To be on the safe side, we immediately took her to a local hospital for a checkup where she was said to be suffering from an extremely mild form of heart failure, but was basically all right. This assured both of us, and I could then proceed with confidence.

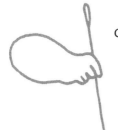

CHAPTER 17

DISEASES OF THE DIGESTIVE TRACT
AND RELATED COMPLAINTS

IN THIS CHAPTER we will discuss a wide variety of diseases of the digestive tract and related complaints, including mouth ulcers, angular cheilitis, glossitis, oral herpes, pancreatitis, stomach and duodenal ulcers, gastritis, loss of appetite, food poisoning, nausea and vomiting, constipation, diarrhea, cholecystisis, gallstones, hepatitis, appendicitis, enteritis, intestinal obstruction, and hemorrhoids. I am including the medical terms here because recently most of the patients coming to my clinic have first been to a physician. They, therefore, arrive with a medical term in hand and often write down the term as their chief complaint.

Nevertheless, it is unwise to rely too much on these diagnoses, as it will prevent treating the patient correctly. As always, it is important to relate the patient's condition to traditional methods of diagnosis and pathology, determine a root pattern, and treat accordingly. This is not to say that there are not specific points that are sometimes useful for treating certain diseases. These, however, should be used selectively according to the pattern. There are also certain patterns that are commonly found with various diseases, and so in this respect, knowing the name of the disease can be of some benefit.

A patient may present with symptoms that include pain in the upper abdomen, heartburn, hiccoughs, loss of appetite, vomiting, diarrhea, constipation, and lower abdominal pain. In this case, if the pathology involved is well understood, it is all right to decide on the pattern and begin treating without knowing the modern medical name for the disease. However, if there is any doubt in the practitioner's mind as to their ability to deal effectively with the problem, then the patient should be referred to a physician for an evaluation. For instance, if a patient presents with vomiting as the chief complaint, questioning should be carefully done to determine the course and, indeed, the cause of the problem. If there is a background of overindulgence in food and drink, there is nothing to be concerned about. However, if the vomiting is possibly caused by food poisoning with the possibility of further vomiting, diarrhea, and dehydration, it is best to send the patient to an emergency facility.

17.1   MOUTH ULCERS AND SIMILAR CONDITIONS

Diagnosis

The topics discussed in this section include ulcers and swellings of the mouth or lips, oral herpes, angular cheilitis, and glossitis. Angular cheilitis, also known as stomatitis and perlèche, is characterized by cracks at the corners of the mouth that may spread to the lips and cheeks. Glossitis, also known as geographic tongue and wandering rash, is an inflammatory disease of the tongue of unknown etiology. Note that ulcers found in the mouth or on the tongue shall all be considered here under the heading of mouth ulcers.

Mouth ulcers can occur as a result of aphthae, Behçet syndrome, diabetes, or leukemia. If the ulcers occur repeatedly, it is a good idea to refer the patient for a medical evaluation, especially because this condition might be an early warning sign of stomach cancer. Aphthae, also known as recurrent aphthous stomatitis, is characterized by small round ulcers that are covered by grayish exudates and surrounded by reddish halos. Sometimes aphthae is associated with a fever, but in most cases, people recover without visiting their physicians. Behçet syndrome is caused by chronic inflammation of the small blood vessels and is characterized by ulcers in the oral and pharyngeal mucous membranes and in the genitalia, followed by erythemic nodes (reddening of the skin), joint inflammation, and fever. While it is valuable to refer these patients to physicians, it is possible to cure the condition with acupuncture and moxibustion (see below). Herpes as well as many other viruses and bacteria (including the causative agent of syphilis) can cause inflammatory responses in the lips and corner of the mouth. In addition, various nutritional deficiencies as well as diabetes can also give rise to small lumps on the lips.

According to traditional medicine, inflammation of the mouth and lips is regarded as a result of heat. When the condition is still relatively mild, the heat is thought to be located in the Small Intestine, Stomach, and Large Intestine. When it becomes chronic or more difficult to treat, the heat is thought to be in the Lungs, Spleen, and Pericardium. The main thing to ascertain is the location of the heat.

The first pattern to consider is Spleen deficiency leading to heat that spreads to the Stomach and Intestines and that causes symptoms such as mouth ulcers; the pattern in this case is that of Spleen deficiency/yin deficiency/heat. Typical scenarios would be a patient who overeats or one who develops, say, swollen lips after recovering from a fever.

The early stages of Behçet syndrome are often a result of Spleen deficiency with heat in the Lung meridian. If the Lung meridian heat enters the Large Intestine meridian, the illness can be cured easily. At this stage there will be mouth ulcers in addition to such symptoms as general lassitude, a variable appetite, constipation, diarrhea, skin eruptions, and cracked lips. However, if the heat continues to move internally, reaching into the Lungs and the other greater yin meridian, the Spleen, then a cure will be difficult. As the disease progresses, the condition evolves into a pattern of Liver deficiency/yang deficiency with overall body chills; the bit of remaining heat is trapped in the Pericardium meridian. At this stage, mouth ulcers will appear and the condition is difficult to cure. However, if the treatment is consistent, a complete cure is possible.

Chronic recurrence of mouth ulcers and angular cheilitis are often caused by Kidney deficiency/yin deficiency/heat spreading to the Stomach, Intestines, Lung, and Spleen meridians. Finally, glossitis is often the result of Liver deficiency/yin deficiency/heat spreading to the Pericardium.

When the overall pulse is forceful and the right distal and medial pulses are readily felt on light pressure, there is yang brightness meridian heat. If a forceful pulse is discerned at the right distal position on firm pressure, there is Lung meridian heat. If the left proximal and right medial pulses are deficient, there is Kidney deficiency with heat in the Spleen meridian. An overall forceful pulse that is coupled to a deficient Spleen pulse is indicative of heat attempting to enter the Spleen meridian. Finally, if the overall pulse is relatively thin, the left proximal and medial pulses are deficient, the left distal pulse is relatively forceful, and the right medial pulse is sunken, thin, and rough, the pattern is that of Liver deficiency/yang deficiency with heat trapped in the Pericardium.

Treatment

The basic treatment is administered according to the pattern where the presence and location of the heat is found by examining the pulse. For Stomach and Large Intestine heat, shunt LI-2, LI-4, LI-10, LI-11, ST-36, and ST-44 if they show tenderness on pressure (see TABLE 17-1); moxibustion may also be used. For Small Intestine meridian heat, SI-1 and SI-3 are shunted. For Lung meridian heat, points such as LU-6 and LU-7 are shunted. Treating LU-7 with acupuncture or moxibustion can sometimes quickly eliminate mouth ulcer pain. For Spleen meridian heat, shunt SP-8 and SP-6. In older texts, HT-7 and PC-8 are recommended, but if the pulse is sunken, thin, and weak, it is inappropriate to shunt these points. In such cases, although heat is definitely found in the Pericardium, cold is nevertheless taking over the body, with the final vestige of yang qi retreating upward and manifesting as heat in the Pericardium. Therefore, it is best to tonify the earth points of the Liver (LR-3) and Kidney (KI-3) meridians to clear this heat.

Table 17-1	Branch Treatment Points for Mouth Ulcers and Similar Conditions
Location	**Points**
ARMS AND LEGS	LU-6, **LU-7**, LI-4, **LI-10**, **LI-11**, ST-36, ST-44, SP-6, **SP-8**, SI-3
ABDOMEN	ST-19, ST-25, CV-4, CV-12
BACK	BL-15, BL-20 to BL-23

Fukuya recommended direct scarring moxibustion (3 to 7 half-rice-grain sized moxa cones) on LR-2 (or LR-3) and a point on the peak of the lateral malleolus, as well as moxibustion at CV-3 and a point one finger width above LI-11. The latter two points are effective in treating mouth ulcers arising from Kidney deficiency and Liver deficiency.

There are also simple but useful methods for treating mouth ulcers with herbs found in older texts. For example, in the seventeenth-century Korean text *Precious Mirror of Oriental Medicine* by Heo Jun, a dough was made of Asari Herba *(sai shin/xì xīn)* that was placed on the navel. An alternative remedy involved chewing some Achyranthis Radix *(go shitsu/niú xī)* and swallowing the extract. Yet another remedy goes all the way back to the *Discussion of Cold Damage* where Zhang Zhong-Jing recommends mixing Pinelliae Rhizoma praeparata *(han ge/bàn xià)* with vinegar in an egg shell, boiling it, and drinking the extract.

If red marks appear after needling a patient with Behçet syndrome, the needling is too deep. In this case, contact needling would be better. If, however, the redness is due to poor radiation of yang qi, which is seen in patterns of Liver deficiency/yang deficiency with heat trapped in the Pericardium meridian, the reddened areas can be removed by applying heat perception moxibustion on top of the spots. To treat repetitive oral herpes, some Edo period texts recommend burning the inflamed spots directly with a hot chopstick. Nowadays, we can use a hot fork, and it does actually work, resulting in a complete cure.

17.2 UPPER ABDOMINAL PAIN

Diagnosis

It is of course better if the patients arrive with a well-defined Western medical diagnosis. If the patient simply arrives with a complaint of upper abdominal pain, we must first be able to uncover the pattern involved. If there is any doubt as to the severity of the problem or if the pain does not respond to acupuncture, the patient should be referred to a physician for a medical evaluation.

The most excruciating upper abdominal pain is that of acute pancreatitis. The pain is constant and severe and extends from the epigastric region to the upper left side of the abdomen and across to the left side of the costal margin. Other symptoms include loss of appetite, fever, and vomiting. Patients try to relieve the pain by hunching the body forward like a shrimp. If you suspect that a patient is suffering from this condition, it is best to get them to a hospital as soon as possible. In my experience it is impossible to stop the pain of acute pancreatitis with acupuncture. I once treated a patient with an extremely high pain tolerance, so high in fact that he gave little indication of having this condition. However, the treatment produced absolutely no change in the pain or in the pulse, a sure sign that I could do nothing for him.

Another condition where severe pain of the upper abdomen is present is a perforated ulcer. The pain can be severe enough to restrict breathing; the pulse will be hollow, rapid, and a little tense. Sometimes the pain may partially subside several hours after the onset of symptoms. However, this condition can readily lead to an elevated temperature and eventually shock. A perforated ulcer can also occur together with peritonitis, giving rise to symptoms such as abdominal swelling, vomiting, and total collapse. When these sorts of symptoms present, the patient must be sent to the hospital.

In any case, whenever a patient presents with nausea, vomiting, severe abdominal pain, and a swollen abdomen, he should be referred for a medical evaluation as soon as possible. If the problem appears not to be that severe and the patient is able to lie face up, needles can be retained on the abdomen, which will usually result in a reduction in the pain. However, if there is no improvement in the pain even while the needles are in place, or the patient cannot even lie face down, then the problem is probably one of the above, in which case acupuncture and moxibustion are inappropriate.

Acupuncture and moxibustion therapy is appropriate for upper abdominal pain stemming from acute gastritis or gastric spasms that are usually accompanied by a bloated feeling and nausea. Similar symptoms can also be caused by gas or other unknown factors, or they can appear while recovering from a fever. We also have the type of pain that can be traced to overindulgence in food and drink and to emotional factors. In any of these situations, if the treatment is appropriate, the pain can be stopped almost instantly.

Upper abdominal pain is also commonly seen in cases of stomach ulcers, duodenal ulcers, and gallstones (see Section 17.7 on Liver and Gallbladder diseases later in this chapter). Although stomach ulcer pain is said to occur after meals and duodenal ulcer pain in between meals, it is often difficult to distinguish between the two, and they are often grouped together under the category of peptic ulcers. With stomach ulcers, the pain is often around ST-20 and ST-21 on the right, while with duodenal ulcers, the pain is often lower around ST-24 and ST-25 on the right. Acupuncture and moxibustion treatment can effect a cure, but if there is hematemesis (vomiting of blood) or blood in the stools, the patient should be referred to a physician.

There are many other diseases of the upper gastrointestinal tract, but regardless of the disease, if the pulse is sunken, thin, tight, and rapid, or if it is sunken, thin, tight, and rough, the treatment should be administered with great care. If this pulse does not change despite the treatment, then the disease is probably serious, perhaps even a hidden tumor.

From a traditional medicine perspective, pain in the upper abdomen is caused by Stomach heat or cold, which in most cases is accompanied by the presence of phlegm. Also, depression resulting from Liver excess can lead to the formation of peptic ulcers. The origin of the heat, cold, and Liver excess is determined by an examination of the pulse, abdomen, and the constellation of symptoms.

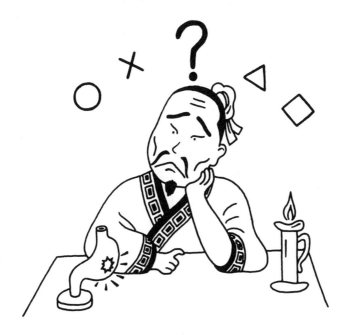

Thinking too much is the cause of ulcers

Acute gastritis is marked by upper abdominal pain and tightness with resistance, and a tender epigastric area. The cause is commonly some problem with diet. If the overall pulse is forceful as well as sunken, wiry, big, or rapid, there is a large amount of heat present. At the same time, if the right medial pulse is found to be wiry and excessive or slippery and excessive when pressed lightly, but deficient when pressed firmly, then the pattern is that of Spleen deficiency with Stomach heat. Spleen deficiency with Stomach heat can be accompanied by bleeding; in this case, the pulse has no force, as seen in a hollow pulse, even if it is big. However, a pulse that lacks force could also indicate the absence of Stomach heat and the possibility of an acute gastric ulcer.

If these same symptoms and abdominal pattern are accompanied by an overall pulse that is sunken, wiry, and deficient and a right medial pulse that is deficient regardless of whether it is pressed firmly or lightly (a sign of an absence of Stomach heat), the pattern is that of Spleen deficiency with Stomach cold. This pattern is commonly seen when there is abdominal pain after recovering from a fever or from eating too much fruit, or in cases of gastritis that have primarily an emotional basis. Finally, if these same symptoms and abdominal pattern are accompanied by nausea and an overall pulse that is sunken, rough, and excessive, and (only) a left proximal pulse that is deficient, then the pattern is Kidney deficiency. This is actually quite common and is due to chilling of the legs or the aftermath of a febrile disease. It is nothing to be really concerned about as there is usually just some trapped gas.

Gastric or duodenal ulcers that stem from a pattern of Spleen deficiency are normally easy to cure. However, ulcers that are a result of Kidney or Liver deficiency with Stomach heat or cold are more difficult to treat. In these cases, the pain occurs after or between meals, and often these patients have already been diagnosed with gastric or duodenal ulcers. If the pulse is big and forceful and the left proximal and right medial pulses are deficient when firmly pressed, the pattern is Kidney deficiency with Spleen and Stomach heat. Rather than causing a lack of appetite, these patients will sometimes have an increased appetite and be prone to overeating.

When the right medial pulse is deficient on firm pressure and it is difficult to decide between Spleen deficiency/yin deficiency/heat or Kidney deficiency/yin deficiency/heat, it is wise to examine the Kidney and Stomach pulses at the feet, near KI-3 and ST-42 respectively. When these are compared, the leg lesser yin pulse should be very slightly floating and smaller than the leg yang brightness pulse. A leg lesser yin pulse that is floating and big indicates Kidney deficiency. The leg yang brightness pulse should be reasonably big and floating, but if it is too big, it indicates Spleen deficiency with Stomach excess heat. Finally, a thin, rough, and weak leg yang brightness pulse indicates simple Spleen deficiency.

An overall pulse that is sunken, weak, and thin reflects the presence of a large amount of cold. If, in addition, the left distal and right medial pulses are deficient regardless of the amount of pressure being applied, the pattern is Spleen deficiency/yang deficiency/cold. If the left distal pulse is especially feeble, the emotions are playing an important role and there is considerable blood deficiency. Conversely, if the left distal pulse is not deficient but the left proximal and right medial pulses are deficient, then the pattern is Spleen deficiency/Kidney deficiency/cold.

If the overall pulse is sunken and thin but the Stomach pulse can be felt on light pressure, there is some heat in either the Stomach or Stomach meridian. However, if the overall pulse is also weak, then this type of Stomach heat should not be cleared by shunting, as a weak pulse is a clear sign of yang deficiency, for which shunting is contraindicated. Similarly, some patients with ulcers present with an overall pulse that is sunken, rough, and thin, which is indicative of a Liver deficiency/yang deficiency pattern. People who suffer from stomach pain when their stomach is empty or when they become irritable often exhibit this pattern. Finally, if the overall pulse is sunken and the left distal and right medial pulses are deficient and the left medial pulse is rough and excessive on firm pressure, the pattern is one of Spleen deficiency/Liver excess/blood stasis. In this state, the static blood collects in the Liver and is not discharged; depression is an overt sign of the constraint.

Obviously, it is quite important to check the abdomen in all of these cases. When there is pain in the upper abdomen and the painful area or the whole abdomen feels good when it is pressed, then the pain is deficient in nature, which is nothing to be overly concerned about. On the other hand, if it is impossible to even touch the abdomen, then the pain is excessive in nature, which can signify the presence of a serious disease.

The epigastric area from ST-21 to ST-24 will be tender to the touch in cases of a gastric or duodenal ulcer. If the muscles of the upper abdominal area are tight overall, the pattern is one of Spleen deficiency/Liver excess/blood stasis with a distinct possibility of ulcers. If there is sudden pain coupled with tension of the abdominal muscles, the condition can be thought of as serious enough to warrant urgent medical evaluation.

Treatment

The root treatment is usually sufficient to treat a nonserious condition and quickly resolve upper abdominal pain. For instance, tonification of K7 and shunting of tender points around ST-36, ST-37, and ST-39 will relieve the pain in cases of upper abdominal pain coming from Kidney deficiency. However, if the treatment consists of this alone, the pain may return at a later date, and so it is important to also treat the abdomen and back areas. Conversely, we may be able to stop the pain by treating the abdomen and back, but in order to prevent it from returning it should be combined with an appropriate root treatment.

The abdomen should be treated before the back by retaining needles at all the painful and tight sites. If this results in borborygmus and the expulsion of gas, the stomach pain is not so serious. If the pain is a little better but still not completely cleared up, contact needling should be applied at ST-19, ST-21, ST-24, ST-25, and CV-14. Again, the pain will be relieved if the treatment is followed by borborygmus.

Any gastrointestinal disease is said to respond to acupuncture at bilateral BL-17, BL-18, and BL-20 (see TABLE 17-2). While this combination is good, reactive points are more likely to be found at BL-20 to BL-23 in difficult cases such as chronic ulcers. BL-17, BL-18, and BL-20 should probably be used to treat relatively acute problems because these points are often reactive in those cases. For gastric pain involving a strong emotional component, the Governing vessel from GV-12 downward is often reactive. Heat perception moxibustion, direct scarring moxibustion, or retained needling can be applied to these reactive points with good results.

Table 17-2	Branch Treatment Points for Upper Abdominal Pain
Location	**Points**
LEGS	ST-32, ST-33, **ST-34**, **ST-36**, **ST-37**, **ST-39**, SP-8
ABDOMEN	ST-19, **ST-20**, **ST-21**, **ST-24**, ST-25, **KI-18**, **KI-21**, LR-13, GB-25, **CV-10**, CV-14
BACK	**BL-17**, **BL-18**, **BL-20**, **BL-21**, BL-22, **BL-23**, BL-49, BL-50

In many Edo period texts there is a section on coughing up blood, vomiting blood, and blood in the stools; these are all indicative of what we would identify today as complications of a gastrointestinal ulcer. It should be noted that blood in the stools can result from hemorrhoids as well as from higher up in the gastrointestinal tract, possibly as a result of an ulcer. The Edo period text *A Collection of Acupuncture and Moxibustion Treasures* recommends LU-9, GV-1, SI-2, CV-9, CV-4, SP-1, BL-20, and BL-18 for vomiting of blood, and BL-23, CV-6, GV-3, SP-6, and GB-39 for blood in the stools. Shukei Suganuma, in *Principles of Acupuncture and Moxibustion*, recommends BL-20, CV-9, BL-62, and SP-9 for vomiting of blood. For blood in the stools, he recommends needling SP-1, ST-36, and BL-62, and the application of moxibustion at SP-6. In *Secret Selections of Acupuncture and Moxibustion*, Kimura Chuta recommends HT-7, CV-12, CV-4, and ST-36 for vomiting of blood, and CV-5, ST-25, GV-20, BL-40, SP-6, and SP-1 for blood in the stools. In *An Anthology of Edified Learning*, Doha Manase recommends direct scarring moxibustion at GV-14 and GV-15 for vomiting of blood from any cause, and direct moxibustion at PC-9, SP-3, BL-35, ST-36, CV-12, and CV-6 for blood in the stools. Important points that I commonly use outside of those used in the root treatment are listed in TABLE 17-2.

Case History

PATIENT: 77-year-old woman

CHIEF COMPLAINT: Six months previously the patient began to feel tightness in her epigastric area, pain in the epigastric region and lower abdomen, and bloating. She was hospitalized for a mass in her abdomen.

VISUAL: She was thin and frail. Her face was pale, but it also had a little luster. Her tongue was moist and pale, indicating a lack of blood, and there was no coating.

SYMPTOMS: She had a reasonable appetite with two bowel movements a day. This patient was the mother of a certain doctor, and for personal reasons she was living on her own.

However, when she became sick, her son moved her close by and admitted her to a local hospital. She was introduced to me by a doctor from that hospital with a diagnosis of pancreatic tumor. The mass, however, was not causing any blockage at the time so there was no sign of jaundice, ascites, or other related symptoms. The mass was expected to increase in size with time.

PULSE: The overall pulse was sunken, thin, and rough with deficiency present in every position except the left medial pulse, which was slightly excessive. Also, the right distal and medial pulses could be discerned with light pressure. The dorsal pedis pulse (near ST-42) was bigger than expected for someone of her condition and age, which meant that she still had a good supply of Stomach qi. Furthermore, she had a good complexion, all of which indicated that her condition would not worsen soon.

ABDOMEN: There was hardness found beneath the right ribs, and a hard lump slightly larger than the size of a clenched fist was found just on the left side of the epigastric region. The lower abdomen was distended overall, with slight pain on pressure below ST-25. When she lay face up, she had a feeling of tightness in her abdomen.

TREATMENT: She was treated for Spleen deficiency/yang deficiency with some heat in the yang brightness meridian that had to be carefully shunted. Needles were retained around the abdominal mass. Heat perception moxibustion was also applied over the mass and at hard spots in the immediate area. To warm up the whole abdomen, salt moxibustion was administered on and around the navel. This was followed by heat perception moxibustion and contact needling at BL-45, BL-17, BL-21, BL-52 and BL-27; this resulted in borborygmus and a reduction in the pain. Finally, a root treatment was performed that consisted of tonifying PC-7 and SP-3; occasionally, KI-3 was also treated.

The above treatment was performed two or three times a week. The episodes of epigastric pain became less and less frequent. Since the patient was feeling better, she requested to be discharged from the hospital and was allowed to do so. However, the referring doctor informed me that the mass had increased in size.

17.3 LOSS OF APPETITE

Diagnosis

Individuals who have weak stomachs or gastric prolapse are prone to losing their appetite if they overeat a little or eat unaccustomed foods. A loss of appetite is also symptomatic of a wide variety of problems, including esophagitis, acute and chronic gastritis, chronic pancreatitis, hepatitis, and even stomach cancer. Individuals suffering from gastric and duodenal ulcers can also present with this symptom, but usually they can finish a meal once they actually start it; there are also those who overeat. Loss of appetite is often accompanied by other symptoms such as a bloated feeling in the epigastrium, heartburn, nausea, hiccoughs, and belching, all of which are considered here.

In the classics, the symptom of food being stuck between the chest and the stomach is called dysphagia occlusion (膈噎 *kaku itsu/gé yē*). While many diseases of the esophagus fall under this rubric, it also includes conditions where the eaten food never seems to be digested properly, leading to a blocked feeling in the upper abdomen. Traditionally, these symptoms are referred to as focal distention (心下痞 *shinka hi/xīn xià pǐ*), fullness (心下痞滿 *shinka hi men/xīn xià pǐ mǎn*), and a stifling sensation in the epigastrium (心下痞悶 *shinka hi mon/xīn xià pǐ mèn*). When these are clearly the result of overeating, the condition is called food damage (食傷 *shoku shō/shí shāng*). Other common symptoms of these problems include hiccoughs, heartburn, acid reflux, and belching.

The causes of these symptoms include consumption of cold or raw foods, nervous strain, good old-fashioned overindulgence in food and drink, and in some cases the aftereffects of a febrile disease. As far as the patterns are concerned, I am sure that most people on hearing that a patient has a loss of appetite will immediately think of Spleen deficiency pattern. For example, there are patients that do not have much appetite but who still finish any meal that they start. It is often difficult to directly elicit this information from the patient. Instead, this type of patient will usually say things like, "I am so tired that I have no appetite" or "I don't feel the need to eat anything." This type of patient is suffering from a pattern of Liver deficiency/yang deficiency/cold. In this condition, there is neither heat nor cold in the Stomach, nor an accumulation of fluids. There is, however, a lack of blood that gives rise to cold; this, in turn, impairs the function of the Stomach. This pattern can be seen in patients with stomach or duodenal ulcers.

Other patients have an appetite but soon become full after eating and are unable to finish their meals. In the Edo period texts, this is termed experiencing hunger without the desire to eat, and results from a pattern of Kidney deficiency/yang deficiency/cold. When the Kidneys are deficient, heat increases to a small extent in the Heart. This steams the Stomach, leading to a feeling of hunger. However, this type of hunger is not the normal hunger experienced when there is sufficient yang qi. Rather, here there is insufficient yang qi in the lower burner. The patient will have a desire for food without the ability to consume or digest it; that is why they soon feel full. Patients suffering from this pattern usually have weak digestion and may suffer from peptic ulcers. Finally, there are patients who have no appetite, are unable to consume food, and cannot really taste their food, as can be seen in cases of hepatitis, febrile disease, or chronic pancreatitis. Such patients have a pattern of Spleen deficiency/Liver excess/heat.

Patients with Spleen deficiency/Liver excess/blood stasis often experience a lot of mental stress that can lead to a loss of appetite, heartburn, and stomachache; they sometimes develop ulcers as well. Others have no appetite but a little bit of food can be consumed and tasted; the pattern is that of Spleen deficiency/yang deficiency/cold. The Stomach itself is cold and there is often fluid accumulation, which is described in the classics as phlegm and thin mucus (痰飲 *dan in/tán yǐn*), or more simply as phlegm. Many of these patients feel nauseous in the morning. A typical example of this are patients who complain of feeling sick while brushing their teeth. Other symptoms include scanty urination, dizziness, but no particular thirst. Individuals who have a weak digestive tract, are beset with an enormous number of worldly cares, or have chronic pancreatitis are prone to developing these symptoms.

Other patients experience a sudden increase in appetite, but after overeating, they have an equally sudden loss of appetite accompanied by epigastric pain and fullness, belching, and abdominal pain. They also have an urgent need to evacuate their bowels immediately after a meal, and the stools are usually soft. These patients suffer from a pattern of Spleen deficiency/yang deficiency/cold, with cold in the Stomach but heat in the Small Intestine. The heat causes the overeating, as it affects the Stomach. Unfortunately, because the Stomach itself has no heat to support the digestive process, the overindulgence in food and drink is followed by a sudden loss of appetite.

Finally, there are patients who present with lack of appetite, lassitude (their legs and arms feel especially tired), heartburn, hiccoughs, abdominal pain, and soft stools (who are nonetheless constipated). This is either a case of Stomach heat or cold. Most people that complain of lassitude have Spleen deficiency/yin deficiency/heat. If phlegm and thin mucus are also present, the individual will also present with nausea, vomiting, dizziness, and scanty urination. Regardless, patients with this pattern are thirsty.

In addition, note that when there is a loss of appetite for whatever reason, a relaxed pulse is a good sign, while a tight pulse is not.

Treatment

The combination of the root treatment plus retained needling on the abdomen and back should result in a return of appetite and control over urination. After this, the branch treatment is performed according to the presenting symptoms, which should further augment the effects of the root treatment.

For acute loss of appetite, BL-17 is useful (see TABLE 17-3). BL-17 can also be used to treat hiccoughs, but it should always be combined with BL-18, BL-20, and BL-21. For chronic weakness of the Stomach and Intestines with a susceptibility to loss of appetite, use BL-20 to BL-22. For loss of vitality, lack of appetite, and weight loss due to Spleen deficiency/yang deficiency/cold, direct scarring moxibustion at LR-13 is very helpful. If, as a consequence, the patient's vitality does not return, the prognosis is poor. If there is phlegm, direct moxibustion should be performed at CV-9.

Table 17-3	Branch Treatment Points for Loss of Appetite
Location	Points
LEGS	**ST-36**, **ST-40**, SP-6
ABDOMEN	**ST-21**, **ST-24**, ST-25, SP-16, **CV-4**, CV-10, **CV-12**, CV-13
BACK	**BL-17**, **BL-20**, **BL-21**, BL-22, BL-23, BL-25, BL-46, BL-47, BL-49, BL-50, BL-52, GV-5

For heartburn due to Spleen deficiency/Liver excess/blood stasis, tonify GB-25 and LR-13 and shunt GB-34. Direct scarring moxibustion at SP-1 is also useful. For hiccoughs in these patients, use BL-17, BL-46, LR-14, GB-24 and ST-19. For hiccoughs, Edo period texts recommend three cones of direct scarring moxibustion at ST-18 on the left side for men, and on the right side for women. If this has no effect, the case is difficult. Fukaya cited a case like this which he dealt with by apparently choking the radial artery of the patient with his hands, resulting in a cure. Direct moxibustion at CV-6, CV-17, CV-12 and LR-14 were also recommended.

Case History

PATIENT: 70-year-old man

CHIEF COMPLAINT: The patient came to the clinic for hiccoughs and lower back pain. The lower back pain started about one week prior to his visit. The incessant hiccoughs began two days before.

BACKGROUND: The patient had a brain hemorrhage 30 years before, an operation for bladder and colon cancer seven years before, and an operation to remove his stomach six years before. At the time of his visit, he was receiving daily injections from his physician for an unknown disease (as far as the patient knew) that was apparently caused by blood acidosis.

VISUAL: The patient looked bloated, with generalized edema and jaundice. His tongue was dry with a yellow coating.

SYMPTOMS: Both the stool and urine were evacuated through artificial openings after his surgeries. He had no appetite, with occasional vomiting and stomachache. He also suffered from insomnia, thirst, numbness and tingling of his legs, a heavy sensation in his head, and tinnitus.

PULSE: The overall pulse was sunken and rapid, the left distal pulse was wiry and deficient, and the left medial and proximal pulses were rough and tight. The right distal pulse was wiry, the right medial pulse was wiry and deficient, and the right proximal pulse was wiry.

ABDOMEN: The abdomen was swollen overall, giving an impression of ascites. The epigastric region was found to be resistant and hard upon the application of pressure. It was difficult to assess the resistance at deeper levels elsewhere on the abdomen because of the ascites.

CONSIDERATIONS: It appeared that the patient was experiencing a relapse of cancer. From the pulse, the cancer appeared to be developing around the bladder or liver. The edema and the jaundice seemed to point toward liver cancer. However, since I was not in contact with his physician, I decided not to alarm the patient unnecessarily and continue quietly with the treatment.

Hiccoughs in patients that have had their stomachs removed can be difficult to treat. The pattern was Spleen deficiency with cold in the Stomach, but heat in the Liver and Kidneys. Because of the weak pulse, I decided not to administer any shunting to relieve the heat.

TREATMENT: The protective qi at PC-7 and SP-3 was tonified. Retained needling and heat perception moxibustion was administered at CV-12, CV-14, CV-9, ST-25, ST-21, and LR-14. After this, retained needling was also applied to the back at BL-17, BL-19 to BL-23, and BL-25. Heat perception moxibustion was also applied to the tight muscles of the lower back. This treatment was performed on three occasions, resulting in a complete recovery of the hiccoughs and the lower back pain.

17.4 VOMITING AND NAUSEA

Diagnosis

It is wise to approach this subject with care, as there are patients with serious diseases that complain of vomiting and nausea. The diseases include many gastrointestinal disorders and many intracranial conditions, such as hemorrhages, tumors, encephalitis, and meningitis. Individuals with menstrual pain, pain from kidney stones, morning sickness, high blood pressure, stiff shoulders, and hot flushes may present with one or both of these symptoms. They are also quite common in motor vehicle accident victims who sustain head injuries; in those cases, there will be nausea, headaches, and lapses of consciousness. Finally, there are cases that are unlikely to be seen in the average acupuncture clinic, such as patients with liver or kidney failure, which include nausea as one of their symptoms.

The types of nausea and vomiting that we will be dealing with here are the more run-of-the-mill types caused by overindulgence in food and drink, a mild case of gastritis, or food poisoning. Care must be exercised if there is a fever accompanying the vomiting or nausea. You may be dealing with nothing more serious than a fever from a common cold, but there is also the possibility that the patient has hepatitis, cholecystisis, or even meningitis. When in doubt, refer the patient to a physician for a medical evaluation.

When patients present with vomiting or nausea, the first thing to do is to question them about the cause. If this proves to be eating or drinking too much, then simply refraining from eating or drinking for awhile will effect a recovery. If the symptoms include diarrhea and stomachache, the food that was eaten was possibly bad and the symptoms are indicative of acute gastritis or enteritis. The most common patterns that are seen in these cases are Spleen deficiency/yang deficiency/cold and Spleen deficiency/yin deficiency/heat.

Then again, it is quite common in the clinic to see cases where there is no known cause for the nausea or vomiting, stomachache, and a feeling of fullness in the epigastric region. If the patient feels better and clearer after vomiting, then the pattern is one of Spleen deficiency/yin deficiency/heat with phlegm and thin mucus. In this case, the patient will have normal thirst and red lips.

If after vomiting the stomach does not feel cleared, then the pattern is that of Spleen deficiency/Liver excess/heat or Spleen deficiency/yang deficiency with phlegm and thin mucus. Liver excess heat is usually accompanied by jaundice—affecting the color of the skin and sclera—as well as possibly fever. If patients with Spleen deficiency/yang deficiency have a dry throat and mouth after vomiting, they are probably recovering. If the patient insists on drinking fluids, they should just be given a small amount of hot water, because drinking too much will again induce vomiting, thereby preventing a recovery. Remember that the dry mouth and throat probably mean that yang deficient patients are starting to regain some internal heat, although it can also mean that they are developing yin deficiency. If at this delicate time the patient is given too much fluids (especially cold fluids), this will overcool the Stomach and push them back into yang deficiency. If the patient is tired after vomiting, has no appetite or thirst, and has pale lips, then the pattern is one of Spleen deficiency/yang deficiency/cold.

In premodern texts, stomachache, vomiting, and diarrhea are described as food-induced damage or food poisoning. In mild cases, vomiting the spoiled food will result in a speedy recovery. In more serious cases, the patient may vomit a number of times and also have diarrhea. If the patient receives treatment and responds, this is all well and good. However, they may still suffer from severe dehydration. The pulse and the lips should be examined carefully. If the pulse is thin and floating and the lips are pale, great caution should be observed. In an extreme case, it could be indicative of heart failure. As noted above, in traditional medicine, vomiting is seen as heat or cold of the Stomach. Often, phlegm is also present. Therefore, food poisoning should be considered and treated with this in mind.

The classics also refer to overturned Stomach (胃反, 胃翻 *han i/wèi fǎn, wèi fān*), which has some overlap with the modern conception of stomach cancer. The characteristic of this disease is the vomiting of food approximately 12 hours later, that is, food consumed in the morning is vomited in the evening and food eaten in the evening is vomited the next morning. If this symptom appears suddenly, it would be good practice to refer the patient to a medical physician for an evaluation.

A pulse that is tight, slippery, and rapid is indicative of blockage caused by food stagnation and heat in the Stomach with phlegm. If this pulse changes and becomes weak and floating, then the yang qi of the Stomach has declined. The condition can worsen, resulting in deficient qi and blood; in this case, the pulse becomes thin, rough, weak, and rapid. If at this time the patient has little or no vitality as well as pale lips, they should be taken to a hospital immediately. On the other hand, if the pulse becomes sunken and soft, the patient is on the road to recovery.

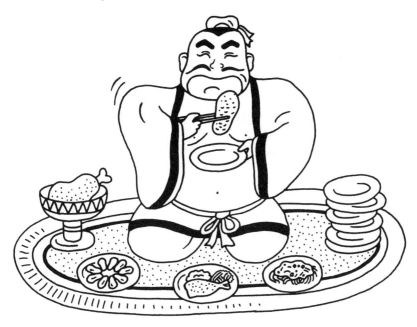

Some people can eat anything and still avoid food poisoning

Treatment

Regardless of the cause, efforts should be made to quell the vomiting and nausea as soon as possible. Treatment of the upper body or the abdomen may result in aggravating the symptoms, and so it is best to first tonify BL-58 or a point just lateral to it. Another possibility is to combine BL-58 with BL-59. Excessive consumption of alcohol or fever that leads to heat in the Liver or Gallbladder, resulting in nausea, should be treated by dispersing GB-41 and/or GB-40.

When performing the root treatment for Spleen deficiency, use PC-6 instead of the standard point PC-7. If CV-3 is tender or there is a pulsation found at CV-9, phlegm is presumably present. Tonify CV-4 and CV-3 to clear the phlegm. The points listed in TABLE 17-4 are treated differently depending on whether the problem is determined to be heat or cold. As always, this means that for cold the points should be needled shallowly and left in for a short time, if at all. For heat they are needled slightly more deeply and left in place longer.

Table 17-4	Branch Treatment Points for Nausea and Vomiting
Location	**Points**
ARM AND LEGS	ST-36, **SP-2, SP-3**, SP-5, **BL-51**, KI-9, TB-6, GB-34, GB-39, **GB-40, GB-41, M-LE-1**
ABDOMEN	ST-19, ST-21, ST-25, ST-27 (left), **KI-21, KI-20**, CV-3, CV-4, CV-6, CV-9, **CV-10, CV-11, CV-16**
BACK	**BL-17**, BL-20, **BL-21 to BL-23, BL-47**, BL-49, BL-50, GB-25, LR-13

With food poisoning, vomiting will continue if there are still remnants of the spoiled food in the system. The beauty of applying retained needling at CV-12, CV-14,CV-15, and ST-25 is that the treatment will cause the patient to vomit if that is appropriate, and cause the patient to cease vomiting when the time is right.

A famous method for treating food poisoning is direct scarring moxibustion at M-LE-1 (裏内庭 *ura nai te/lǐ nèi tíng*), located on the underside of ST-44. These points are usually found to be rather insensitive to heat when there is food poisoning; moxibustion is performed until the heat is felt. Another method is to place salt in the navel and perform moxa on it until the heat penetrates into the lower abdomen; this can be used to stop vomiting and diarrhea.

Case History

PATIENT: 56-year-old woman

CHIEF COMPLAINT: At lunch the patient ate some shellfish cooked in their own shells. An hour afterward, she began to vomit and have diarrhea. She tried to treat herself by drinking plum wine and the extract of sour plum, but to no avail.

VISUAL: The lips of the patient were a bright red, indicating heat.

SYMPTOMS: The diarrhea was preceded by epigastric and abdominal pain.

ABDOMINAL: Pain on pressure was noted at CV-12, ST-25, ST-19, and ST-21. The heat was so intense that it felt as if it was overflowing from her body.

TREATMENT: The first thing I did was to retain needles at points on the abdomen. If there was anything left of the shellfish, it would either be rapidly vomited or expelled through the stool. I decided to adopt this strategy because the patient was strong, with a large amount of heat in her Stomach and Intestines. After a short while, she asked to be allowed to go to the toilet where she proceeded to vomit and have diarrhea. After returning from the toilet, I again retained needles at points on her abdomen with the same result: abdominal pain, vomiting, and diarrhea (thankfully, the latter two occurred in the toilet!) This process occurred three times, after which the vomiting and diarrhea ceased, but there was still stomach pain and a blocked feeling in the epigastric region.

The root treatment consisted of tonifying PC-6, SP-4, and GB-41. Retained needles were placed at BL-23, BL-25, BL-58, and BL-59, and direct moxibustion was applied at M-LE-1. Around a hundred cones of moxa were applied before the patient finally felt the heat. She went home and rested, and that evening began to feel hungry; she ate some rice porridge with no adverse effect. After that, she made a full recovery.

17.5 LOWER ABDOMINAL PAIN

Diagnosis

Patients that come in with lower abdominal pain should immediately be asked a number of questions, the foremost of which is the location of the pain, trying to identify the affected organ. For instance, is it the colon, uterus, or kidneys? In this section, the discussion is limited to lower abdominal pain from intestinal problems. Pain from kidney stones is discussed in the next chapter, while pain associated with menstrual problems is discussed in Chapter 19.

It is also important to ascertain the history of the pain. Has it occurred before or is this the first occurrence? Is the pain constant, or does it occur intermittently? Of course, other factors, including the presence of absence of an appetite, fever, and thirst as well as the condition of the urine and stool, should be determined. In addition, there are patients who are predisposed to developing abdominal pain even though they may not present with this problem at the time of the consultation. It is important to determine the nature of that pain and its probable cause.

After the questioning phase, the pulse and the abdomen should be examined. The facts can be collected into a working hypothesis that should be discussed with the patient. In addition, the practitioner must decide if the condition constitutes a serious disease, as defined in Western medical terms. Of course, the practitioner must also think in terms of excess, deficiency, heat, and cold, and must determine the pattern.

Some patients complain of abdominal pain despite having no intestinal disease. These patients are suffering from cold; this condition falls under the traditional disorder known as bulging or bulging accumulation (疝 *sen/shàn* or 疝積 *sen shaku/shàn jī*), which refers to bulging and cramping pain in the lower abdomen and inguinal areas. When this occurs in men, there is commonly a cramping pain in the testicles. Women often become quite needlessly worried, as the problem has nothing to do with their reproductive organs. Since the pain in the inguinal area happens after long periods of standing, giving patients this information will help them understand that the condition is a result of cold and will help reduce their anxiety. Bulging disorders fall under the rubric of Liver deficiency/yin deficiency/heat.

There are individuals who have weak Intestines and who tend to easily get abdominal pains; often, they make their situation worse by overindulging in fruit as well as cold food items and drinks. Warming their abdomens will make the pain disappear. They also usually feel better after bowel movements, which are typically very loose. However, patients with intermittent pain will often not feel better immediately after a bowel movement because of the presence of a significant amount of either heat or cold in their intestines. These patients suffer from a pattern of Spleen deficiency. In these individuals, an attack of intermittent abdominal pain is usually nothing to worry about. The pain may simply be caused by gas in their intestines, or constipation. If the pulse is sunken, wiry, and big and the patient is thirsty, the pattern is one of Spleen deficiency/yin deficiency. If the pulse is sunken, thin, and deficient but the patient has no thirst, then the pattern is one of Spleen deficiency/yang deficiency.

If the pain starts soon after the ingestion of food, then food poisoning is quite likely (see the preceding section). If the food poisoning is accompanied by abdominal pain, diarrhea, and vomiting, then the patient has developed enteritis. This is best treated using the protocol for a pattern of Spleen deficiency/yin deficiency or Spleen deficiency/yang deficiency.

A constant pain that is in a fixed location may indicate a serious condition. In children, it could be a sign of an intussusception, the prolapse of one part of the intestine into the lumen of an adjacent part, while in adults, it may be a sign of torsion in the intestines. There may also be stool blocking the intestines and causing the pain, possibly as a result of colon cancer. Whenever you suspect a serious disease or are just unsure, it is wise to refer the patient for a medical evaluation. Having said this, there are also cases where this kind of pain may simply be due to something like the person becoming cold.

It is important to determine whether heat or cold is producing these abdominal pains. If cold is the culprit, then the pulse will be floating, big, and deficient, or sunken and deficient. Of course, a sunken pulse is preferable, and the prognosis for a patient with a floating, big, and deficient pulse is not good. A sunken and tight pulse can be taken to indicate that the cold is particularly strong. Obviously, the patient will not have, for example, thirst, which is associated with heat, but instead will have a lack of appetite and often diarrhea. The pattern is one of either Spleen deficiency/yang deficiency/cold or Spleen deficiency/Kidney deficiency/cold.

If heat is the culprit, there will be a feeling of fullness and fever with an inability to pass stool or gas. Another possibility is that there is fever with diarrhea, in which case the abdominal pain may remain constant. If the pulse is sunken and excessive, the pattern is one of excess heat with Spleen deficiency/yang excess/heat, but if the pulse is sunken and wiry, then the pattern is Spleen deficiency/yin deficiency heat.

A feeling of fullness and distention commonly appears together with abdominal pain, which is a consequence of trapped heat trying to make its way outward. Therefore, the stronger the feeling of distention, the more heat there is trapped in the Intestines. Furthermore, if the distention does not change after the passing of stools, the pattern is that of Spleen deficiency/yang excess/heat. On the other hand, if the distention is reduced after the passing of stool, the pattern is one of Spleen deficiency/yin deficiency/heat.

If the abdomen is pressed firmly and there is severe pain, the condition is called pain from excess (or excessive pain) and indicates the presence of trapped heat as a result of either Spleen deficiency/yang excess/heat or Spleen deficiency/yin deficiency/heat. If, on the other hand, the abdominal pain actually improves with pressure, the condition is called pain from deficiency (or deficiency pain), probably as a result of either Spleen deficiency/yin deficiency/heat or Spleen deficiency/yang deficiency/cold.

Pain in the lower right quadrant of the abdomen that is preceded by abdominal discomfort and nausea may point toward appendicitis. A test for appendicitis would consist of pressing and releasing the McBurney point; an increase in pain is indicative of appendicitis, but this test is far from foolproof and is insufficient to make this diagnosis. It is possible to treat appendicitis with acupuncture and moxibustion, but even in Japan, it is best to check with the patient and/or family before proceeding with the treatment. It is usually more prudent to send the patient to an acute care facility. A rapid pulse is indicative of suppuration, which requires surgery. The pattern that is often seen in cases of appendicitis is that of Spleen deficiency/Liver excess/blood stasis. However, pain in the ileocecal region that is not associated with appendicitis is often the result of Spleen deficiency/Liver excess/blood stasis.

Abdominal pain that is accompanied by constipation is usually relieved when the stool is passed. If, however, there is an intestinal obstruction, then not even gas can be passed. When this condition worsens, the patients will actually begin to vomit, but it is unusual to see untreated cases in an acupuncture clinic. Usually, they are already under the supervision of a physician for other related problems, and so if they appear at all, it is usually because they have found no relief from their physicians. These patients can sometimes be helped by acupuncture and moxibustion; the relevant pattern is commonly Spleen deficiency/Kidney deficiency/cold or Liver deficiency/yang deficiency/cold.

Chronic intestinal diseases include ulcerative colitis and Crohn's disease. I have only seen about 10 such cases myself. They will usually have been diagnosed by a physician before visiting an acupuncturist, and so we do not need to worry about identifying these diseases in detail. In my experience, these patients have a pattern of Liver deficiency/yang deficiency with heat in the chest. This is a terminal yin disease with heat in the chest. The chest includes the Heart and, by means of their interior-exterior relationship, also heat in the Small Intestine.

Treatment

The only way to cure pain from heat is to shunt the pain from the meridians with excess. For example, appendicitis is treated by shunting LR-8, ST-36, and ST-37 and by administering retained needling or contact needling over the painful area. Another method is to perform direct scarring moxibustion on CV-6 until the heat is felt. In cases of yin deficiency heat, yang excess heat, or heat in the chest from Liver deficiency/yang deficiency, use heat perception moxibustion. For Spleen deficiency/yang deficiency and Spleen deficiency/Kidney deficiency patterns, direct scarring moxibustion using around 10 half-rice-grain sized moxa cones is performed at CV-4, CV-6, and CV-7. Other points are shown in TABLE 17-5 and are selected based on whether heat or cold is present.

Table 17-5	Branch Treatment Points for Lower Abdominal Pain
Location	Points
LEGS	ST-33, **ST-36 to ST-38, ST-40, SP-3**, SP-6, SP-8, **KI-3**, KI-7, LR-1, LR-4, **LR-8**
ABDOMEN	**ST-13, ST-22, ST-25**, SP-16, SI-26, KI-14, **KI-16, CV-4, CV-6**, CV-7, **CV-8, CV-9**, CV-18
BACK	BL-18, BL-20, **BL-21, BL-22, BL-25, BL-27**, BL-33, BL-52

Case History

PATIENT: 28-year-old mother of one

CHIEF COMPLAINT: Five years before the patient had an operation on her ovaries after suffering from a miscarriage. From that time onward, she became prone to intestinal obstruction, which would cause abdominal pain, an inability to pass either gas or stool, followed finally by vomiting. She would take pain medication, suffering for one day until she found relief by passing stool the following day. Recently, the duration of the pain and discomfort began to increase to three or four days.

VISUAL: She was thin with a small frame. She had a moist tongue and a shiny complexion with a superficial redness, suggesting a condition known in the *Discussion of Cold Damage* as 'face made up with yang' (面載陽 *men sai yo/miàn dài yáng*). It is called 'made up with yang' because the yang qi that is normally present in the interior has been pushed out by overabundant internal yin qi, causing it to appear on the surface; this type of redness is not a normal, healthy phenomenon. Her abdomen, by contrast, showed a lack of luster.

SYMPTOMS: She had stiff shoulders, headaches, and lower back pain. She also had occasions when she collapsed, presumably from anemia. Her lips were dry but she was not thirsty. Her legs were cold but her hands were uncomfortably hot. Although she had a tendency toward constipation, she experienced diarrhea during menstruation. She had little appetite but once she began a meal she was able to finish it. Her periods were painful and her stools were loose during this time.

PULSE: The overall pulse was sunken, rough, and thin. The left distal pulse was a little more forceful than normal, and the left medial and proximal pulses were deficient. The right distal pulse was a little forceful, the right medial pulse was rough, and the right proximal pulse was rough and deficient. Both the left and right distal pedis pulses (which reflect the yang brightness pulse, and is taken at ST-42) were faint, and both the left and right posterior tibialis pulses (which reflect the lesser yin pulse, and is taken at KI-3) were rough and faint.

ABDOMEN: The upper abdomen and the ileocecal region were tight, and pulsations were felt around CV-12. In addition, the lower abdomen was cool in general.

CONSIDERATIONS: On the day of the treatment, the patient had been suffering from abdominal pain and could not pass gas or stools. From the state of her appetite and the occurrence of diarrhea during her period, I concluded that she had a pattern of Liver deficiency/yang deficiency. The rough and thin pulse, especially one that was marked as deficient at both the Liver and Kidney positions, confirmed the diagnosis. The resistance to pressure at the ileocecal region was also seen as representative of chronic cold and of a Liver yang deficiency pattern.

TREATMENT: Contact needling was performed on the abdomen at various points, including CV-12, ST-21, ST-25, and CV-4. The needling was followed by borborygmus, which resulted in an immediate lessening of the pain. The root treatment consisted of tonification at KI-3, LR-3, SP-1, GB-40, and GB-41. In addition, needles were retained on the back at BL-18 and BL-20 to BL-23. This treatment cleared the pain and allowed the patient to pass gas. Thereafter, the patient received treatment whenever the pain appeared, which was approximately once a month, and over time, she regained her health.

17.6 CONSTIPATION AND DIARRHEA

Diagnosis

Let us first consider the 'image,' that is, the physiology, of the Intestines in traditional medicine and then use this information to help us understand the pathology of constipation and diarrhea. The Intestines are connected to the skin. The surface of the skin opens and closes appropriately to discharge yang qi outward. The same process occurs in the Intestines, thus allowing it to regulate the yin and yang. From this we can see why the Lungs and the Large Intestine are paired and why changes in yin and yang in the Intestines adversely affect the actions of the Intestines. Thus, an increase in yin qi in the Intestines cools the Intestines, making it easier for stool to pass, while an increase in yang qi in the Intestines heats the Intestines, making it more difficult for stool to pass.

Ingested water is absorbed in the Stomach and Intestines, especially the Small Intestines, and is excreted from the Bladder. The Spleen helps prepare the water (and food) that is received by the Small Intestine; the Small Intestine is therefore dependent on the proper functioning of the Spleen. This is why Spleen deficiency results in a decrease in urination and a tendency toward diarrhea.

The Kidneys, which control the Bladder, are located in the lower burner. The other thing to remember is that the Kidneys are surrounded by the Intestines. Therefore, when the Kidneys are deficient and produce heat, the heat enters the Bladder, increasing its activity and leading to excessive urination. This, in turn, depletes the fluids of the Intestines, which gives rise to constipation. On the other hand, if the Kidneys have too much fluid, the lower burner becomes cold, giving rise to diarrhea. Finally, deficiency of the source qi of the Triple Burner results in a decrease in both urination and defecation. This brief overview of the functioning of the Intestines explains the pathology of constipation and diarrhea in, say, those individuals with constitutionally weak Intestines and also those cases that recover naturally. However, if the situation worsens to where the level of heat and cold significantly increases, then it is necessary to treat the patient to achieve a recovery.

CONSTIPATION

In general, constipation will occur when there is a large amount of heat in the Intestines because heat increases absorption of the water from the lumen. The source of the heat is often a febrile disease. It is often difficult to lower a fever that is accompanied by constipation, which is seen in patients who have pneumonia or some forms of meningitis; these patients should be observed and treated with the utmost care. In such cases, the pattern is Spleen deficiency/yang excess/heat. Enemas and laxatives are often used to induce bowel movements, but it is best not to do this unless the patient does not suffer from chills (which, combined with feverishness, is the cardinal sign of an exterior condition); if that is the case, then a laxative can be used.

Constipation can sometimes persist even after a fever has abated, and overeating can also be a very simple cause of constipation. The type of constipation usually encountered after overeating or after a fever has dissipated is associated with a pattern of Spleen deficiency/yin deficiency/heat or Spleen deficiency/Liver excess/heat. The *Discussion of Cold Damage* provides a very detailed description of how to treat constipation that appears after a fever.

Constipation can also result from yin deficiency, which dries up the fluids in general and causes heat to spread to the Intestines. Yin deficiency heat can be produced by Liver, Kidney, or Spleen deficiency. The type of constipation that is found in cases of hemiplegia is often a result of Liver deficiency/yin deficiency or Kidney deficiency/yin deficiency. Spleen deficiency/yin deficiency leads to constipation that is accompanied by abdominal pain and fullness, which, as noted above, can result from overeating or can occur after a febrile disease has abated.

Constipation can also result when the Intestines become cold. Normally, this would result in diarrhea. However, if there is constipation, the condition is difficult to resolve; intestinal obstruction, which can be life threatening, is an example of this type of constipation. The patterns associated with this type of constipation will all be yang deficiency cold patterns.

Constipation can occur even when there is no heat or cold, but only qi deficiency. A deficiency of Lung qi can lead to a cascade of events. Initially, the deficiency of Lung qi leads to a deficiency of the exterior (greater yang) yang qi. This results in a deficiency of yang qi in the Bladder, causing excessive urination. The loss of bodily fluids, in turn, depletes the fluids of the Intestines, which gives rise to constipation. Usually, Lung deficiency leads to diarrhea, and so the above scenario is generally only temporary. Naturally, the treatment should be for Lung deficiency, and this type of constipation is not life threatening.

Blood stasis can also result in constipation. Blood stasis can be caused by heat affecting the blood and a simultaneous lack of fluids, both of which leads to hard, dried out stools. This will obviously increase the probability of having constipation and preclude the possibility of having diarrhea. The pattern will either be one of Spleen deficiency/Liver excess/blood stasis or Lung deficiency/Liver excess/blood stasis. This type of constipation can occur after a febrile disease or as a result of constitutional factors. The constipation itself is not life threatening, but it may be indicative of a serious disease.

DIARRHEA

In the past, what we now refer to as diarrhea was divided into two problems: dysenteric disease (痢病 *ri byō/lì bìng*) and draining diarrhea (泄瀉 *setsu sha/xiè xiè*). Dysenteric disease includes symptoms such as the passing of blood and pus along with tenesmus and abdominal pain. In modern medical terms, it would include diseases such as dysentery and typhoid. Draining diarrhea refers to a condition where any consumed food simply passes quickly through the system, giving diarrhea with little abdominal pain as well as scanty urination. Regardless of the traditional or modern diagnosis, the main thing is to think in terms of hot and cold and treat accordingly.

Chills, fever, and diarrhea with little abdominal pain is indicative of heat trapped in the yang brightness meridian. This heat is not being discharged from the surface, and because of this, it enters the Intestines and causes the symptoms. The pattern is one of Lung deficiency/yang brightness meridian excess/heat.

Watery diarrhea, without the accompanying chills, fever, or abdominal pain, can be a result of Kidney deficiency, which causes the Intestines to become cold, thereby adversely affecting water metabolism. Many premodern texts mention that rebellious qi (逆気 *gyaku ki/nì qì*), which is a reversal of the normal movement of qi, can also give rise to a relatively painless form of diarrhea. In this state, the yang qi collects in the upper body, leaving the lower body cold. This leads to blood rushing to the person's head as well as diarrhea; the treatment should be for a Kidney deficiency pattern.

Heat from Lung deficiency/yang brightness meridian excess/heat can enter the Intestines, leading to fever, abdominal pain, diarrhea, and tenesmus. The abdominal pain, fever, and diarrhea may be present from the very beginning of the disease, as seen in, say, enteritis. There are also cases of enteritis that do not include a fever, in which case there will be abdominal pain and the passing of soft stools after eating. The abdominal pain will usually subside after the bowel movement unless there is an extreme amount of heat in the Intestines, in which case there may be no change. The combination of tenesmus and soft stools leaves the patient with a feeling of retained stools and a corresponding increased urge to defecate (but not urinate).

There are also individuals who, because of their constitution, tend to defecate immediately after a meal. In these cases, the stools will be soft, and there will be a feeling that not all of it has been expelled. The pattern is treated as one of Spleen deficiency/yang deficiency/cold with heat in the Small Intestines. These cases can also be thought of as a type of terminal yin disease where both the lower and middle burners are cold and where heat collects in the upper heater, including the Heart. Because of its interior-exterior relationship with the Heart, the heat spreads to the Small Intestine, where it irritates the Intestines and causes the sufferer to feel a false sense of hunger. In these cases, if they eat what would normally be considered an average size meal, the Spleen is stressed, leading to diarrhea. If the condition persists, there will be a seemingly paradoxical total loss of appetite. Individuals who constitutionally have a large amount of heat in the Intestines often say that they feel better after passing the diarrhea. Interestingly, if these individuals suffer from constipation, the heat in their Intestines will induce pain because there is no outlet for its discharge. This phenomenon is often seen in individuals that drink a large amount of alcohol. This pattern is treated as one of Spleen deficiency/yang excess/heat.

There are also cases where the diarrhea is derived from cold in the Intestines, which is often seen during the course of febrile disease. Paradoxically, while there may be a fever as measured by a thermometer, nevertheless the patient's hands and feet are cold. Additional symptoms include a lack of appetite, possible abdominal pain, undigested food particles in the stools, and a high number of episodes of diarrhea, with each episode resulting in a corresponding decrease in the vitality of the patient. This is a serious condition that sometimes requires emergency treatment. It can also be a bit confusing for the patient because, while the fever has abated, the diarrhea has nevertheless not ceased, and while there is no fever or chills, the patient will nevertheless be cold to the touch. The pattern is one of Spleen deficiency/yang deficiency, Spleen deficiency/Kidney deficiency, or Kidney deficiency/yang deficiency.

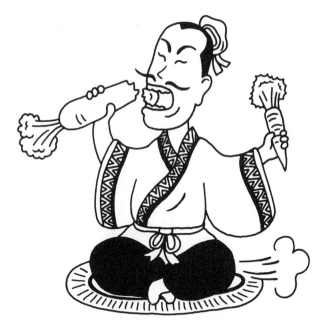

The best thing for constipation are vegetables

Another case of yang deficiency is when the blood is insufficient leading to cooling which causes diarrhea. This pattern can be identified by diarrhea that occurs during menstruation. This type of diarrhea is treated as a Liver deficiency/yang deficiency pattern. Sometimes, acute cases of Liver deficiency/yang deficiency can present with vomiting, diarrhea, chilled hands and feet, and heat in the chest that will lead to palpitations. It is important to stop the diarrhea as soon as possible as the condition may become life threatening.

Treatment

Constipation

Use LU-5 to treat constipation due to Lung deficiency with attendant qi deficiency. Ideally, tonifying this point should initially result in rumbling in the intestines followed by a bowel movement soon after. For constipation from Spleen deficiency, tonify SP-2, and if there is abdominal pain, add SP-4. When there is a large amount of heat in the Small Intestine, BL-40 is shunted. For Spleen deficiency/Liver excess/heat and blood stasis, LR-8 is shunted. In addition, retained needling can be applied to the lower left quadrant at SP-13 and SP-14. If the abdomen is found to have hard, stiff areas and blood stasis is suspected, needle head moxibustion can also be applied to the stiff areas. Additional points are identified in TABLE 17-6.

Table 17-6	Branch Treatment Points for Constipation
Location	**Points**
ARMS AND LEGS	**LU-5**, ST-40, **BL-50**, **BL-56**, **BL-57**, BL-60, KI-3, KI-4
ABDOMEN	**KI-16**, KI-18, CV-5, **CV-12**
BACK	BL-21, BL-29, BL-30, BL-33

The Sawada school of moxibustion has an alternate location for HT-7, locating it on the ulnar side of the tendon; the point is effective for treating constipation from Spleen deficiency. This point is useful because it is halfway between the Heart and Small Intestine meridians; the point therefore promotes the flow of qi in the Small Intestine and regulates heat and cold in the Stomach and Intestines.

Diarrhea

Tonify KI-7 and KI-8 for diarrhea from Kidney deficiency. Tonify SP-1, KI-3, and LR-3 for Liver deficiency/yang deficiency, especially the first point. It is essential to tonify SP-6 for Spleen deficiency diarrhea. Use BL-17, BL-18, and BL-20 for acute diarrhea, and use BL-20 to BL-23 for chronic diarrhea (see TABLE 17-7). Other points which are useful for diarrhea in general are BL-27, GV-3, and M-BW-16.

For chronic diarrhea, perform direct scarring moxibustion at GB-25 and/or LR-13. For diarrhea from Liver deficiency/yang deficiency, perform direct scarring moxibustion at CV-4 to CV-6. For every type of diarrhea, salt moxibustion on the navel is also effective.

Table 17-7	Branch Treatment Points for Diarrhea
Location	**Points**
ARMS AND LEGS	LI-3, ST-41, **SP-8**, BL-63
ABDOMEN	ST-21, ST-22, **ST-25, SP-14**, CV-8
BACK	**BL-25, BL-28**, BL-35, BL-47 to BL-49

17.7 LIVER AND GALLBLADDER DISEASES

Diagnosis

In this section we will discuss acute and chronic forms of hepatitis, cholecystitis, and gallstones (cholelithiasis). However, other liver and gallbladder diseases can also be treated using acupuncture and moxibustion; for example, I have also treated patients with cirrhosis, liver cancer, fatty liver, and obstructed bile duct. Most of these diseases are difficult to cure with modern medicine as well as with acupuncture and moxibustion. However, some cases will result in a complete recovery. Furthermore, if the chosen treatment protocol is correct, we can expect a definite increase in survival time and improvement in the quality of life of cirrhosis and liver cancer patients.

In premodern texts, jaundice (黄疸 *ō dan/huáng dǎn*) and flank pain (脇痛 *kyō tsū/xié tòng*) are the terms that correspond best to the medical terms liver disease and gallbladder disease, respectively. In Zhang Zhong-Jing's *Essentials from the Golden Cabinet*, jaundice is further subdivided into five types: yellow jaundice (黄疸 *ō dan/huáng dǎn*), black jaundice (黒疸 *koku dan/hēi dǎn*), jaundice from sexual overindulgence (女勞疸 *jo rō dan/nǔ láo dǎn*), alcoholic jaundice (酒疸 *shu dan/jiǔ dǎn*), and grain jaundice (穀疸 *koku dan/gǔ dǎn*). Yellow jaundice and grain jaundice are thought to be related to the medical disease hepatitis A. Alcoholic jaundice refers to alcoholic hepatitis. Black jaundice can appear in any type of chronic hepatitis where the skin darkens. Finally, the pain felt from cholecystitis and gallstones falls under the rubric of flank pain.

All these different types of jaundice have Spleen deficiency with water stagnation as their basic pathology. The symptoms are said to develop when heat is added, producing damp-heat disease. The same state can also be caused by Kidney deficiency, which is the case for jaundice from sexual overindulgence or overwork. In this case, therefore, Kidney deficiency/yin deficiency produces heat that spreads to the Spleen, creating a disease state that is little different from hepatitis in modern medicine.

We can see, then, that the basic pathology for hepatitis is Spleen deficiency. Because the Spleen becomes deficient, heat builds up in the Liver and Gallbladder. In the early stages of the disease, the pattern is Spleen deficiency/Liver excess/heat, and the symptoms include fever, general lassitude, vomiting and nausea, lack of appetite, constipation, yellow, dark urine, and jaundice. At this stage the color change is not marked, and so it is easy to miss. If you suspect something, check the whites of the eyes.

The abdomen will normally feel hot from above and below the angle of the right ribs to the epigastric area around the point CV-14; in addition, there will be marked pain on pressure in this area. This is known classically as suffering and fullness in the chest and ribs, and is described in Chapter 8 here. Cases of chronic hepatitis where this fullness is not present are more likely to progress to cirrhosis. The pulse is wiry, big, and rapid, or sunken, rough, excessive, and rapid. The right medial pulse is deficient on firm pressure, while the left medial pulse is excessive.

It is possible to treat this condition with acupuncture and moxibustion, but it is often better if the patient has a thorough medical workup first. The more marked the jaundice and the greater the level of heat, the easier it is to cure the condition. When the color is not so marked, as is commonly the case with chronic hepatitis, a cure will take more time.

While acute hepatitis A almost never leads to chronic hepatitis, the Spleen deficiency/Liver excess/heat pattern can become chronic and lead to a pattern of Spleen deficiency/Liver excess/blood stasis or Lung deficiency/Liver excess/blood stasis. This change occurs because the Liver blood, which held the heat, cools down, congealing in the process and thereby leading to the formation of blood stasis. However, it should be noted that while chronic hepatitis cases often begin with elements of blood stasis and end up as Liver excess/blood stasis, in those individuals who constitutionally have only a small amount of blood stasis, a pattern of Liver deficiency/yin deficiency will develop instead.

An abdominal examination in cases of chronic hepatitis will reveal increased muscular resistance in the area below the right ribs, which is a sign of Liver excess/blood stasis. As the blood stasis progresses, the muscular resistance will spread to the epigastric region. If the condition worsens still further, ascites will develop. The overall pulse will become sunken, rough, and excessive at this stage.

As noted above, there are some patients with chronic hepatitis who do not develop a Liver excess/blood stasis pattern; actually, they exhibit a Spleen deficiency/yang deficiency/cold pattern. When these patients are treated, their pattern usually changes to that of Spleen deficiency/Liver excess/blood stasis with Liver heat. If a blood test is taken at this stage, the measures of their liver function will appear to temporarily worsen, but with continued treatment, the Liver heat will diminish as the patient is led gently toward recovery.

For patients with cholecystitis or gallstones, the main symptom will be pain in the upper abdomen. If the area over the gallbladder is pressed, the patient will experience pain and will also vomit, and so the problem is often quite easy to identify. This can be treated well with acupuncture and moxibustion. However, if there are large gallstones, the treatment can be difficult, and so surgery is recommended in these cases.

People with gallstones usually present with a Spleen deficiency/Liver excess/heat pattern. However, if patients with gallstones exhibit a Liver deficiency/yang deficiency/cold pattern with a sunken, thin pulse, then the gallbladder itself has been damaged. Consistent pain can indicate the development of peritonitis, and the patient should be sent to an emergency facility immediately. This is common among patients who have been consistently taking pain medication to manage their gallstone pain.

Treatment

Whatever the type of hepatitis, the areas around LR-14, GB-24, and ST-19 should be very carefully examined and treated. In addition, there are two off-channel points that are important for these patients. M-LE-23 (胆囊穴 *tan no ketsu/dǎn náng xué*, the 'gall bladder point') is located 1-2 units below GB-34, and N-LE-14 (肝炎点 *kan en ten/gān yán diǎn*, the 'hepatitis point') is located 2 units directly above the medial malleolus (see TABLE 17-8). On the back, BL-18 to BL-21 and areas on the inside and outside of these points are often tender on pressure. Retained needling or direct scarring moxibustion is applied to these points. If the condition is chronic, then the tenderness on pressure is not so pronounced; instead, hardness and resistance will be the main findings. In this case, the use of needle head moxibustion is recommended. For gallbladder disease, shunt SP-1.

Table 17-8	Branch Treatment Points for Liver and Gallbladder Diseases
Location	**Points**
ARMS AND LEGS	ST-36, SP-1, SI-4, **LR-3, LR-4, LR-8**, M-LE-23, N-LE-14
ABDOMEN	**ST-19**, ST-20, ST-21, **ST-25, GB-24**, LR-13, **LR-14**, CV-6 CV-9, CV-12, CV-14
BACK	**BL-17 to BL-21**, BL-23, BL-43, **BL-48**, GV-6

Fukaya recommended direct scarring moxibustion at SP-6 to SP-8 in cases of hepatitis, as these points will show tenderness on pressure. It is to be expected that the Spleen meridian will be tender in these cases, and applying moxibustion at the tender points will result in a tonifying action on the Spleen. However, if the Liver heat or blood stasis is not removed at the same time, a cure will be difficult.

Case History

PATIENT: 41-year-old man

CHIEF COMPLAINT: He came to see me for hepatitis C that he contracted as a result of a blood transfusion. The patient underwent a total of nine or ten operations for hemorrhoids, but received no relief. On the last occasion, there was a surgical error, resulting in a large loss of blood. It was at this point that the patient received a blood transfusion that caused him to experience palpitations and resulted in the hepatitis C.

VISUAL: The patient had a good physique but was a little on the thin side. The tongue had no moss on it. There was a strong smell of medication emanating from the whole of the patient's body. There was one small spider angioma on his chest, and his palms were red.

SYMPTOMS: These included an overall lack of energy, alternating diarrhea and constipation, reduced appetite and lack of ability to taste food, insomnia, and bleeding from his hemorrhoids and gums. He also had headaches, a tendency toward palpitations, a skin rash that appeared throughout his body in the spring, lower back pain, and a prostate condition that gave him pain on urination. Hospital tests revealed significantly elevated liver enzymes and a platelet count of 70,000.

PULSE: The overall pulse was big and wiry with deficiency on firm pressure at the left proximal and right medial positions.

ABDOMEN: There was no pain or fullness in the chest or flanks. However, the liver was swollen about two finger widths larger than normal, and was a little hard. The chest was hot to the touch with pain on pressure along the Kidney points on the chest. There was also pain on pressure on the inguinal areas that wrapped around to the lower back.

TREATMENT: In this case, the hepatitis was evolving into cirrhosis. The pattern was thought to be Spleen deficiency/yin deficiency without pain and fullness in the chest and flanks, but with some heat in the Liver. At the same time, there was also yin deficiency of the Kidneys that, when it came to the fore, resulted in symptoms such as palpitations, lower back pain, and pain on urination.

To start with, I tonified PC-8, SP-2, LR-4, ST-36, and BL-40, and shunted GB-41. I also retained needles at LR-14, ST-19, CV-12, CV-4, and ST-25. The hard, stiff areas of the back were treated with heat perception moxibustion, and needles were retained at the deficient areas. Because the patient occasionally complained of palpitations beneath the ribs, I also tonified KI-7. To treat his high blood pressure, direct scarring moxibustion at ST-36, ST-35, and ST-40 was applied successfully. To treat the prostate inflammation, direct scarring moxibustion was applied at BL-43, LR-1, and LR-5, with good results.

The above treatment was continued for 10 years, after which he had a tendency toward high blood pressure, irritability, stiff shoulders, and a heavy feeling in his head. However, all the other symptoms had disappeared. The rash that would appear in the spring had also disappeared, and there was no more hemorrhaging. His platelet count had risen to 90,000 and the spider angioma and the red palms had disappeared. Interestingly enough, his liver enzyme levels and other blood test values had not changed much at all.

17.8 HEMORRHOIDS

Diagnosis

Included under this general heading are hemorrhoids, anal fissures, prolapsed anus, and anal fistulas. In every case, the cause is heat in the Large and Small Intestines. The origin of the heat as well as the amount of heat are important considerations. Of course, the patient should be advised concerning lifestyle changes, as excessive amounts of alcohol, food, work, sitting, and sex will tend to make the hemorrhoids worse.

Let us first consider the case where the problem is caused by a pattern of Spleen deficiency/Liver excess/blood stasis, resulting in poor blood flow to the Intestines because of a large amount of blood stasis. This pattern is commonly seen in cases of acute and chronic hemorrhoids, and increases the incidence of anal fissures. There are also times when qi stagnation can cause hemorrhoids. This is not so surprising when we consider that poor circulation of Lung qi can lead to heat accumulation in the Intestines.

Because of the interior-exterior relationship between the Lungs and Large Intestine, any Lung heat can spread to the Large Intestine, making the hemorrhoids worse. In this situation, the patient should be treated for a Spleen deficiency/Lung heat or Liver deficiency/Lung heat pattern. These patterns are commonly seen in cases of acute hemorrhoids and bleeding hemorrhoids. There are also cases where Lung heat is the precipitating factor for the formation of anal fistulas; these cases are often chronic in nature.

When the intestines become lax, losing their natural tonus, the result is a prolapse of the anus. A common pattern seen in chronic conditions is Spleen deficiency/yang deficiency. As the problem becomes more chronic, there is less heat, and the condition progresses to one of Spleen deficiency/yin deficiency.

The prognosis for hemorrhoids can be estimated to some extent by the pulse. A sunken, small, excessive pulse is better than a floating, weak pulse, which indicates yang deficiency. The latter indicates hemorrhoids that are more difficult to cure.

Treatment

A root treatment must be performed after determining the pattern. This works on the cause of the problem, but it is usually not enough to cure the hemorrhoids. It is also important to carry out an appropriate branch treatment according to the pattern (see TABLE 17-9). Among the large number of branch treatments available for treating this condition, direct scarring moxibustion at LU-6 is very popular in Japan. This is effective when Lung heat is responsible for the hemorrhoids, regardless of whether or not they are bleeding. In addition, acute cases generally respond well, but if there is no pain felt on pressure at LU-6, the treatment will not be effective.

Table 17-9	Branch Treatment Points for Hemorrhoids
Location	Points
HEAD	**GV-20**
ARMS AND LEGS	**LU-6, ST-32, SP-6, BL-36**, BL-37, BL-40, **BL-56 to BL-58**, KI-7, **GB-31**, points on the ulnar side of crease of proximal interphalangeal joints
BACK	**BL-20, BL-30 to BL-35**, BL-54, **GV-1, GV-4**, GV-12 to GV-14

Another equally well-known point is GV-20. Since the Liver meridian goes up to this point, it can be used to treat hemorrhoids that are caused by blood stasis, anal prolapse, and bleeding hemorrhoids. This point, too, is effective when there is pain on pressure; direct scarring moxibustion should be performed using about seven rice-grain sized moxa cones. If there is no luck with either LU-6 or GV-20, points that are painful on pressure on the lower back can sometimes be treated with success.

There are also some other points known to be especially effective. One is found by measuring the distance between PC-7 and the tip of the middle finger. This length is then used to measure from the tip of the coccyx up along the Governing vessel, and the point is marked. From here, two points, 1 unit to the left and 1 unit to right of this point, are noted, as well as a point 2 units above the point first marked on the Governing vessel. Direct scarring moxibustion at these three points is useful for any type of hemorrhoids.

For hemorrhoids due to qi stagnation, tender points found between GV-9 and GV-12 should be treated. Points between GV-1 and GV-4 can also be checked for tenderness and treated. Another line to be checked is between BL-20 and BL-30, or just outside of this line. These tender points can be used to treat any type of hemorrhoids.

Among problems related to hemorrhoids, anal fistulas are often the most difficult to treat. In premodern texts, direct scarring moxibustion (50 to 100 cones) was recommended directly on the hemorrhoid itself. If this is impossible, moxibustion can be used to fumigate the area of the hemorrhoid. Heat perception moxibustion is also good. Another method that was recommended is to mix some powdered aconite or garlic with some of the patient's own saliva and knead it into a paste. This is then placed over the hemorrhoid and moxibustion is performed on it until the paste dries out. This is repeated two or three times. Direct scarring moxibustion at GV-1, SP-5, and BL-36 was also recommended.

I personally have never performed direct scarring moxibustion at GV-1, but I found that moxa head needling at this point was effective. Another point that is good for anal fistulas is found 2 units below SP-6; around seven cones of direct scarring moxibustion are applied.

Finally, anal prolapse can be treated using GV-12 to GV-14 by selecting the most tender points and applying direct scarring moxibustion until the tenderness diminishes or disappears.

delivered to the Kidneys, leading to puffiness. From this, we can see why the Kidneys are likened to water, while the Spleen is classically likened to an earthen dike or embankment. The Kidneys are also said to be the gateway to the Stomach, which basically means that if the Kidneys are deficient, the Stomach will be deficient, and vice versa. From the above pathology, it is clear that water qi diseases should in general be treated as a pattern of Kidney deficiency/yin deficiency/heat.

Phlegm and thin mucus disease occurs when the Spleen is deficient, which affects the absorption of water by the Stomach and Intestines, thereby leading to a buildup of water. We can further subdivide these problems into phlegm and thin mucus. Phlegm is basically the product of water and heat from any source.

For instance, we can say that phlegm plays a role in the development of urinary problems if they arose as a result of Spleen deficiency/yin deficiency heat spreading to the Kidneys and Bladder and causing a buildup of water. At the same time, heat can spread to the Lungs and the Liver simultaneously. This pattern is often seen in nephritis or nephrosis. My brother (Takio Ikeda) commented on this to me when he said "The Spleen has the capacity to push out water, [and] so Kidney disease should be treated by tonifying the Spleen." Thin mucus, by contrast, is caused by Spleen deficiency coupled to deficiency of the yang qi of the Stomach and Intestines, causing a buildup of water. It is common to find this pattern in congestive heart disease and also in cases where there is unexplained puffiness of the face.

As we have seen above, nephritis and nephrosis can be a result of either Kidney deficiency/yin deficiency/heat or Spleen deficiency/yin deficiency/heat. Distinguishing between the two should be based on the symptoms and the pulse, but can be quite difficult in practice. In the classics, there is a school of thought that edema is due to Spleen deficiency (e.g., Chapters 29 and 45 of *Basic Questions)*, and there is another school that says it is due primarily to Kidney deficiency (e.g., Chapter 34 of *Basic Questions*, Chapter 2 of the *Divine Pivot*, and Chapter 40 of the *Classic of Difficulties)*.

What we can say is that when edema is present, a floating and big or flooding pulse, or a floating, big, and deficient pulse will likely be present, all of which indicate a preponderance of yang qi. Cases of nephritis with Kidney deficiency/yin deficiency/heat typically have an appetite and sometimes also have high blood pressure. On the other hand, cases of nephritis where the pulse is sunken, fine, thin, and deficient, and that also have gastrointestinal symptoms as well as poor urine flow, are caused by a pattern of Spleen deficiency/yin deficiency or Spleen deficiency/yang deficiency. In either case, if the left proximal pulse is hard, the prognosis is poor.

Cases of acute nephritis can also be caused by Spleen deficiency/Liver excess/heat. In this case, the pulse would be sunken, wiry, and excessive. Also, the number of people with kidney failure that are on dialysis machines is growing recently. These patients tend to have pulses that are difficult to read and therefore pose problems in determining the pattern. Based on my experience, they typically have either a Spleen deficiency yin/deficiency or Spleen deficiency/yang deficiency pattern.

In those cases where there is kidney disease as well as high blood pressure, concentrate on improving the health of the kidneys and the blood pressure will take care of itself. There is no need to emphasize treating the high blood pressure during your selection of points.

Finally, in such classics as *Essentials from the Golden Cabinet*, terms such as distention, fullness, and drum-like distention (鼓脹 *ko chō/gǔ zhàng*) are used to describe disease states when the abdomen is big and full like a drum and the face, eyes, arms, and legs are also puffy. Ascites, which can be seen in cases of cirrhosis, is perhaps one such disease state. Temporary improvement in the condition can be obtained by using the treatment for Spleen deficiency/yang deficiency/cold pattern. If there is some Liver heat rising to the surface, then a Spleen deficiency/Liver excess/heat pattern treatment protocol should be followed.

Treatment

The simplest way to treat edema is to administer direct scarring moxibustion to the heels at M-LE-5 (失眠 *shitsu min/shī mián*); the point, which can be translated as 'insomnia,' is located at the center of the heel on the bottom of the foot. This point is useful when there is a Spleen deficiency with Kidney and Bladder heat. Although the moxibustion is applied until heat is felt (a tonifying technique), it is most effective when it builds up to the point where it can radiate out and have a shunting effect on the Kidneys. This requires that moxibustion be repeated a number of times until the patient feels the heat. It is often the case that one heel takes more cones than the other. Remember that the entire sole of the foot, including the heel, is thought to be connected with the Kidneys.

If too much heat is applied or it does not radiate outward, there can be problems. I remember on one occasion when a patient with a pattern of Kidney deficiency/yin deficiency/heat decided to perform moxibustion on his legs and did so to the extent that he was then unable to stand up. Admittedly, he did select about 20 sites on which to perform his "labor of love," and only two of those points were M-LE-5. However, it demonstrates that we should be aware of the pattern when performing moxibustion.

Another way of dealing with edema is to perform direct scarring moxibustion or needle head moxibustion on points surrounding the navel. Different practitioners recommend various measurements around the navel, including 1.5 and 2.2 units. I personally prefer using CV-9, which is 1 unit above the navel, as a yardstick, and so I take the lower, left, and right points all at 1 unit from the navel, as well as CV-9, and apply moxibustion there. If this proves to be ineffective, I locate ST-25 and take points 2 units above and below the navel, as well as ST-25, and apply moxibustion there.

There are some patients with swollen, puffy faces who have nothing abnormal when tested biomedically. These patients are best treated for a Spleen deficiency/yang deficiency pattern using ST-42 in addition to the basic root treatment points. Other points that may also be useful are ST-40, ST-41, and ST-43. There are other patients who suffer from swollen legs in the evenings. These conditions normally respond well when they are treated for either Liver deficiency/yin deficiency or Kidney deficiency/yin deficiency. A number of these patients will present no irregularities when they are tested, but nevertheless they urinate too infrequently, a condition which would have been considered a type of leg qi disease in older texts. In this condition, the legs are painful and weak. The older texts recommend leg qi eight point moxibustion (see Chapter 14), which consists of direct scarring moxibustion at GB-31, ST-32, ST-35, M-LE-16, ST-36, ST-37, and GB-39. For patients with ascites, administer moxibustion at CV-9, GV-13, GV-12, and the point found in the gap between the fourth and fifth spinous processes, that is, the point between GV-11 and GV-12. Other useful points for edema are summarized in TABLE 18-1.

Table 18-1	Branch Treatment Points for Edema
Location	**Points**
LEGS	ST-36, SP-6, **SP-9**, KI-7, **KI-8, M-LE-5**
ABDOMEN	**ST-28, KI-14, KI-16**, GB-25, GB-28, CV-5 to CV-7
BACK	BL-17, **BL-20, BL-21**, BL-23, **BL-25, BL-27, BL-28**, BL-30, BL-49, BL-50

Case History

PATIENT: 60-year-old woman

CHIEF COMPLAINT: The patient's chief complaint began as gestational nephritis and became worse at some point later in her life. Fifteen years before, she was found by chance during a routine examination to have high blood pressure and protein in her urine. While she was not in good condition at the time of this examination, it was thought that acupuncture treatments had prevented her from deteriorating further. Unfortunately, the patient lived too far away to come in for regular acupuncture treatments and did not have sufficient funds for herbal medicine. Recently, her blood pressure and the amount of protein in her urine increased, and so she came to me to mark some points for moxibustion treatment at home for her condition.

VISUAL: She had a small frame but was slightly obese and had especially marked fluid buildup in her legs. There were no significant changes in the tongue.

SYMPTOMS: Her appetite, stools, and sleeping were all normal. Her urine was a little scanty, and she had a dry mouth.

PULSE: The pulse was sunken, wiry, and a little hard. However, it was difficult to discern because of the fluid stagnation.

TREATMENT: The patient had taken Eight Ingredient Pill (八味丸 *hachi mi gan/bā wèi wán*), better known outside of Japan as Kidney Qi Pill (*jīn guì shèn qì wán*), with reasonable results, and so it was thought that she was Kidney deficient. When I pressed along the Kidney meridian, she felt pain at KI-8. Since the patient wanted to do some moxibustion on herself at home, I selected left and right KI-8 and instructed her to burn 7 to 20 half-rice-grain sized moxa cones directly on each point.

Apparently, the patient did not feel the heat of the moxibustion, and so she burned 30 to 40 cones on each point for the next two months. At the end of that time, she no longer had protein in her urine, her blood pressure dropped to 124/70mmHg, and her renal function had returned to normal. This was an amazing result, and I was just as surprised as the patient!

18.2 ABNORMAL URINATION

Diagnosis

Abnormal urination includes a variety of symptoms such as inability to urinate, insufficient urination, excessive quantity or frequency of urination, difficulty urinating, bloody urine, urine containing pus, painful urination, and a sense of retained urine. The symptom of not being able to urinate or of insufficient urination can occur together with other acute symptoms such as violent vomiting, diarrhea, or sudden low blood pressure. Cases that do not quickly respond to acupuncture and moxibustion should be treated as very serious, as there is a real possibility that a problem exists that could lead to renal failure. These patients are best served by referring them quickly to a medical physician. Of course, an inability to urinate can also be caused by such problems as prostatic hypertrophy, kidney stones, and tumors, which for the most part are not acute conditions.

Excessive urination is associated with conditions such as hydronephrosis (also known as hypokalemic nephrosis or osmotic nephrosis) and chronic nephritis. Again, if you have any doubts, refer the patient to a medical physician. Having said this, excessive quantity and frequency of urination can also result from chilling of the body (see Section 19.1). Difficulty in urinating can also be caused by such diverse conditions as a kidney stone, enlarged prostate, and even tumor. Symptoms such as blood and pus in the urine, painful urination, and a sense of retained urine are present in conditions such as cystitis, urethritis, pyelonephritis, and kidney stones. Of course, painful urination and a sense of retained urine can also be indicative of pregnancy or a nervous disorder. In rare cases, they can be due to bladder cancer, uterine fibroids, or cancer affecting the pelvis.

We will now take a look at the diagnosis and treatment of these various conditions. Many of them are included under the rubric of the traditional term 'painful urinary dribbling' (淋病 *rin byō/lín bìng*), which is generally thought to be a result of heat collecting in the Bladder, causing the urine to dribble out and to be at least somewhat turbid. There are six types of painful urinary dribbling conditions:

1. Hot painful urinary dribbling (熱淋 *netsu rin/rè lín*). Here the urine is reddish and turbid, with intense pain. The modern day equivalent is cystitis or urethritis.

2. Painful bloody urinary dribbling (血淋 *ketsu rin/xuè lín*). The urine is bloody, and there is pain in the urethra. The modern day equivalent is again cystitis or urethritis.

3. Stony painful urinary dribbling (石淋 *seki rin/shí lín*). There is pain in the urethra, and the urine may appear to contain sand or gravel. The modern day equivalent is of course kidney or bladder stones.

4. Qi painful urinary dribbling (気淋 *ki rin/qì lín*). The urine is turbid and painful to pass, and the urine flow is always poor. The modern day equivalent is mild cystitis or prostatic hypertrophy.

5. Cloudy painful urinary dribbling (膏淋 *kō rin/gāo lín*). The urine becomes thick and cloudy almost to the point of resembling paste. A modern day equivalent would be urethritis.

6. Consumptive painful urinary difficulty (勞淋 *rō rin/láo lín*). There is a sudden desire to urinate and urinating is uncomfortable. In addition, there is a lack of sexual desire and no emission of semen; the condition manifests when the body is tired. A modern day equivalent would be prostatitis or prostatic hypertrophy.

Looking at the above list, we can see general similarities between these traditional terms and modern disease categories. Cloudy painful urinary dribbling relates to urethritis, which leads to pus in the urine. Consumptive painful urinary dribbling often represents prostatitis or prostatic hypertrophy. Stony painful urinary dribbling is of course related to kidney or bladder stones. Hot painful urinary dribbling and painful bloody urinary dribbling usually occur in those with cystitis or urethritis. Qi painful urinary dribbling also usually occurs in those with mild cystitis, but also can manifest in men with prostate hypertrophy. There are also cases where there may be blood in the urine, without any pain or particular discomfort, due to over-sweating or excessive worry. Even though this does not fit the definition of painful urinary dribbling, for treatment purposes we can assume that there is heat lodged in the Bladder.

It is best to inquire of individuals who suffer from urinary difficulties whether they have been examined by a physician, and whether there is any chance of a sexually transmitted infection. Regardless, if there is pus in the urine and pain on urination, it is best to refer them to a physician. However, there are cases where tests reveal no irregularities; indeed, women who suffer from repeated bouts of cystitis often test negative for a bacterial infection and are diagnosed as having nongonorrheal urethritis, with the main symptom being a sense of retained urine. This sort of problem is very effectively treated with acupuncture and moxibustion. Chronic gonorrhea that has not responded to antibiotics can fortunately also be treated effectively with acupuncture and moxibustion.

Cystitis and urethritis give rise to varied, readily identifiable symptoms such as blood and pus in the urine, pain on urination, a sense of retained urine, cloudy urine, and frequent urination. However, when these conditions become chronic, the main symptoms become the sense of retained urine and pain on urination; blood in the urine often cannot be seen by the naked eye.

With acute cases of pyelonephritis, even if there are chills, there will be fever as well. The condition is, therefore, sometimes mistaken for a cold, but cases of pyelonephritis also present with lower back pain and blood in the urine. There are occasions when it is difficult to see the blood in the urine with the naked eye. However, if there is a fever with lower back pain, pyelonephritis should be suspected, especially if the patient has a history of the disease. Chronic pyelonephritis presents with no symptoms or only a mild fever with lassitude and lower back pain. There may also be a decline in renal function.

The back pain associated with kidney stones may be so severe that even breathing is difficult. Also, referred pain may be present in the lower abdomen around the inguinal area. The pain is due to stone particles that are traveling through the ureter and that reach the intersection of the ureter and the abdominal aorta. Since this junction is a little narrower than the rest of the ureter, stone particles lodge there, giving rise to pain. Alternatively, in some cases the stones have moved through this area and are lodged instead in the tissue located at the entrance to the bladder; the pain is much less severe in these cases. After moving into the bladder, everything will be normal in most cases, with the particles being expelled upon urination within two or three days. There are some cases, however, where stone particles are formed within the bladder itself and become lodged in the urethra, causing blood in the urine. However, since blood in the urine may also be indicative of bladder cancer, it is advisable to refer the patient to a physician for an examination.

Kidney stones seem to be more common in people who consume lots of sweet or spicy products, or who stand for long periods during their work (acupuncturists beware!) There are even those that appear to suffer from them regularly every few years. First-timers are naturally unsure about what is happening and therefore are rather anxious. Typically, the pain begins after urinating first thing in the morning. If the pain is severe enough, there will also be a feeling of nausea; under these conditions, the patient may also experience difficulty urinating and/or blood in the urine. If the stone particles are small, the resulting blood may not be visible to the naked eye, but the last part of the urine stream may be visibly red. Patients who repeatedly develop kidney stones often have generalized edema and elevated blood pressure.

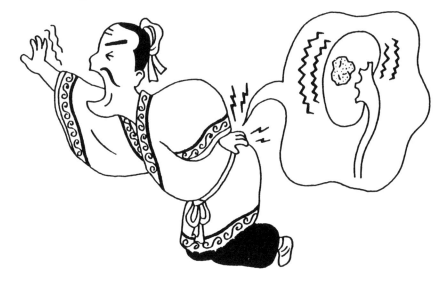

Kidney stones are incredibly painful

All of the above disorders can be considered and treated as Bladder heat, where the root of the heat can vary; Kidney deficiency/yin deficiency/heat, Spleen deficiency/yin deficiency/heat, and Spleen deficiency/Liver excess/blood stasis are the most common patterns. An accompanying fever and acute onset of symptoms often points toward Spleen deficiency with Bladder heat. A chronic condition with diarrhea or soft stools but a strong appetite is often indicative of Kidney deficiency/yin deficiency with Bladder heat. Normally, poor urinary function goes hand in hand with a tendency toward diarrhea. If instead of this there is constipation or hard stools, then the pattern is probably Spleen deficiency/Liver excess/blood stasis. We have noted that gonorrhea is often accompanied by blood stasis.

The pulse for these conditions is generally sunken and wiry, or sunken, rough, and tight overall. However, when there is a large amount of heat, the pulse will be rapid and the proximal pulses will be tight. A floating, big pulse indicates that the symptoms may be severe but the recovery should be relatively easy. On the other hand, when the pulse is deficient, thin, and rough, the recovery will be difficult. An examination of the abdomen will often find pain on pressure at CV-3. Also, in cases of chronic urethritis or cystitis, there may be a thin, palpable, pencil-like line below the navel running vertically along the Conception vessel.

Treatment

Of course, it is important that the root treatment be administered, but it is also imperative that the heat in the Bladder be removed. BL-40 and BL-58 can be used to remove Bladder heat, but it is good to shunt CV-3 and KI-12 as well. When blood stasis is involved, it is necessary to use points on the Liver meridian, for example, press LR-3, LR-5, and LR-8, and shunt those that exhibit pain. If the problem is chronic, direct scarring moxibustion or needle head moxibustion can be used. In TABLE 18-2, I have listed a number of points that should be used according to the pattern. The guiding principle, however, is that if there is no hardness or pain on pressure, then using the point will have no effect.

Table 18-2	Branch Treatment Points for Abnormal Urination
Location	Points
LEGS	SP-3, SP-8, SP-9, KI-2, KI-5, KI-6, **KI-7, KI-8**, GB-41, LR-3
ABDOMEN	ST-25, KI-12, GB-29, **CV-3**, CV-4, **CV-5, CV-7**, CV-12
BACK	BL-23, BL-25, BL-27, BL-28, BL-32, BL-33, BL-48, BL-52 to BL-54, M-BW-16

For chronic cystitis and urethritis, Fukaya suggested using scarring moxibustion on the pair of points SP-6 and GB-39, as well as ST-39 and KI-9. In this method, the heat from the points is made to penetrate from one side toward the other. For painful urinary dribbling, the early nineteenth-century text *Selected Interpretations of Famous Family Moxibustion Methods* recommends finding a hard and tender point between ST-36 and ST-41 and treating it with direct scarring moxibustion until heat is felt. Another method from the same book measures the width of the patient's mouth with a piece of string. One end of this length of string is then placed at the tip of the coccyx, the string following the course of the Governing vessel, and the other end is marked. Another piece of string is used to measure the length from the edge of the mouth to the bottom of the nose. This length is then halved and placed perpendicular to the Governing vessel with its middle on the previously marked point, so that the two ends of the string are equidistant to the point and parallel to the torso. Direct scarring moxibustion is applied to these three points.

The easiest way to work on the pain accompanying kidney stones is to ask the patient to lie on their side, with the painful side uppermost. The painful area is then pressed vigorously, helping to dislodge the stone particles and thus allowing them to descend. Another method is to find the hard painful points on the lower back with the patient lying face down if possible, and perform moxa head needling at these points. For chronic kidney stones, it may take up to a 100 cones of direct scarring moxibustion before heat is felt. Also, the point SP-3 often exhibits hard nodules on the side where the lower back has pain, in which case it is also treated with direct scarring moxibustion.

Case History

PATIENT: 45-year-old single woman

CHIEF COMPLAINT: Several days before, the patient started to experience chills and fever as well as spontaneous pain on the right side from the lumbar area down through the inguinal area. The urge to urinate was unaffected, but the intense pain caused her to vomit.

VISUAL: The patient was thin with a pale, poor complexion. The tongue was dry with no coating.

SYMPTOMS: Apart from the chief complaint, there was no change in her stool or urine; there was a lack of appetite.

PULSE: The overall pulse was rapid, wiry, and thin. The left distal and right medial pulses were deficient on firm pressure, although the right medial pulse could be felt on light pressure. The left medial pulse was wiry and excessive. When pressed lightly, the right medial pulse could be felt. In addition, the dorsal pedis pulse (at ST-42) was floating and big, while the tibialis posterior pulse (at KI-3) was wiry and therefore normal. The pattern was, therefore, Spleen deficiency/Liver excess/heat with a little bit of heat in the Stomach.

ABDOMEN: The right inguinal area and the right lower back at BL-22, BL-23, and BL-26 exhibited pain on pressure. The rectus abdominus muscles were tight on both sides, and a pulsation was noticeable on the left side of the navel.

TREATMENT: Although the patient had not received the appropriate tests, it was obvious to me that she was suffering from kidney stones. The chills and fever she was displaying meant that she probably had a pattern of Spleen deficiency/Liver excess/heat. I began the treatment by tonifying PC-7 and SP-3, followed by contact needling to the areas on the abdomen and lower back that were painful on pressure.

After the treatment, the chills had disappeared. That night, at around 2 AM, the pain became very intense, and the patient went to a hospital, receiving an intradermal pain killer. After that, she passed urine, and the stone was also ejected, resulting in immediate pain relief. The next morning, the patient felt sluggish and had a fever with a slight cough. The treatment this time consisted of tonifying PC-7 and SP-3, shunting GB-41, and contact needling on the back, abdomen, legs, and arms. This treatment resulted in the fever coming down to normal. However, the patient took a bath two days later, got chilled, and the fever came back. The same treatment was repeated for three consecutive days, resulting in a complete recovery.

18.3 NOCTURIA

Diagnosis

Both prostatitis and prostatic hypertrophy can lead to abnormal urination, especially an increase in urinary frequency at night. In the past, these diseases were connected with painful urinary dribbling (see the previous section), but that is not completely satisfactory, as they deserve a more thorough discussion. At the same time, other problems marked by frequent urination without pain, frequent and copious urine, and incontinence will also be discussed here.

Pain on urination and the feeling of retention of urine even though the frequency of urination is high, are usually indicative of pregnancy or a nervous disorder. In rare cases it can be due to bladder cancer. Other possible etiologies are problems that result in an increase in pressure on the bladder, such as uterine fibroids or cancer affecting the pelvis.

Prostatitis can be caused by a variety of infectious agents and can get worse after such things as a poorly performed hemorrhoid operation. Also, there are cases where men with a history of tuberculosis develop the symptoms of prostatitis in old age, including pain and discomfort extending from the anus to the rectum, pain in the perineum, pain on urination or defecation, urethral pain after urination, blood stained sperm, increased frequency of urination, and diarrhea. In some cases, there may be fever as well.

With an enlarged prostate, there will be poor urinary flow, a sense of retained urine, and nocturia. As the condition worsens, there will be anuria, a lack of urination, the early signs of which may occur in some men as early as 50 years of age. A sure sign of the onset of an enlarged prostate is standing in front of a urinal and taking a long time to urinate.

When there are prostatic problems, the urine cannot be fully expelled. This naturally leads to an increase in the frequency of urination. At night, the yang qi moves internally, and because of this, the heat in the Bladder and the Kidneys increases, causing an increase in volume and frequency of urination. With these problems, there will always be heat in the Bladder, but the pattern is often that of Liver deficiency/yin deficiency/heat or Kidney deficiency/yin deficiency/heat. A few patients may show a pattern of Spleen deficiency/Liver excess/blood stasis, in which case the pulse is sunken; if heat is present, the pulse will be slippery and rapid. Finally, problems with the prostate reveal a specific peculiarity on abdominal examination: the area above the pubic symphysis will have an increase in resistance to pressure accompanied by pain.

There are also cases where the act of urination itself is normal, but there is an increase in the frequency and volume of urination. This condition is a result of cold, and the relevant patterns are Lung deficiency/yang deficiency, Spleen deficiency/yang deficiency, and Kidney deficiency/yang deficiency. The patient will be incontinent if the cold worsens.

Treatment

In TABLE 18-3, I have again listed a number of points that should be used in addition to a root treatment for nocturia. Of course, the patient will need lifestyle advice, as alcohol and overindulgence in sex are contraindicated for both prostatitis and enlarged prostate conditions, causing even more heat to accumulate in the prostate.

Table 18-3	Branch Treatment Points for Nocturia
Location	**Points**
LEGS	ST-36, SP-9, BL-60, **LR-1**, **LR-3**, **LR-5**, LR-8
ABDOMEN	**CV-3 to CV-5**, CV-6
BACK	BL-22, **BL-23**, BL-27, **BL-28**, BL-30, BL-31, **BL-32**, **BL-33**, BL-35, **BL-52**, GB-25, GV-2

Fukaya recommended SP-8, SP-6, and GB-39 for difficulty urinating. For an enlarged prostate, Fukaya recommended moxibustion at, say, CV-3, GB-31, BL-37, a point just lateral to BL-37, BL-40, and BL-36. He also recommended moxibustion at BL-22, BL-27, and CV-3 for retention of urine.

I have found that direct moxibustion at LR-1, LR-5, BL-43, and CV-3 is effective for discomfort from prostatic hypertrophy or prostatitis. It is best to use 3 sesame-seed sized moxa cones on LR-1 and 7 to 10 half-rice-grain sized moxa cones on the rest of the points. Needle head moxibustion to the lower back and sacrum is without doubt the best thing you can do.

For cases of excessive urination due to a cold pattern, performing the appropriate root treatment will result in a cure. If there is incontinence, the branch treatment becomes important, for example, burn a large number of moxa cones on CV-3 to CV-5 and BL-23. Another good choice would be to do moxibustion on LR-1. I have successfully treated cases of bladder paralysis that lead to incontinence by using needle head moxibustion on CV-4, BL-23, BL-28, and BL-30

Case History

PATIENT: 55-year-old man

CHIEF COMPLAINT: The patient originally complained of lower back pain, but he was referred to my clinic by a patient who had been treated for and recovered from an enlarged prostate. He wanted the same results if that was possible.

VISUAL: The patient had a very solid build. His eyes were large (Liver excess constitution), and there did not appear to be anything drastically wrong with him. The tongue was unremarkable.

SYMPTOMS: There were no irregularities in his stool. There was an increase in the frequency of urination with only a very small amount of urine being passed each time. He had a sense of retained urine and normally had to get up to urinate once during the night. He enjoyed drinking alcohol.

PULSE: Although he was of solid build, his overall pulse was sunken, rough, and thin. It was, however, not rapid. When pressed firmly, the left proximal and medial pulses were deficient.

ABDOMEN: The area below the navel along the Conception vessel was lacking in tone, being rather flaccid. The rectus abdominus muscles along the Stomach meridians were tight on both sides. There was also tightness and discomfort in the epigastric region. Since the patient still had an appetite, this was thought to be a reflection of deficiency heat from the Kidneys.

TREATMENT: The patient was treated for a pattern of Liver deficiency/yin deficiency. KI-10 and LR-8 were tonified, followed by needle head moxibustion at GV-2, BL-30, BL-25, and BL-23. At the same time, needles were retained at BL-60, which is useful for lower back pain, but also an absolute necessity when dealing with urogenital problems. This treatment was repeated twice, leading to a complete cure of the condition, probably because the treatment was started early.

18.4 SEXUAL DYSFUNCTION

Diagnosis

The Kidneys store fluids as well as yin qi, which is responsible for both hardening and compacting. When the fluids and yin qi are functioning correctly, the fire at the gate of vitality descends from the Heart and causes the Kidneys to perform properly, including in the matter of sexual performance. Problems with sexual performance therefore imply a decrease in the fire at the gate of vitality, the fluids, yin qi, or both fluids and yin qi.

A decrease in the fluids and yin qi will lead to the production of heat from deficiency and a corresponding increase in Heart heat, which can cause premature ejaculation. If the condition worsens further, the patient will have nocturnal emission of sperm or spermatorrhea. This is different from the nocturnal emissions seen in young people who are overflowing with vitality; here, they are due to deficiency heat and are indicative of a pathological condition such as is sometimes seen in cases of prostatitis or epididymitis. If the deficiency heat increases still further, the penis becomes rigid and cannot be retracted to its normal state, which is known as priapism.

These problems are usually caused by overindulgence in sex, which leads to an exhaustion of the Kidney fluids and which in turn produces heat from deficiency. The pattern is that of either Kidney deficiency/yin deficiency or Liver deficiency/yin deficiency. With this problem, the libido is still healthy, but sexual performance declines to the point of impotence. The pulse is big and slippery, or wiry and often a little bit rapid. If the rapid pulse can be resolved, then the premature ejaculation and spermatorrhea will be cured.

If someone in the above state continues to overindulge in sex, the fluids of the Kidneys become even more depleted, causing the fluids of the bone marrow and brain to dry up. When this happens there will be forgetfulness and the onset of dementia. If the depletion of Kidney fluids continues further, the fire at the gate of vitality also decreases, resulting in the disappearance of the libido as well as spermatorrhea, an obvious decline in sexual performance! If this happens in young people, it is a serious problem that can be remedied by tonifying the Kidney fluids and the fire at the gate of vitality. In other words, this type of problem should be treated as a pattern of Kidney deficiency/yang deficiency/cold.

Sometimes young men lose their libido, but it is not really a decline in sexual performance. Rather, the symptom is that of nervous erectile dysfunction. This type of impotence comes from depression that is not due to a deficiency of Lung qi but rather to a blockage in the Liver. In this case, the radiation of yang qi from the blood of the Liver is insufficient, leading to Liver excess/blood stasis. Thus, this condition can be successfully treated as a Spleen deficiency/Liver excess/blood stasis or Lung deficiency/Liver excess/blood stasis pattern.

Male infertility, in other words, low sperm count, is usually accompanied by a general lack of vitality. In my experience, it is often seen in overweight patients with a pattern of Kidney deficiency/yin deficiency/heat. The pulse is often big, wiry, and deficient.

Women do not often complain of performance problems, but they may say that sex is not enjoyable and that the whole process is more trouble than it is worth. Treatment based on a pattern of Liver deficiency/yang deficiency/cold or Lung deficiency/Liver excess/blood stasis is usually successful for these women.

The fluids secreted by women during sexual arousal and intercourse are derived from sweat, which is in turn derived from blood. If a woman sweats too much, she will develop blood deficiency and she will lack sufficient amounts of sexual fluids, resulting in sex that is painful and not enjoyable. Inadequate secretion of sexual fluids can also be caused by blood stasis, because the constraint will cause the overall blood flow to be poor.

The classics discuss a set of diseases known as deficiency consumption (虚劳 *kyo rō/xū láo*) and deficiency harm (虚損 *kyo son/xū sǔn*). These diseases are caused by overwork and exhaustion; they can be divided into five types and are described in Chapter 23 of *Basic Questions* as follows:

1. Prolonged physical activity that damages the Liver

2. Prolonged use of the eyes that damages the Heart

3. Prolonged sitting that damages the Spleen

4. Prolonged sleeping that damages the Lungs

5. Prolonged standing that damages the Kidneys

Let me simply explain the pathology behind consumption as we now understand it. The most common cause of consumption is overindulgence in sex, which is treated as a pattern of Kidney deficiency. A patient who is overweight and looks reasonably forceful, but who is easily tired, also has a Kidney deficiency pattern. The next most common form of consumption is caused in those engaged in work that uses their arms, legs, and hands while sitting for long periods, such as office workers or taxi drivers. This is treated as a Spleen deficiency pattern, which produces, for example, weakness of the arms and legs or general lassitude brought on by hot weather.

Generally speaking, if the patient's chief complaint is feeling tired, the pattern is probably that of Kidney or Spleen deficiency. If the patient complains more of mental or emotional fatigue, the pattern is probably that of Lung or Liver deficiency. Any damage to the Heart would be treated by following a Kidney deficiency pattern protocol.

Treatment

For premature ejaculation, get the patient to sit cross-legged on the floor and mark a point three finger widths up from the floor along the Governing vessel. In this way, if the patient has an increased lumbar lordosis, this point will be closer to the coccyx, and if the patient has a decreased lumbar lordosis, the point will be closer to the lumbar spine. Mark two points located three finger widths to the left and the right of this initial point. Also mark another two points located two finger widths above these two points. Perform direct scarring moxibustion on these four points as well as LR-8, CV-6, and CV-7.

For the usual case of impotence, BL-23, BL-31, BL-33, GV-4, CV-6, KI-2, and LR-1 are good. In my experience, needle head moxibustion at points that include BL-23, BL-28, and BL-30, and a proper root treatment, will definitely result in a cure. Impotence due to depression is treated well with Governing vessel points such as GV-8 to GV-12 (and other tender points on the Governing vessel) as well as SP-6, BL-18, GB-39, and LR-14. If the root treatment is correct, it does not matter if the branch treatment is a little bit off the mark; the treatment will still be effective.

For epididymitis, direct scarring moxibustion at LR-1 and TB-4 is effective. For nocturnal emissions, needling or moxibustion at BL-43, GV-11, GV-10, GV-9, and LR-8 is effective. Other good points to treat using moxibustion are BL-20, BL-13, BL-23, CV-6, and ST-36. Acupuncture should be performed at CV-4, LR-8, KI-2, KI-12, and SP-6. For forgetfulness, use points such as BL-17, BL-18, BL-13, BL-20, BL-23, GV-4, and ST-25.

When there is consumption due to Kidney deficiency/yin deficiency, direct scarring moxibustion should be administered at BL-23. Consumption due to Kidney deficiency/yang deficiency is best treated with direct scarring moxibustion at CV-4. Consumption as a result of Spleen deficiency/yin deficiency is treated with direct scarring moxibustion at BL-20. Consumption due to Spleen deficiency/yang deficiency is treated with direct scarring moxibustion at BL-21 and BL-22, and salt moxibustion at CV-8.

In addition to the above points, see TABLE 18-4 for a list of points that are useful for a variety of sexual dysfunctions. However, these points should be considered in terms of yin deficiency or yang deficiency; tonification or shunting of the protective qi or nutritive qi should be carefully administered according to the patient's underlying problem. For example, use KI-1 and KI-2 for yin deficiency, and KI-3 and tender points on the Triple Burner meridian of the leg (first discussed in Chapter 4) for yang deficiency.

Table 18-4	Branch Treatment Points for Sexual Dysfunction
Location	**Points**
LEGS	KI-1 to KI-3, Triple burner meridian of the leg
ABDOMEN	**KI-12, CV-2 to CV-6**
BACK	**BL-23, BL-25, BL-29, BL-30, BL-34, BL-53, BL-54** (all needle head moxibustion)

CHAPTER 19

WOMEN'S DISEASES

T HERE ARE MANY gynecological and obstetrical diseases, and most of them require the assistance of a physician in their examination and treatment. The type of diseases we will consider here are those that are not regarded as diseases as such by gynecologists, or that are recognized as a disease, but do not respond well to Western medical treatment. I have divided the diseases under the following headings:

- *Cold extremities.* In itself, this does not constitute a disease per se, but it is often the chief complaint. This complaint is more common in women than men, and is one that can be treated with great success using acupuncture and moxibustion.

- *Problems of the female genitals.* The topics in this section include menstrual irregularities, menstrual pain, vaginal discharge, irregular bleeding, infertility, and uterine fibroids. While some cases of menstrual pain can be traced to medically defined disorders, such as endometriosis, there are also many cases that have no known medical diagnosis. In these cases, acupuncture and moxibustion are particularly effective. Vaginal discharge and irregular bleeding can be caused by sexually transmitted diseases or uterine cancer, and so the patient should be referred to a gynecologist for the appropriate tests, and should get acupuncture in conjunction with any biomedical treatment, if that is appropriate. Finally, the use of medication to induce ovulation is often successful in treating infertility, but acupuncture and moxibustion is also effective, even in cases where the reason for the infertility is unknown.

- *Problems that arise during pregnancy.* This includes, to some extent, morning sickness. They are treated effectively using acupuncture and moxibustion, which can also be used to promote a safe birth.

- *Postpartum problems.* The topics in this section include insomnia, headaches, diarrhea, and insufficient lactation. They are treated effectively using acupuncture and moxibustion. Although mastitis and uterine prolapse are not always postpartum-related, they are nevertheless also discussed in this section.

- *Menopausal problems.* These conditions are commonly known in Japan as problems of the blood pathway (血の道 *chi no michi*). Although there is no specific strategy for treating menopause per se, acupuncture and moxibustion can be effective at treating the various symptoms associated with menopause.

19.1   COLD EXTREMITIES

Diagnosis

Although some men suffer from this problem, cold extremities are much more common in women. This is because cold extremities are commonly caused by blood stasis or blood deficiency, both of which are much more likely to develop in women secondary to menstruation and childbirth.

COLD EXTREMITIES AS A RESULT OF BLOOD STASIS

As we saw in Part One, there are basically two types of blood stasis patterns: Spleen deficiency/Liver excess/blood stasis and Lung deficiency/Liver excess/blood stasis. A pattern of Spleen deficiency/Liver excess/blood stasis is more likely found in acute conditions, and so it is more common in younger women (see Chapter 9). A pattern of Lung deficiency/Liver excess/blood stasis is more likely found in chronic conditions, and so is more common in middle-aged and elderly women (see Chapter 10).

When there is blood stasis, the blood becomes trapped inside; therefore, the circulation of blood and qi on the outside of the body is impaired. This usually causes chilling of only the lower body and hot flushing of the upper body. The person is basically hot on the inside but cold on the outside. Accompanying symptoms include a large appetite, constipation with hard stools, and increased frequency of urination.

Those with Lung deficiency/Liver excess/blood stasis are often overweight and have edema. Even though they are overweight, they feel cold and are often overly sensitive to both heat and cold. They are sensitive to cold because they have a large amount of water located on the outer surface of their bodies, which leads to poor circulation of qi, making them more susceptible to cold in cold environments. They are sensitive to heat because they have trouble radiating and dispersing heat from the body surface, preventing them from cooling off in hot environments.

The overall pulse for a patient with cold extremities who presents with a pattern of Spleen deficiency/Liver excess/blood stasis is sunken, rough, and fine. When they present with a Lung deficiency/Liver excess/blood stasis pattern, the pulse will be sunken, wiry, and slippery, and the left medial pulse will not disappear even if it is pressed firmly. In both cases, abdominal diagnosis will reveal that the area below and to the sides of the navel is hard as well as painful on pressure. This is due to blood stasis.

COLD EXTREMITIES AS A RESULT OF BLOOD DEFICIENCY

The two relevant patterns are Liver deficiency/yin deficiency/heat and Liver deficiency/yang deficiency/cold. Those with a Liver deficiency/yin deficiency/heat pattern have cold extremities yet also experience hot flushes, which is typical of Liver yin conditions where alternating chills and fever can lead to heat going up from the feet, leaving the lower extremities cold. In cases of yin deficiency, the heat is palpable. For example, those with a Kidney deficiency pattern have hands and feet that feel warm to others, while in cases of blood stasis, there is only a subjective feeling of heat. Patients with Liver deficiency/yin deficiency/heat can also experience a sensation of heat in the hands and feet, as there is a deficiency of both the Liver and the Kidneys.

Chills without flushing can occur as a result of a lack of blood; the pattern in this case is Liver deficiency/yang deficiency/cold. The condition is characterized by coldness of the entire body. If the patient begins to menstruate because her blood is already deficient, then her blood will become even more deficient, resulting in even further chilling, as evidenced by diarrhea. In addition, the appetite will be poor because the cold affects the Stomach from outside. However, the inside of the Stomach is unaffected, and so there is no production of phlegm or thin mucus, which means that there is not a complete loss of appetite. Rather, the patient can finish a meal once it is begun.

The pulse for Liver deficiency/yang deficiency is sunken, rough, and thin, and the left medial and proximal pulses will be deficient on firm pressure. A pattern of Liver yang deficiency reveals a thin layer of muscular tension in the upper abdomen but no resistance or pain on pressure at deeper levels. The pulse for Liver deficiency/yin deficiency is big, relative to that of yang deficiency, but when it is pressed firmly, it is found to be deficient. A Liver yin deficiency pattern reveals an abdominal picture that is characterized mainly by an increase in resistance from the left hypochondria inferiorly.

OTHER TYPES OF COLD EXTREMITIES

Yang deficiency patterns, such as those involving Spleen deficiency/yang deficiency/cold, Kidney deficiency/yang deficiency/cold, and Lung deficiency/yang deficiency/cold, all give rise to cold extremities to some extent. When these patterns are acute in nature, chills are the main characteristic; however, here we will concern ourselves with chills that are mainly due to constitutional factors or that have become chronic in nature. In any case, the main distinguishing feature that we are looking at is one of chilling throughout the body, both inside and out. The patient should be questioned whether both the hands and feet feel cold. If the feet are cold but the hands are still all right, then the condition is probably not that of yang deficiency, but is more likely due to either blood stasis or yin deficiency.

A pattern of Spleen deficiency/yang deficiency/cold results in a reduced appetite and diarrhea with fatigue that increases after bowel movements. In addition, more saliva than usual collects in the mouth, and the patient urinates copious amounts of pale urine. A pattern of Kidney deficiency/yang deficiency/cold will result in cold throughout the entire body, with the lower back being especially cold as well as sore. There will also be copious urination, which often leads to constipation. The patient will have a good appetite but will be unable to finish a meal once it is begun. A pattern of Lung deficiency/yang deficiency/cold results in an aversion to cold, rather than actually feeling cold. This type develops a runny nose and sneezing at the first hint of cold. This is commonly seen in people with Lung-deficient type constitutions. If such people just exercise, improving the circulation of their qi, they will not complain of cold extremities. For details concerning the pulse and abdominal findings associated with each of these patterns, the reader is referred to the relevant chapters in Part One.

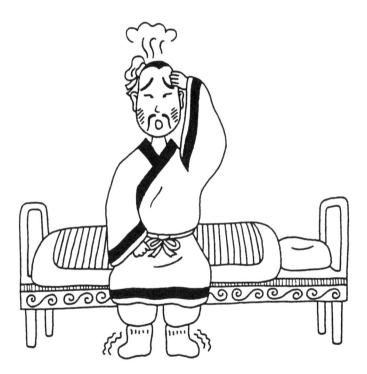

Cold feet with a hot head

Some medical conditions include cold extremities as part of their symptom picture, including Raynaud's disease, arthritis, and heart disease. Raynaud's disease can be cured by treating it as a Kidney deficiency/yin deficiency/heat pattern. Arthritis and heart disease are best treated as patterns of Spleen deficiency/yang deficiency/cold. With heart disease, the patient may also require Western medical treatment.

Treatment

Chills and hot flushes caused by yin deficiency or blood stasis should be treated by retaining needles on the back and at the Triple Burner meridian of the leg (see Chapter 4), BL-59, and BL-60. This will warm the legs and lessen the hot flushing. The only proviso is that if the root treatment is incorrect, it will be difficult to warm the legs. Chills that do not respond to retaining needles on the Bladder meridian are often caused by yang deficiency. For Kidney deficiency/yang deficiency/cold, use KI-3 and KI-7; for Spleen deficiency/yang deficiency/cold, use ST-42; and for Liver deficiency/yang deficiency/cold, use LR-3.

If the root treatment is correct but the patient still does not warm up, we have to think a little more about the branch treatment; general branch treatment points are set forth in TABLE 19-1. Usually, moxa head needling at SP-6 is good, but sometimes it can be contraindicated in some yang deficient patients, as this will cause radiation of yang qi, thereby further increasing the chills. Cold extremities caused by yang deficiency/cold patterns also respond well to direct scarring moxibustion at CV-4 to CV-6. Cold extremities caused by blood stasis require moxa head needling on the hard areas on the abdomen, and on the lower back from BL-23 downward. Cold sensations in general respond best to moxibustion. For cold sensations below the waist, use ST-33 and GB-38, and for cold sensations below the knees, use GB-33 and GB-34. For cold extremities experienced after an abortion or miscarriage, use GB-21. Chills with hot flushes can be treated with direct scarring moxibustion, needling, or moxa head needling at ST-36. In yin deficient conditions when the feet are not cold but instead experience annoying hot sensations, use KI-1 and KI-2.

Table 19-1	Branch Treatment Points for Cold Extremities
Location	**Points**
LEGS	ST-33, ST-36, **SP-6**, GB-33, GB-34, GB-38
ABDOMEN	**ST-25, CV-4 to CV-7**
BACK	**BL-22 to Bl-24**, GB-30, **GV-3**

19.2   PROBLEMS OF THE FEMALE GENITALS

Diagnosis

In this section we will discuss a variety of problems related to the female genitals that are often responsive to acupuncture, including irregular menstruation, painful menstruation, vaginal discharge and abnormal bleeding, infertility, and uterine fibroids. The most common patterns include Liver deficiency/yang deficiency/cold, Liver deficiency/yin deficiency/heat, Liver excess/heat, and Liver excess/blood stasis.

IRREGULAR MENSTRUATION

The following conditions fall under the rubric of irregular menstruation:

- *Menstruation that is late and scanty.* The pattern is often one of Liver deficiency/yang deficiency or of blood stasis, which can be differentiated by the pulse. If the menstrual bleeding is scanty during a woman's early years, she will at a certain stage in her later years become obese, because menstrual blood is derived from the fluids and scanty menstrual bleeding results from a failure of the fluids to be changed into blood; the net gradual buildup of fluids will result in a gradual increase in weight. This condition is often seen in women that complain of weight gain after a drop in their bleeding. The pattern is often that of Lung deficiency/Liver excess/blood stasis, and women with this pattern often go through menopause earlier than usual.

- *Heavy menstruation, that is, large amounts of blood and long duration of bleeding.* Women that menstruate heavily often have a pattern of Liver deficiency/yang deficiency/cold, in which case their hands and feet will be cold and they will have the other signs and symptoms of yang deficiency, including a sunken, rough, thin, and deficient pulse.

- *Premature menstruation.* Premature menstruation is often caused by a pattern of yin deficiency/heat.

- *Amenorrhea.* Women who suffer from amenorrhea are often seeing their gynecologists, and many are not ovulating. Proper treatment can correct this condition. The pattern is most often that of Liver deficiency/yang deficiency/cold. Women who are anorexic or who are particularly nervous may also develop amenorrhea; this should also be treated as a pattern of Liver deficiency/yang deficiency/cold. Some women who develop amenorrhea have an extremely weak Spleen and Stomach, in which case they should be treated for Spleen deficiency/yang deficiency/cold.

- *Nosebleeds in place of menstruation.* Some young women may suffer from nosebleeds that often occur in place of menstruation; by itself, the nosebleeds are nothing to worry about. However, these women should be carefully examined to see if their menstruation is delayed, which would be a sign of a Liver deficiency/yang deficiency/cold pattern, or if there is any other reason for their nosebleeds.

PAINFUL MENSTRUATION

Painful menstruation in younger women is either a Spleen deficiency/Liver excess/blood stasis or Liver deficiency/yang deficiency/cold pattern. Painful menstruation in a sexually active woman is either a Liver deficiency/yin deficiency/heat or Spleen deficiency/Liver excess/blood stasis pattern.

Endometriosis is a relatively common cause of painful menstruation. Painful menstruation can also occur when a fever or cold is contracted at the onset of a menstrual period. When this occurs, the woman will often develop pain during her menses even if she had never experienced any such problem before. The pattern is often that of Spleen deficiency/Liver excess/heat.

Abdominal pain that is not associated with a woman's menstrual cycle and is not due to enteritis is often caused by cold. This can be successfully treated with a Liver deficiency/yang deficiency/cold pattern protocol. There may be times when the patient may not respond well to treatment because of diseased ovaries. In that case, the patient should be referred to a gynecologist. Also, much less common but something to watch out for is ectopic pregnancy, which usually manifests as spotting and cramping after a missed period. In my experience, there may be more pain in the morning. The pulse will be sunken and tight. If you have any suspicion of an ectopic pregnancy, refer the patient immediately to an acute medical facility.

VAGINAL DISCHARGE AND ABNORMAL BLEEDING

A clear discharge that stains the underwear a yellow color is usually nothing to be concerned about. This discharge is due to cold and is best treated as a pattern of Liver deficiency/yang deficiency/cold. A milky or brownish colored discharge that is definitely not connected to the patient's period should be referred to a gynecologist because the discharge might be emblematic of a sexually transmitted disease. Nevertheless, it is possible to treat this condition with acupuncture and moxibustion, for example, trichomonas vaginitis and candida infections are best treated as a pattern of Spleen deficiency/Liver excess/blood stasis.

If the discharge immediately follows the passage of menstrual blood, making it difficult to distinguish between the two, then it is associated with Liver deficiency/yin deficiency/heat or Spleen deficiency/Liver excess/blood stasis. Women with significant blood stasis may have two periods a month. However, women who present with irregular bleeding should be referred to a gynecologist for a checkup because of the possibility of uterine fibroids or uterine cancer.

INFERTILITY

There are various reasons for infertility. However, if the patient is ovulating and if there is no problem with her male partner, then acupuncture and moxibustion should be able to successfully treat her condition. The most common pattern is Liver deficiency/yang deficiency/cold, and the next most common is Spleen deficiency/Liver excess/blood stasis, followed by Liver deficiency/yin deficiency/heat. Other yang deficiency cold patterns, such as Spleen deficiency/yang deficiency/cold and Kidney deficiency/yang deficiency/cold, can also cause difficulties in conception, probably because of a basic lack of bodily strength, a fact which has to be dealt with. It is commonly believed that working women are also less able to conceive, again possibly because they are often relatively tired.

Another possible reason for infertility is poor sexual technique or lack of basic knowledge about sex. In the past, there have been cases where women believed that in order to become pregnant all they had to do was fall asleep in the arms of their lovers. In other cases, the patients had a simplistic belief that as long as sperm entered their vaginal tract, they would automatically become pregnant. Sometimes it is necessary to counsel a couple that they need to make sure that the woman is sufficiently stimulated so that her Bartholin's gland is excreting fully before coitus to maximize the chances of conception.

Pulse diagnosis can provide one method of evaluating a woman's fertility. A woman is able to conceive when her overall pulse is relaxed and full of Stomach qi and her proximal pulses are neither excessive nor deficient. Naturally, one of the goals when treating a woman for infertility is to obtain such a pulse.

Uterine Fibroids

A relatively common patient inquiry concerns uterine fibroids. As no one wants to undergo surgery unless it is absolutely necessary, most patients would prefer to clear up the condition with acupuncture, moxibustion, and herbs. However, uterine fibroids are quite difficult to successfully cure. Therefore, if the case involves prolonged bleeding and subsequent anemia, I often recommend surgery. Also, if the location of the fibroid is such that it compresses the rectum or bladder, again it is best to have surgery, sooner rather than later.

In cases of prolonged bleeding, acupuncture and moxibustion can help the patients recover from the ensuing anemia sufficiently to allow them to have the surgery. Under these conditions it is best to treat using a protocol for Liver deficiency/yang deficiency/cold or Spleen deficiency/Liver excess/blood stasis.

Treatment

For irregular menstruation, the root treatment should be administered according to the appropriate pattern. In addition, the points listed in Table 19-2 should be checked for pain on pressure; those that are painful should be added to the treatment. This will usually result in a cure. However, if there is blood stasis, the number of points that will require shunting will naturally increase. On the other hand, if the problem is a result of yang deficiency, the treatment will consist essentially of tonification.

For menstrual pain, just leaving needles in place at SP-6 is often enough to stop the pain. If this is insufficient, then select points from Table 19-2. When the menstrual pain is accompanied by heat, LR-14 should be shunted. For endometriosis, Bl-31 to BL-34 should be used.

For Trichomonas vaginitis and candida infections, LR-8 should be shunted. If there is a lot of vaginal discharge, LR-5 should be shunted and scarring moxibustion should be applied at SP-5 and KI-3. Alternatively, apply scarring moxa to the 'inner' GB-37 point, which is found on the medial aspect of the leg at the same height as GB-37.

For infertility, midline flow moxibustion (see Chapter 14) can be performed using 20 to 30 half-rice-grain sized moxa cones. Alternatively, scarring moxibustion can be performed at SP-6, CV-2, GV-4, and BL-23 with seven half-rice-grain sized moxa cones on each point.

Table 19-2	Branch Treatment Points for Problems of the Female Genitals
Problem	Points
IRREGULAR MENSTRUATION	**ST-25**, ST-28, ST-29, SP-6, **SP-10**, KI-11, KI-13, **GB-26**, GB-31, GB-39, LR-6, LR-8, LR-9, **CV-3**, **CV-6**
PROFUSE MENSTRUATION	**SP-1**, SP-5, SP-6, KI-3, LR-2, **CV-7**
AMENORRHEA	ST-25, ST-30, SP-6, BL-22, BL-24, **KI-5**, **GB-41**, GV-4, CV-3, **CV-4**, CV-6, CV-12
MENSTRUAL PAIN	**ST-35**, ST-36, **SP-6**, **SP-10**, SI-26, BL-25, LR-3, **LR-5**, LR-9, CV-6, CV-7
LOWER ABDOMINAL PAIN	GB-27, GB-28, **LR-5**, **LR-8**, LR-12
VAGINAL DISCHARGE	ST-28, **SP-6**, BL-27, BL-32 to BL-34, **KI-12**, **GB-26**, **LR-6**, GV-1, GV-3, **CV-2**, CV-4, CV-5, CV-7
UTERINE BLEEDING	SP-6, BL-55, KI-2, KI-6, GB-34, LR-1, LR-3, LR-5, LR-6
INFERTILITY	**ST-27**, **ST-28**, SP-5, **SP-6**, **BL-23**, BL-31, BL-33, KI-2, **GV-4**, **CV-2**

Case History

PATIENT: 22-year-old unmarried woman

CHIEF COMPLAINT: This patient came to the clinic for menstrual pain and associated lower back pain, coupled with nausea.

VISUAL: Her cheeks were red but her lips were pale, giving me an uneasy feeling. She was of normal build with a little bit more water in her tissue than usual.

SYMPTOMS: She would often catch cold. She had an appendectomy three years previously.

She wrestled during her student years, resulting in residual sciatica on the right side. Her stools were generally hard, but they softened during menstruation. She had scanty urination three times a day and no appetite.

At the time of her visit to the clinic, she had been suffering from a fever with nausea and diarrhea for a week. She took some over-the-counter cold medication. Two days previously, she began to experience menstrual pain, and on the morning of the visit, it worsened; she took some over-the-counter pain killers, but to no avail.

PULSE: The pulse was sunken, rough, and tight. The left medial pulse was excessive and the right medial pulse was deficient.

TREATMENT: The pulse as well as her cold led me to believe that I was dealing with menstrual pain related to a Spleen deficiency/Liver excess/blood stasis pattern. In this case, retaining needles at SP-6 points bilaterally is usually enough to quell the pain. However, this had absolutely no effect on her pain whatsoever. After this, I jumped right in and placed retaining needles at BL-23, BL-27, and BL-28 without performing a root treatment. After 10 minutes, she complained of feeling chills and a worsening of the pain. This was probably caused by heat pooling in the uterus, leaving the rest of the body cold. I probably should have treated this patient for yang deficiency from the very beginning.

I regretted not having fully examined her pulse and abdomen, but after a more thorough examination, I decided that her pattern was that of Spleen deficiency/Kidney deficiency/cold. I tonified KI-3, but with no result; in fact, the chills became worse, and she began to lose her vitality. This was a terribly wrong treatment, so I had no other choice but to request a doctor acquaintance of mine to give the patient an injection to stop the pain. Two days later, while I was away from the clinic, one of my students treated the patient in my absence. According to the records, chills were no longer present, but she complained of lower back pain. The treatment consisted of tonifying PC-7 and SP-3, followed by retaining needles in the back associated points. After 10 minutes, the patient complained of abdominal pain and a cramping and numb feeling from the left lower back along the Gallbladder meridian on the left leg. Remember that among her original complaints, she mentioned that she was suffering from right-sided (but not left-sided) sciatica.

The patient received Do In massage for her lower back pain, as well as herbs; however, Poria and Licorice Decoction (茯苓甘草湯 *buku ryō kan so tō/fú líng gān cǎo tāng*) had no effect. Almost predictably, the local doctor acquaintance had to be called in, and she was once again given an injection for the pain. After this, she slept for a while and upon wakening, went to the toilet and urinated. This was followed by a resumption of the chills, numbness of the leg, lower back pain, and abdominal pain, which became worse. Her temperature was checked and found to be 37.4°C, indicating a mild fever.

The injection was given once more, and she fell asleep. Later, in order to ask a member of her family to collect her, she was asked to give her family's telephone number. She seemed strangely unsure whether to give the number or not; it turned out that she had in fact run away from home. She was living on her own, the landlord being her uncle. He was asked to come and collect her, and he explained that she had lived with her older sister and mother but had had an argument and ran away from home.

Five days later, there was a telephone call from the patient requesting treatment for abdominal pain. However, as she had already finished menstruating, I advised her to have a checkup with her gynecologist. Another five days passed, and I received information to the effect that she had gone to the gynecologist as I suggested, but the abdominal pain did not diminish. The pain was so intense that she lost consciousness, stopped breathing, and had to be rushed by ambulance to the local state hospital where she was admitted for two days. At this point I realized that this young lady's abdominal pain was due to hysteria, and in reality she wanted to return home to her mother. I talked to the patient about this and advised her to resolve her dispute with her mother and return home.

The next day she came to the clinic complaining of menstrual pain. She had returned to her mother's place and the pain was less than before. She also had lower back pain. I treated her for a pattern of Kidney deficiency/yang deficiency/cold. I simply tonified KI-7 and did some contact needling around the lower back, resulting in an immediate cessation of pain. After this, she no longer suffered from menstrual pain.

19.3   PROBLEMS OF PREGNANCY AND CHILDBIRTH

Diagnosis

A woman is able to conceive when her overall pulse is relaxed and full of Stomach qi and her proximal pulses are neither excessive nor deficient. Naturally, one of the goals when treating a woman for infertility is to obtain such a pulse. When conception does occur, the pulse changes: the overall pulse becomes somewhat rapid and slippery, with the right distal pulses being slightly deficient and the proximal pulses starting to become excessive.

A rough, thin, sunken, and rather slow pulse during pregnancy indicates that there is a possibility of miscarriage, as the pattern is one of Liver deficiency/yang deficiency/cold. Women with a Lung deficiency constitution are also more liable to miscarriage. Although the young people of today prefer thin underwear, it is important to keep the lower body warm, and so 'sensible' underwear should be recommended.

After conceiving, women often experience morning sickness. If they have a large amount of phlegm and thin mucus, the problem can get quite severe. On the other hand, those that have little phlegm and thin mucus can escape quite lightly and not suffer much from morning sickness. Treatments aimed at a pattern of Spleen deficiency/yang deficiency/cold or Spleen deficiency/yin deficiency/heat are commonly used for this problem.

Some pregnant women have difficulty urinating and have edema of the lower limbs, which can occur in the absence of a serious renal problem. Sometimes the water that builds up in this state can engulf the Lungs and cause coughing. There are even cases where the patient develops kidney stones (see Chapter 18) during pregnancy. From a traditional medicine perspective, this condition is caused by heat building up in the Bladder, with the pattern being that of Kidney deficiency/yin deficiency/heat.

Some pregnant women become more prone to catching colds because of the imbalance in the distribution of heat: heat gathers on the inside of the body, leaving correspondingly less yang qi on the outside of the body. Colds during pregnancy are commonly treated as a Lung deficiency/yang deficiency/heat pattern. Other problems often associated with pregnancy include constipation (Chapter 17), hemorrhoids (Chapter 17), and lower back pain (Chapter 14).

Wang Shu-He in the *Pulse Classic* discussed the meridians that nourish the fetus at different stages during pregnancy. In ancient China as well as in Japan today, the gestational period is counted as 10 months and not nine, as in the West. The list is as follows:

First month	Liver
Second month	Gallbladder
Third month	Pericardium
Fourth month	Triple Burner
Fifth month	Spleen
Sixth month	Stomach
Seventh month	Lung
Eighth month	Large Intestine
Ninth month	Kidney
Tenth month	Bladder

Note that in this scheme the Heart and Small Intestine meridians are associated with pregestational menstruation and postpartum breast milk.

This way of looking at pregnancy is exactly right in many ways. For instance, if the Liver meridian is not functioning properly, conception is difficult. During the fifth and sixth months of pregnancy, when the Spleen and Stomach meridians are particularly active, we normally see an increase in appetite of the mother. We also know that in the last stages of pregnancy, moxibustion at BL-67 can be effective in helping with difficult births or breach positions of the fetus.

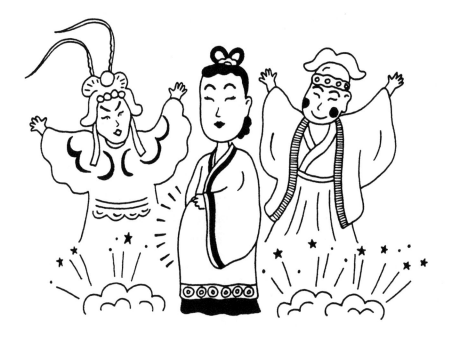

Pregnancy is not a disease

Treatment

It is said that scarring moxibustion at M-LE-1 (裏内庭 *ura nai te/lǐ nèi tíng*) is good for morning sickness, but I have not found it to be particularly useful. I have found that it is more effective to treat hard points located just lateral to BL-58 until they soften. I also personally do not treat points on the upper body if there is nausea, as I believe that these disperse the yang qi, which is a very precious commodity for pregnant women. However, Fukaya, the master of moxibustion, recommended scarring moxibustion at GV-11, GV-10, CV-18, and CV-17.

As a preventive measure against miscarriage, salt moxibustion is recommended at CV-8. This is done by burning moxa cones on a bed of salt that has been packed into the navel until the patient feels the warmth. The treatment can be done either before conception or during the pregnancy. Edema during pregnancy can be treated by scarring moxibustion at SP-6; however, I find that KI-8 is more effective. Colds during pregnancy are treated as a pattern of Lung deficiency/yang deficiency/heat. After the root treatment, contact needling should be administered on the upper back and shoulders. At the same time, tonifying LU-5 and shunting LI-4 will also deal with the stiff shoulders that develop secondary to a cold during pregnancy.

Applying scarring moxibustion at SP-6 is a well-known technique for nourishing the fetus and encouraging the health of the mother. To my knowledge, the first person to present this publicly in modern times was Ishino Shinyasu, a doctor who published an article on this subject in the *Journal of the Japanese Oriental Medical Society* in 1960. It was also mentioned in Edo period texts. The technique should begin in the third month of pregnancy. If the mother feels good during the treatment, 30 to 50 moxa cones can be safely burned. However, if the point location is incorrect, the treatment can feel very hot to the mother. This is a sign to stop and relocate the point again. This is true for moxibustion in general during pregnancy.

Scarring moxibustion at SP-6 is also effective for constipation, hemorrhoids, and lower back pain during pregnancy. If the hemorrhoids do not respond to the treatment, then administer scarring moxibustion on LU-6 instead; if the constipation does not respond to the treatment, then administer scarring moxibustion on SI-4 instead. The pattern that is commonly seen in cases of lower back pain is Liver deficiency/yin deficiency/heat. In addition to the root treatment, contact needling and heat perception moxibustion over the local area, plus needling to BL-58 and BL-59, should be performed. During pregnancy, I do not retain needles in the lower back.

If the birth looks as if it is going to be delayed, I usually recommend that the mother take leisurely walks, as this helps the fetus to descend and encourages a safe birth. If this is ineffective, the fetus is either in a breach position or this is the mother's first baby, both of which can result in a difficult birth. Scarring moxibustion using three to five moxa cones at BL-67 should be administered to facilitate the birth.

19.4 POSTPARTUM PROBLEMS

Diagnosis

There are many types of postpartum problems that can be effectively treated with acupuncture and moxibustion. The most commonly seen problems are headaches, insomnia, stiff shoulders, insufficient lactation, fever, diarrhea, hemorrhoids, emotional disturbances, and dizziness. As noted at the beginning of the chapter, although mastitis and uterine prolapse are not always postpartum-related, they are nevertheless also discussed in this section.

In many Edo period texts, a moderate, slippery pulse is considered a healthy sign during the postpartum period while a wiry, big, and excessive pulse or a rough and urgent (extremely rapid) pulse is considered to be unhealthy. A moderate, slippery pulse reflects the presence of heat, which is to be expected because in a normal birth, the mother will be lacking in blood and this will cause some heat from deficiency to be produced. However, if there is too much deficiency heat, the pulse becomes wiry, big, and excessive. On the other hand, if deficiency heat is not produced, the pulse will become rough and extremely rapid as the last remnants of heat collect in the chest as part of a Liver yang deficiency pattern.

When there is a lack of blood, we are talking about Liver deficiency, but if there is too much deficiency heat, it will rise up to the head and cause fever, headaches, insomnia, dizziness, eye pain, and emotional disturbances. Another possibility is that the deficiency heat will enter the yang brightness meridian, leading to mastitis, or enter the yang brightness Large Intestine organ, leading to hemorrhoids and abdominal pain. Alternatively, the deficiency heat may enter the blood and cause blood heat, which represents a shift from Liver deficiency/yin deficiency/heat to Liver excess heat; both patterns give rise to the same sort of symptoms. In fertile women, the most common presentation is that of Spleen deficiency/Liver excess while in older women, Lung deficiency/Liver excess is more common. Over time, the Liver excess/heat will lead to blood stasis.

On the opposite end of the scale, if someone has very little deficiency heat, they become blood deficient and thus suffer from chills. The pattern is that of Liver deficiency/yang deficiency/cold and is characterized by symptoms such as feeling cold, diarrhea, lack of appetite, abdominal pain, insomnia, headaches, hot flushes, dizziness, and uterine prolapse.

Other postpartum symptoms can all basically be dealt with effectively by treating them as a pattern of Liver deficiency/yin deficiency/heat, Spleen deficiency/Liver excess/heat, or Liver deficiency/yang deficiency/cold.

Treatment

Traditionally, Japanese women used their eyes as little as possible after giving birth because mothers in the postpartum period develop blood deficiency, which makes the eyes—the sensory organ of the Liver—vulnerable. Doing things like reading the newspaper and watching television could often result in eye strain and pain as well as headaches. Shunting LR-14 can treat headaches and fevers that result from Liver excess. Insomnia in these patients can be treated using scatter needling on the temples. This vulnerability extends even to their later years when they are more likely to suffer from cataracts as a result of the overuse of their eyes during this period. All of this should be explained clearly to every pregnant woman so that she knows to use her eyes as little as possible after giving birth.

Lack of breast milk is a problem for some mothers but is usually dealt with effectively by treating any hard points on the medial aspect of the shoulder blades (around BL-42 and BL-43) and on the chest (LU-1, SP-20, and around SP-21) as well as by treating posterior HT-1 (後極泉 *ushiro kyoku sen/hòu jí quán),* which is located by palpating the area just posterior to the axillary crease and finding a hard, painful nodule. Some mothers who suffer from poor breast milk flow immediately decide to put their babies on formula. This is actually not such a good idea because the baby will become more susceptible to infections and the mother will also be more likely to suffer from mastitis. Mastitis is also best treated by working on any hard points on the medial aspect of the shoulder blades and on the chest, as well as doing moxibustion (two to three cones) locally. (See the cautionary note below concerning moxibustion.) Of course the root treatment is also very important, and in most cases, the presentation is one of Liver deficiency/yin deficiency/heat, with the heat going into the yang brightness meridian.

Table 19-3	Branch Treatment Points for Postpartum Problems
Problem	Points
INSUFFICIENT LACTATION AND MASTITIS	LU-1, LI-8, LI-10, SP-20, SP-21, SI-1, SI-2, SI-11, BL-42, BL-43, CV-17, posterior HT-1
HEADACHES	GB-41, LR-14
MENTAL-EMOTIONAL DISORDERS	LI-4, SP-6, TB-6, GV-12, GV-20, CV-6
DIZZINESS	ST-36, SP-6, KI-1, PC-8, TB-3, TB-6
ABDOMINAL PAIN	SP-6, CV-2 to CV-5, CV-7
INSOMNIA	GB-40, GB-41
HEMORRHOIDS	LU-6, GV-20
UTERINE PROLAPSE	SI-8, BL-31, LR-1, LR-8, CV-3
FEVER	LR-14
LEG PAIN	Points 5 units lateral to CV-12

Moxibustion administered on a postpartum mother runs the risk of increasing the heat trapped in the woman's body. If there is blood heat, moxibustion will feel hotter than usual. The same thing applies to the use of moxibustion during menstruation: it feels much hotter than usual. In these cases, be careful when applying scarring moxibustion in order not to cause blood heat.

Case History

PATIENT: 40-year-old woman

CHIEF COMPLAINT: The patient gave birth 14 years prior, but directly after doing so, she felt that she had lost her sanity. She would utter strange things and was unable to reply satisfactorily to questions that were put to her. She received psychiatric treatment at that time and recovered. Recently, however, she became extremely sensitive to anything that was said about her, and was unable to control herself. She had a persecution complex. She felt restless and compelled to make phone calls here and there. She was known for being silent with people but would talk incessantly to her husband. Whenever she displayed this manic-type behavior, she would lose her appetite.

VISUAL: Her build was average, and her tongue showed nothing unusual. Her eyes were small in comparison to the rest of her face, and had a preoccupied look about them.

SYMPTOMS: The patient was on antianxiety medication from her psychiatrist; as a result, her appetite was good. She suffered from constipation, insomnia, tinnitus, stiff shoulders, and hot flushes. She did not have cold hands or feet.

PULSE: The left distal pulse was sunken, wiry, and deficient; the left medial pulse was sunken, rough, and excessive; and the left proximal pulse was wiry and deficient. The right distal pulse was wiry and forceful; the right medial pulse was somewhat deficient; and the right proximal pulse was wiry and normal.

ABDOMEN: CV-14 and the area below the ribs on both sides displayed muscular resistance, with the right side having the stronger resistance. On either side of the navel, spreading as far away as the area above the McBurney point, there was resistance to pressure that was indicative of blood stasis. In addition, both flanks were tight, and there was resistance and pain on pressure at the pubic symphysis and the left and right inguinal areas.

TREATMENT: I was undecided whether to treat for Spleen deficiency/Liver excess/blood stasis or Lung deficiency/Liver excess/blood stasis. I decided to treat for the latter. I tonified KI-10 and shunted LR-8. I then retained needles at the hard areas of the abdomen and back. During the treatment, the patient did not speak at all apart from extremely curt replies to my questions. Needling on the back, arms, and legs caused some involuntary movements by the patient.

Two weeks later, the patient displayed severe pain on pressure at SP-6 and SP-8 and also below the right side of the ribs. The left proximal pulse still showed deficiency, and the left medial pulse was excessive. However, the right distal and medial pulses were normal, and the overall pulse had quickened, developing a rapid quality. This meant that the pattern was still that of Lung deficiency/Liver excess/blood stasis but that the blood stasis had lifted somewhat, resulting in some heat returning to the Liver. I thus shifted my treatment, tonifying KI-7 and shunting LR-2. This treatment was repeated about six times, causing the Liver excess pulse to change to a Liver deficiency/yin deficiency pulse. At the same time, she began, bit by bit, to talk. The subjects ranged from the differences she had with her mother precluding her visiting her hometown to how tired she was but was putting on a brave face.

From this time on, I treated her for a pattern of Liver deficiency/yin deficiency, tonifying KI-10 and LR-8. I also retained needles at areas of deficiency of nutritive qi (that is, the hollow areas) on the abdomen and back. Apart from this shift, I did not do anything special, and treated the patient once a week. After six months of this regime, her vitality returned, and after another four months, she was able to take part-time employment. However, because of her Liver deficiency/yang deficiency constitution (her smaller than normal eyes revealed this), I cautioned her not to overdo it. At this point, the treatment was discontinued.

19.5 MENOPAUSAL PROBLEMS

Diagnosis

This set of problems is commonly known in Japan as problems of the blood pathway (血の道 *chi no michi*). The gynecologist would group the various symptoms into what is termed menopausal syndrome because these symptoms tend to occur before or after menopause. The other reason is that there are so many symptoms that do not fit neatly under any other disease category; it is easier to label it all under menopause. However, among those women suffering from menopausal symptoms, there are those who are obviously suffering from emotional and psychiatric problems, and so in extreme cases, they should also be referred to a physician.

Menopausal women often complain of a variety of symptoms. It is very important to attentively listen to all of the complaints because this in itself is an important part of the treatment. Even if you feel that the patient is completely unwarranted in her fears, it is important not to criticize her in any way and not to laugh at any thing she may say. If the patient gets the feeling that she is not being taken seriously, you will find that she will not appear for her next appointment and you will not be able to help her.

If you convince the patient that she is not suffering from anything life threatening and gain her confidence, then, if she can feel even temporary relief from her symptoms with the treatment, she will start to believe in the treatment process. However, you must understand that if you enter into this relationship, you might receive telephone calls at any time of the day or night from the patient asking such things as whether it is all right to have a bath, eat at a certain time, or defecate in a certain way. With this method, it may really take a long time before it can be said that the patient is cured.

The point is that the only way to approach perimenopausal symptoms is to silently and attentively listen to everything the patient has to say while treating her to the best of your ability. Then it is up to the patient to become aware of her emotional state on her own. All we can do is wait and not become entangled in the patient's complaints. While, of course, the symptoms of the patient are important, we must be clear and decide on the pattern. Once this is done and the general direction of treatment is apparent, it is important not to shift and change the diagnosis with every new complaint.

Complaints often heard from menopausal women include headaches, a heavy sensation in the head, hot flushes, cyclical hot and cold sensations, stiff shoulders, insomnia, depression, irritability, a feeling of uneasiness, emotional upset, palpitations, loss of appetite (but food can be consumed once a meal is started), diarrhea, constipation, irregular bleeding, menstrual pain, lower back pain, lower abdominal pain, and cold legs. These symptoms usually do not register as any specific disease from a medical perspective, and the various laboratory tests and imaging studies will come back as normal. These tests, in fact, can be a disservice to the patient. Given their age, if enough tests are done, there will be at least one test that is abnormal, no matter how trivial or irrelevant the finding. For example, if the patient has slightly elevated blood pressure, she will be pronounced as suffering from hypertension. Often in these cases, the medical treatment will make the woman feel worse and have no positive effect on her long-term health.

Table 19-4	Branch Treatment Points for Perimenopausal Problems
Problem	**Points**
HEAVY HEAD, PAIN, AND FLUSHES	ST-36, SP-6, BL-10, GB-20, GB-38, GB-40, GB-41, GV-15, GV-17, GV-20
INSOMNIA	BL-2, GB-4, GB-40, M-BW-35, points along Governing vessel that are painful to pressure
ALTERNATING FEVERS AND CHILLS	GB-38 to GB-41
STIFF SHOULDERS	SI-11, BL-42, BL-43, GB-21
PALPITATIONS AND CHEST DISTRESS	KI-7, CV-4
LOSS OF APPETITE	SP-1

Many women who suffer significantly from menopause have some sort of domestic problem and are unable to express it verbally or choose to express it through one of the symptoms described above. Therefore, when treating these women, it is important to let them have their say and listen to everything in a nonjudgmental manner. Finally, most of the women should be treated for Liver deficiency/yin deficiency/heat or Lung deficiency/Liver excess/blood stasis.

Treatment

Let me first start by saying that there is no special treatment for this problem. So we go back to the basics: carry out the root treatment. Next, we examine the organ-meridian system and determine which ones have been infiltrated by heat or cold. This is done by carefully locating hard areas and those that are painful on pressure and treating them, most commonly using retained needling, moxa head needling, and scarring moxibustion. Contact needling can be used, but is not as effective as the other methods. Commonly used points for specific problems are noted in TABLE 19-4.

Case History

PATIENT: 55-year-old woman

CHIEF COMPLAINT: The patient came to the clinic because she suffered from tinnitus, occipital headaches, facial edema, irritability that was marked by an inability to accomplish tasks, stiff shoulders with tension rising up through the neck, hot flushes of the head, palpitations, night sweats, and pain, numbness, and weakness of the right side of the body.

SYMPTOMS: Apart from the chief complaints, she had cold feet, urinated frequently yet had a feeling of retained urine, sweated easily from the upper body, found it difficult to fall asleep, and felt thirsty. Her appetite and stools were normal.

VISUAL: She had a good build and was slightly overweight. Her skin was darker than average. Her tongue was dry with sticky saliva. Her movements were slow and clumsy.

PULSE: The left distal pulse was sunken, wiry, and forceful; the left medial pulse was sunken, wiry, and excessive; and the left proximal pulse was deficient. The right distal pulse was wiry and forceful; the right medial pulse was wiry and deficient; and the right proximal pulse was also wiry.

ABDOMEN: The chest felt warm, and the area beneath the right ribs exhibited resistance, pain on pressure, and some water retention, that is, there was suffering and fullness in the chest and ribs (see Chapter 8). In addition, the left side of the abdomen was tight and cramped, the navel showed resistance and pain on pressure, and the Gallbladder meridian demonstrated marked pain on pressure.

TREATMENT: After I examined the patient for the first time, I referred her to a neurologist for possible brain damage because the movements of her whole right side were so cumbersome and slow. The results showed, however, that there were no irregularities.

The patient insisted that her present condition started after a traffic accident she had five years before; however, the symptoms were not typical of such an event.

I believed that I was dealing with a menopausal condition and that the correct pattern would have been Spleen deficiency/Liver excess/blood stasis but for the fact that both the right and left distal pulses were strong. I therefore chose to treat for a Lung deficiency/Liver excess/blood stasis pattern. I began by tonifying KI-10 and shunting the Liver using LR-8, and the Gallbladder using GB-38. I also applied moxa head needling to SP-6 and to the right GB-30.

After this treatment, the strong distal pulses faded, and because of this, I treated her at the next visit for a Spleen deficiency/Liver excess/blood stasis pattern by tonifying PC-6, SP-4, and SP-2 and shunting GB-41, LR-2, and TB-3. I repeated this treatment for about three months on a more or less daily basis. Depending on the day, the painful areas of the patient changed, and so I would palpate these areas for the most painful points and retain needles or apply moxa head needling to these points. The most commonly used points were ST-36, SP-6, BL-23, BL-25, and GB-30.

She responded well and recovered to the point where her symptoms had almost disappeared. At this point, I decided that it was no longer necessary for her to come into the clinic and that she could be treated by a member of her family at home. I marked the points GV-12, BL-13, BL-18, BL-23, and BL-52 and instructed them to burn 20 rice-grain-sized cones of scarring moxibustion on each point. The patient reported that she felt no heat from the moxibustion whatsoever. The moxibustion was continued for one week at home, and I was very surprised to see that all of her symptoms had completely disappeared. Moxibustion at the last stage of the treatment process seemed to have finished things off nicely. However, I believe that moxibustion would not have been appropriate while the distal pulses were still strong in the early stages of the treatment.

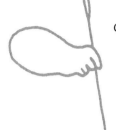

CHAPTER 20

NEUROLOGICAL AND
PSYCHOLOGICAL DISORDERS

THIS CHAPTER DISCUSSES a wide variety of emotional, neurological, and psychiatric diseases, including dizziness, insomnia in its various forms, depression, mania, schizophrenia, obsessive-compulsive disorder, headaches, and seizure disorders. However, not all of these conditions should be treated with acupuncture and moxibustion. Neuroses can range from simple and easy cases to those that do not respond very well to acupuncture and moxibustion treatment. When dealing with emotional and nervous problems, it is important to have the relevant knowledge and training in mental health; otherwise, the encounter can be extremely difficult. This is especially true when dealing with schizophrenia: things may temporarily appear to be going well, but a mistake in the treatment approach can make the patient's condition worse. It is necessary to refer these patients to a psychiatrist. Another example is depression, which can range from simply feeling a little bit down to real full-blown depression. The former is not so much of a problem, but the latter is extremely difficult, carrying with it a distinct possibility of suicide. If considerable care is not taken, grave mistakes can occur. Thus, although acupuncture and moxibustion are good treatment modalities, if there is any doubt, the patient should be referred to the relevant specialist.

Full-blown manic behavior is difficult to handle, and, again, it is best to leave this type of patient to a psychiatrist. Even those who present with what appear to be simple cases of insomnia or headaches may actually be concealing the fact that they are suffering from depression or other emotional disorders. Also, there are those who have been through the hospital system without success and ask to have their insomnia cured. Of course, we should get as much information from the physicians and psychologists about the status and history of the patients, but there are times when we have to make an educated guess about what is going on. Therefore, it is best to have some knowledge to call upon.

When there is no underlying serious disease, problems such as headaches, heavy-headedness, and hot flushes respond very well to acupuncture and moxibustion. However, there may be patients who present with these symptoms that are suffering from high blood pressure or even subarachnoid hemorrhage, conditions that may require medical treatment.

As far as seizures are concerned, almost every patient suffering from this disease is on medication and does not often present with this symptom as their chief complaint. If the patient appears to have clouded mental capacity, you are probably dealing with a serious case of epilepsy. The treatment of epilepsy is discussed in the classics, but I have not dealt with enough of these patients to profess any real confidence in how best to treat them.

20.1   DIZZINESS

Diagnosis

Patients often present with symptoms including dizziness, light-headedness on standing, and instability. There are many possible causes, including exhaustion, anemia, low blood pressure, high blood pressure, menopause, Menière's disease, chronic inflammation of the middle ear, and brain tumors.

Light-headedness on standing that is caused by anemia is often not so problematic, but if the anemia is significant, it will require appropriate treatment. If the condition is caused by high or low blood pressure, usually the instability is mild enough that the patient can stand up. Menopause-based conditions commonly exhibit light-headedness and instability on standing rather than dizziness.

Dizziness can range from a mild disturbance to a debilitating condition. We will limit the discussion here to cases that range from mild to instances where the patient cannot get up ('prostrating vertigo'). The latter condition is often seen in cases of Menière's disease, which is characterized by recurrent prostrating vertigo, progressive (fluctuating) hearing loss, possible nausea, and tinnitus. The causes of the disease are not well understood by Western medicine. Also there is dizziness or vertigo whose cause is said to be unknown, but this is often due to exhaustion.

Most patients with dizziness will have had a medical evaluation prior to visiting an acupuncture clinic, and so it is always a useful exercise to ask what diagnosis they were given. However, if they have not been evaluated by a physician, it may be a good idea to refer them initially for a medical checkup because it is possible that the dizziness is caused by a serious condition that is outside our scope of practice, such as a brain tumor or subarachnoid hemorrhage. In these cases, the dizziness is often accompanied by difficulty in walking a straight line, vomiting, and/or an excruciating headache.

In premodern texts, various terms are used for dizziness, each with a slightly different meaning, including 冒眩 (*bō gen/mào xuàn*), 目眩 (*moku gen/mù xuàn*), 頭眩 (*zu gen/tóu xuàn*), and 眩暈 (*gen un/xuàn yùn*). The character common to all of these terms is 眩 (*gen/xuàn*), which means to be dazzled, as if the light is too bright for the eyes. This is a type of visual disturbance resulting in dizziness. Another common character is 暈 (*un/yùn*), which means faint or light-headed. Together they make up perhaps the most common term for dizziness: 眩暈 (*gen un/xuàn yùn*). In the sixth-century text *Discussion of the Origins and Symptoms of Disease* by Chao Yuan-Fang, the pathology of this condition is described as follows:

> Wind dazzling is caused by a deficiency of blood and qi, [and arises] when the wind pathogen enters the brain and tugs on the visual system. The essential qi of the five yin and six yang organs all flow into the eyes; the blood, qi, and vessels all meet and go upward, becoming part of the brain, and exit via the neck. The deficient body will be afflicted by the wind pathogen, and if this enters the brain, it will cause the brain to spin and the visual system to cramp. When the visual system is cramped, it will cause [a sensation of being] dazzled. The pulse will be flooding and big, and if it is long, this means wind dazzling. If there is a floating pulse affecting the yang meridians [the Yang Linking vessel and Gallbladder meridians], there will be dizziness.

In section 38 of the same text, discussing eye diseases, the author states:

> The eyes represent the flowering of the essences of the five yin and six yang organs and are the location where the ancestral vessels [宗脈 *sō myaku/zōng mài*] gather. The essence of the sinews, bones, blood, qi, and meridians all join and become the visual system. This system goes upward into the brain. If the organs are deficient and the wind pathogen exploits this deficiency, it will follow the visual system and enter the brain, causing it to spin, cramping the visual system, and [causing] minute eye movements and [a sensation of being] dazzled.

The wind pathogen can be taken to mean that the Liver is deficient and produces heat. In the passage above, a pattern of Liver deficiency/yin deficiency leads to heat that moves from the brain to the eyes and causes dizziness.

The Edo period text *Principles of Acupuncture and Moxibustion* observes that, "If there is no phlegm, there will be no [sensation of being] dazzled. When the phlegm is in the upper area and [there is] fire below, if the fire flares upward, it disturbs the phlegm." In this passage, the author is saying that dizziness will result when the "fire below"—the heat generated by Kidney deficiency/yin deficiency or Liver deficiency/yin deficiency—acts on the large amount of phlegm in the "upper area"—the Stomach.

Another Edo period text, the *Pulse Method Handbook*, explains things this way:

> Obese, pale-skinned people have a large amount of dampness, and phlegm collects in the upper body. This is caused by the fire below; the phlegm rises upward with the fire. So if there is no phlegm, there cannot be [a sensation of being] dazzled. Thin people have a lack of Kidney water, and so the ministerial fire flares up and causes dizziness. When the wind pathogen is dominant, [it will feel like] there are earth tremors. When fire receives wind, [it will feel like] there is a swirling blaze.

Those who have a tendency to retain a large amount of phlegm and are obese become

Kidney deficient, which causes deficiency heat to rise up, leading to the sensation of being dazzled. In this case, "ministerial fire" refers to the deficiency heat created by Kidney yin deficiency. "Wind pathogen being dominant" refers to deficiency heat produced by Liver deficiency/yin deficiency. When this is combined with Kidney deficiency, the result is fire receiving wind, which leads to dizziness.

When I read these classical texts and combine them with my own experience, I conclude that dizziness is usually caused by either a pattern of Liver deficiency/yin deficiency/heat, Liver deficiency/yang deficiency/cold, or Spleen deficiency/yin deficiency/heat. The dizziness that originates from a pattern of Spleen deficiency/yin deficiency/heat is caused by deficiency heat spreading to the Gallbladder meridian. In addition, there are cases of dizziness that result from a sudden drop in yang qi. This is not discussed in detail here because it is not common.

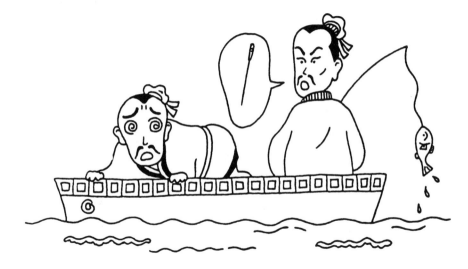

Acupuncture is effective for motion sickness

Treatment

Anemia is a common cause of dizziness, particularly when the symptom is that of feeling light-headed. Women tend to suffer from this more than men because of their menstrual bleeding and because of various problems associated with the lower burner, for instance, hemorrhaging from fibroids. When the patient is anemic, the anemia must be treated. If there is no other complicating disease, acupuncture and moxibustion can effectively treat the anemia. There is no special method for treating anemia; we just determine the pattern, treat to the best of our ability, and the anemia should clear up. The most common pattern for this type of problem is Liver deficiency/yang deficiency/cold. For the branch treatment, perform scarring moxibustion at such points as SP-6, BL-18, BL-20, and BL-22.

When the patient is experiencing dizziness, first retain needles at the abdomen, head, arms, and legs. However, if the patient has a pattern of Liver deficiency/yang deficiency/cold, you must be careful when retaining the needles: do not use too many needles, and keep them in place for only a short time.

A point that is often used for dizziness is GV-23. Another point on the head that can be used is *to yo* (当陽), which is an extra point that is found halfway between GB-15 and GB-16; it can be thought of as GB-15.5. The interesting thing about this point is that if a needle is retained at *to yo,* both the Liver and the Gallbladder pulses will become larger. Other useful points are listed in TABLE 20-1.

Table 20-1	Branch Treatment Points for Dizziness
Location	Points
ARMS AND LEGS	Yin deficiency: **ST-36, TB-3, GB-38, GB-39, GB-41** Yang deficiency: **ST-42, BL-62, BL-63, GB-40** Spleen deficiency/yin deficiency with Gallbladder heat: **GB-38, GB-41**
HEAD	**GB-4**, GB-13, **GB-15, GV-20**
NECK	BL-10, GB-12, **GB-20, TB-17**
ABDOMEN	**ST-21**, ST-25, **CV-4, CV-12**, CV-13, **CV-14**
BACK	BL-14, **BL-18, BL-20**, BL-45, GV-13

Case History

PATIENT: 63-year-old woman

CHIEF COMPLAINT: Three years before, the patient began to experience occasional bouts of dizziness. She went to the hospital and underwent various tests, including an MRI. Nothing abnormal was found. A month prior to her visit the dizziness returned, most often in the morning. The dizziness made it difficult for her to walk.

VISUAL: Her complexion was dark but without any luster. She looked nervous. Her tongue was dry and lacked a coating. She had long narrow eyes.

SYMPTOMS: The sides of the abdomen were sensitive and twitching. The area from the inside of the shoulder blades to the neck was stiff. The right arm was cramping from LI-15 downward. Her legs were cold, and she had cramps around GB-41, sometimes making it difficult to walk. She passed hard stools once every two to three days. She was not clear about her urination, but she did have to get up once a night to urinate. Her appetite was fine, but she admitted to domestic problems that made her irritable and unable to sleep on occasion. She had a thirst and drank a large amount of tea. She also used her hands a great deal.

PULSE: The left distal pulse was sunken, wiry, and forceful; the left middle pulse was sunken, tight, and deficient; and the left proximal pulse was sunken, tight, and deficient. On light touch, the Gallbladder pulse was deficient. The right distal pulse was sunken, wiry, and forceful, and the right medial and proximal pulses were sunken, rough, and thin.

ABDOMEN: The middle of the chest felt warm, and the epigastric area from CV-12 to CV-14 showed resistance on pressure. There was cramping on both the left and right flanks of the abdomen. There was pain on pressure on the left and right inguinal folds right up to the top of the iliac crest. Finally, there was a thin, hard line below the navel on the Conception vessel.

PALPATION: There was pain on pressure along the leg pathways of the Gallbladder meridian, and the inside of the right scapula was extremely stiff, with indurations.

CONSIDERATIONS: The long, narrow eyes indicate a Liver deficiency constitution. Looking at the signs and symptoms, we can see that there is an irregularity in the Gallbladder meridian. While the Gallbladder pulse is not floating, the symptoms do include thirst and constipation. The forceful left and right distal pulses and the heat in the chest are indicative of a Liver deficiency/yin deficiency/heat pattern, which could explain the dizziness. The left middle and proximal pulses are both sunken and tight, suggesting a lack of fluids. However, the fact that the Gallbladder pulse is not floating indicates that the heat has not invaded the Gallbladder meridian, but is instead stuck in the chest. The resistance found in the epigastric region is due to phlegm and thin mucus, and the thin, hard line below the navel on the Conception vessel is indicative of Kidney deficiency. (I forgot to check this with the patient, but this probably reflects a history of bladder infections.) Therefore, from the above, I surmised that this patient with a Liver deficiency constitution had become pathologically Liver deficient, producing deficiency heat. The phlegm and thin mucus then caused the heat to stick in the chest, causing dizziness.

As far as the prognosis is concerned, if the pulse becomes softer overall and the Gallbladder pulse appears, the patient should recover. At the same time, if we could remove the resistance in the epigastric region and the stiffness from the inside of the scapula, things would be perfect.

TREATMENT: Needles were retained at CV-14, CV-12, ST-19, ST-25, and CV-4 on the abdomen as well as *to yo*, GV-23, and TB-17. The root treatment consisted of tonifying

KI-10, LR-8, GB-38, and GB-41. Needles were also retained at stiff points found on the inside of the scapula where the nutritive qi was deficient.

Following treatment the patient felt good, saying she felt like her blood vessels had expanded. The next day, after the same type of treatment, she felt better, although she did complain of slight dizziness two days after that. By the second week of treatment, she had made a complete recovery. Her Gallbladder pulse was easily discernible on light pressure, the resistance in the epigastric region had diminished, and the hard, thin line below the navel had disappeared.

20.2 INSOMNIA AND MENTAL AND EMOTIONAL DISORDERS

Diagnosis

The conditions discussed in this chapter are somewhat wide-ranging and would not be classified together in a textbook on modern medicine. They are placed together here in part because people who suffer with mental and emotional disorders are themselves not aware of their problems and only know that they have trouble sleeping. It is the insomnia that brings them to our clinics. In addition, their pathologies are quite similar and can be treated by acupuncture and moxibustion using similar methods.

INSOMNIA

In traditional medicine, insomnia is intertwined with the imagery used to describe the yin and yang organs. The processes of sleep and sleep disturbances are dependent on the circulation of yang qi and blood as follows:

• The yang qi generated by the Spleen and the Stomach rises to the Lungs from which it is circulated throughout the body. During the day, this yang qi circulates through the yang areas, animating areas that include the head, eyes, and other sensory organs. At night, the yang qi enters the yin areas, resulting in sleep. However, if for some reason the yang qi does not enter the yin areas, there will be some leftover yang qi in locations such as the head and eyes, causing insomnia.

• Blood is the other half of the equation. The Liver is said to store blood. During the day, blood and qi are circulated to locations as needed. At night, the blood returns to the Liver. If for some reason the blood cannot return to the Liver, then insomnia results.

Based on these pathways, I will explain various types of insomnia as well as some commonly seen psychiatric disorders. Note that, regardless of the type of insomnia, the right proximal pulse will be stronger than usual and the overall pulse will often be rapid. Even if a patient complains of insomnia, if the pulse is not rapid, the patient is in all probability sleeping but does not feel rested.

Difficulty in falling asleep: This is caused by the yang qi not entering into the yin areas, usually as a result of the yang qi being stuck in yang meridians, especially in the head. Once the yang qi eventually enters into the yin areas, sleep will follow. An example of this state is the intake of alcoholic beverages to such an extent that the person gets tipsy. After this state wears off, the individual will be unable to sleep because the hot qi from the alcohol still resides in the head.

The method for curing this problem is to tonify the deficient meridians and to shunt the affected yang meridians. The only problem is that if the diagnosis is incorrect, the treatment will have no effect whatsoever. Normally, it is effective to treat for Spleen deficiency by tonifying the Pericardium and Spleen meridians followed by shunting the yang qi of the yang brightness meridians into the yin areas. With this type of insomnia, patients will commonly feel sleepy after meals since the yang qi is gathering in the Stomach, 'stealing' the available yang qi from the head; the lack of yang qi in the head makes the person feel sleepy.

Awakening during the night: In this case, heat is already present inside the body, most commonly in the Heart or Lungs, probably as a result of deficiency heat from Liver deficiency/yin deficiency or Kidney deficiency/yin deficiency spreading to the chest. At night, the yang qi moves to the inside and combines with this heat, resulting in a large amount of internal heat that moves up to the head and eyes, thereby activating them.

Unable to sleep at all: Here, there is simply not enough blood and so it is unable to return to the Liver. This type of pathology is often seen in cases of postpartum or postoperative insomnia. This is, of course, best treated as a pattern of Liver deficiency/yin deficiency/heat or Liver deficiency/yang deficiency/cold.

After sex, the participants usually sleep because stress has been relieved, and they feel relaxed. In some cases, this is not the case, and they cannot sleep even after sex. This is again because of a lack of blood. People with this pattern who exercise and think too much can also suffer from sleeplessness. Anything that leads to exhaustion of the blood can generate total sleeplessness.

Waking up early: This is common among the elderly because they are yin deficient and therefore produce a large amount of deficiency heat. It is the outward and upward movement of this heat that causes them to wake up early.

Excessive dreaming and not feeling rested after sleeping: This is often seen in people with constitutional Liver deficiency who tend to have long, narrow eyes or small eyes. In addition, their ears are folded sharply at the first fold—the antihelix—and when viewed from behind, this fold juts out beyond the helix. They are usually very positive about their work, requiring that it be done systematically and exhaustively; otherwise, they are dissatisfied and can become irritable. Their brain may also be whirring away 24 hours a day, and they therefore find it difficult to relax. Another way of looking at it is that these people live their lives and usually manage to maintain their balance within the constraints of a Liver deficiency pattern.

This type of background makes them prone to insomnia. When this constitutional tendency becomes pathological, they have many dreams and do not feel rested after sleeping. If they continue to exert themselves, their blood deficiency can worsen to the point where they become unable to sleep whatsoever. When this happens, the sides of the rib cage are cold because their Gallbladder qi is not being circulated.

The discussion above provides a brief explanation of the pathology of insomnia. Sometimes modern medicine makes a connection between these types of problems and mental and emotional diseases. For this reason, I will briefly discuss the differentiation of depression, mania, schizophrenia, and obsessive-compulsive disorder. Insomnia due to significant mental and emotional disease should be treated by someone with adequate training and ability in treating mental health.

MENTAL AND EMOTIONAL DISORDERS

Depression: Many people tend toward depression rather than suffer from outright depression. More often than not, we are likely to see these types of patients in our clinics rather than those who have been diagnosed as depressed by a psychiatrist or psychologist.

There are many reasons for depression. Someone moves to a new area and finds it difficult to fit in and therefore feels depressed. Another person has been involved in various volunteer activities but does not feel appreciated; consequently, the person feels depressed. A person moving into old age who experiences a symptom such as incontinence can also become depressed.

Depression can be thought of as an extreme form of exhaustion. Sufferers want to be liberated from this situation, but even though they want to make a go of it, they just do not have the energy to do so. Unfortunately, well-meaning friends, often with the best of intentions, encourage them to do their best, extolling them to cheer up and get well as soon as possible. Even at home, families may rebuke the sufferers. Consequently, the depressed individuals feel even more depressed and under pressure to do something that they are incapable of doing. They feel that they want to die but do not have the energy to do so. Some depressed individuals may actually commit suicide after they build up some energy as a result of receiving therapy. This means that we need to be especially vigilant with these patients and maintain a good connection with them.

Depressed patients are not expressive facially or verbally and often want to die. It is important to be attentive and confirm these tendencies so that you can immediately refer suicidal patients to the appropriate practitioners and support organizations. Also, you must definitely refrain from trying to cheer or pep up these patients. They are exhausted both mentally and physically and so should be encouraged to rest and take it easy. If you feel confident enough to be part of their treatment team, you must tell the patient that they can call at any time if they feel suicidal. It you cannot do this or are too uncomfortable with this responsibility, do not treat these patients. The patterns that most commonly correspond with depression are Spleen deficiency/yang deficiency/cold, Spleen deficiency/Liver excess/blood stasis, and Lung deficiency/Liver excess/blood stasis.

Mania: Either as a disease itself or part of a bipolar manic-depressive disorder, mania is treated as a pattern of Spleen deficiency/Stomach excess/heat. Recently, people with this condition are often under the care of specialists. Therefore, it is unusual for us to see someone in their manic state in the clinic. Still, even when the sufferer is under medication, they may nevertheless exhibit manic symptoms if, say, they are traveling and become excited or overindulge in alcohol. They are usually very big eaters and like to sing. It is best to leave these cases to a specialist, but sometimes these patients can be treated to good effect. However, I am not sure whether a complete cure can be achieved.

Schizophrenia: These patients experience a range of hallucinations and delusions and may claim to have had contact with aliens or feel qi so strongly that they are unable to live a normal life. If a patient begins to say things that go way beyond the bounds of common sense, you may suspect schizophrenia. Sometimes it can be difficult to distinguish between neurosis and schizophrenia.

With schizophrenia, there may be visual and auditory hallucinations, or the patient may start to talk to himself. When this occurs, it is best to refer the patient to a specialist. Without special psychiatric knowledge, it would be reckless folly to take on cases like these.

Obsessive-compulsive disorder: While patients with an obsessive-compulsive disorder may know on some level that the focus of their fixation is trivial, nevertheless they still become obsessed. This is common among people that know themselves well internally. There is no desire to commit suicide and no visual or auditory hallucinations. Having said this, these cases can be difficult to deal with, and if you lack confidence, refer the patient to a specialist. The important thing is to listen attentively to the patient.

Treatment

Retain needles at BL-2 and GB-4, as well as on the abdomen, to treat insomnia, schizophrenia, or obsessive-compulsive disorder. Another method includes performing contact needling to the temples around M-HN-9 (太陽 *tai yō/tài yáng*). On the legs, shunt the Gallbladder meridian (GB-38 or GB-41). On the upper back, needle or treat with heat perception moxibustion painful spots between GV-9 and GV-12, and apply retaining needles at points such as BL-13 to BL-15 as well as points between the scapulae. The latter will help the patient sleep.

Liver excess is a characteristic of depression. By means of the controlling cycle of the five phases, Spleen deficiency is the most common root pattern. The root treatment for depression is to tonify PC-6 and SP-4. This is a variant of the root treatment using the connecting points in order to tonify not only the yin meridians (Spleen and Pericardium here), but also their yang counterparts (Stomach and Triple Burner). This approach is often used for stubborn diseases.

In the elderly and in patients with long-standing depression, there can also be Kidney deficiency, which leads to a Lung deficiency/Liver excess presentation.

The branch treatment consists of treating muscular resistance found below the ribs with moxa head needling or heat perception moxibustion. For manic disease, if it is possible, thicker Chinese needles should be retained to shunt LI-4 and ST-36. If the patient settles down sufficiently, the area of the forehead should be shunted. Other branch treatment points for all these conditions are listed in TABLE 20-2.

Table 20-2	Branch Treatment Points for Insomnia and Mental and Emotional Disorders
Location	**Points**
ARMS AND LEGS	ST-36, ST-38, SP-1, SP-9, BL-37, BL-38, BL-40, BL-55, BL-57, KI-1, **M-LE-5**
HEAD	GB-11, **GV-17, GV-20**, GV-24
ABDOMEN	GB-26, CV-6, **CV-12**, CV-13
BACK	**BL-13, BL-14, BL-17**, BL-18, BL-19, **BL-42**, BL-43, BL-45, GB-20, GB-21, **GV-9 to GV-12**

Case History

PATIENT: 26-year-old male public official

CHIEF COMPLAINT: This patient obsessed over things to such an extent that he lost his appetite and thus lost weight. He also suffered from insomnia.

VISUAL: There was nothing particularly evident in his face. However, I had been treating this patient from the time he was a child, so I could see from his complexion that he had lost some vitality and weight.

SYMPTOMS: He had always had a weak Stomach and Intestines and was prone to diarrhea. Apart from this, there was nothing unusual. The thing that was bothering him had to do with his car. He became obsessed with the idea that when he drove on gravel, the stones displaced by the motion of the car would hit innocent pedestrians and perhaps cause an accident. As a result, he stopped driving his much-cherished car. He was an exceptionally bright and serious student, and when he began working, I well remember cautioning him not to take things too seriously at work.

PULSE: The overall pulse was sunken, wiry, and strong; it also had a tense, rough quality.

ABDOMEN: The rectus abdominal muscles were tight on both sides, and there was a feeling of fullness and stiffness in the epigastric region.

TREATMENT: I decided to treat the young man for a pattern of Spleen deficiency/yin deficiency/heat, and therefore tonified PC-6 and SP-4. For the branch treatment, I retained needles in the painful points found by palpating the upper part of the Governing vessel—from GV-9 to GV-14—as well as BL-20 to BL-22.

After a few treatments, he began to sleep better and started to regain his appetite. He did not, however, recover enough to drive again. Because he had a very loving and supportive family who lived in comfortable circumstances, it was hard for him to become independent. After approximately a year of treatment, he resumed driving.

20.3 HEADACHES

Diagnosis

Headache, heavy-headedness, and flushes appear as symptoms in a variety of diseases, for instance, hypertension, subarachnoid hemorrhages, brain tumors, and even fevers associated with infections. Flushes are a common symptom of menopausal problems. The type of headache, heavy-headedness, and flushes we will consider here are those that occur despite the absence of any particular disease.

In traditional medicine, these symptoms are thought to reflect the circulation of yin and yang qi. Yin and yang qi circulate through the body by means of the yin and yang meridians, respectively, and balance between the two is maintained by the rising of the yin qi and the sinking of the yang qi. However, yang has a tendency to rise and yin a tendency to sink. Because of this state of affairs, when the yin and yang balance is disrupted, the yang qi remains up while the yin qi remains down, resulting in symptoms such as cold feet, heavy-headedness, and flushing of the head. To effectively treat this condition, the circulation of the yin and yang qi should be renormalized. To accomplish this, one portion of the yang qi is discharged from the head, allowing the other part to descend to the lower burner; the yin qi in turn rises to the upper part of the body. This approach is very useful in the diagnosis and treatment of conditions affecting the head.

The first task is to identify the meridian with the trapped qi. This can more or less be determined by questioning the patient concerning the headache. For migraines, it is the lesser yang meridian; for frontal headaches, it is the yang brightness meridian; for occipital headaches, it is the greater yang meridian; and for headaches located at the top of the head, it is the Liver meridian. The affected meridian can be deduced from the routes of the meridians and the nature of the headache.

There are times, however, when the patient complains of pain throughout the entire head. It is important to know why these headaches manifest in these areas. On such occasions, we query the patient regarding the type of pain and the timing of the pain. Also, we examine the abdomen and the pulse to obtain confirming information to solidify the diagnosis.

There are headaches caused by blood stasis; they typically begin at night. The patient may also feel that the head is caught in a vise. This condition is treated as a pattern of Spleen deficiency/Liver excess/blood stasis, and mainly the Liver and Gallbladder meridians are used in its treatment. Migraines can be mistaken for blood stasis headaches, but migraines are commonly a result of a pattern of Liver deficiency/yin deficiency/heat.

Occipital headaches often occur in conjunction with stiff shoulders. In its acute form, this is best treated as Lung deficiency. In its chronic form, it is usually best treated as a pattern of Kidney deficiency. Frontal headaches are caused by Spleen deficiency with heat in the yang brightness meridian. Frontal headaches can also occur as a result of Spleen deficiency/yang deficiency/cold. This commonly occurs when the Stomach is cold. In such cases, the yang qi of the yang brightness meridian cannot return to the Stomach, thus leaving heat stuck in the Stomach meridian.

Heavy-headedness, where the whole head feels heavy, is caused by a large amount of phlegm and thin mucus, and is best remedied by tonifying the Spleen and Stomach. This should cause the circulation of yang qi to improve, clearing the phlegm and thin mucus and lightening up the head. The pattern is that of Spleen deficiency/yang deficiency/cold. Flushes and overall headaches are commonly caused by either a Kidney deficiency or Liver deficiency pattern with deficiency heat.

Treatment

In addition to treating the basic pattern, it is also important to consider the branch treatment to the head in terms of deficiency and excess. There are occasions when touching the head can cause the pain to increase; sometimes even lightly touching the hair can elicit pain. These are symptomatic of an excess pain condition, which means that even if the pattern is one of yang deficiency, the branch treatment should consist of shunting the painful areas of the head using a reasonably thick Chinese needle or a thicker than usual Japanese needle; this will probably result in a little bit of pain.

By contrast, if touching the painful area feels good, the condition is one of deficiency pain. This is often effectively treated by retaining needles at the painful sites. Sometimes the area may feel puffy to the touch, in which case scarring moxibustion in the form of three to five half-rice-grain sized moxa cones should be applied, with good results.

Pain in the area around GV-20 is commonly caused by blood stasis. Depending on the severity of the pain, this can be treated by pricking the painful area to let out a few drops of blood.

It is all very well to treat the head, but if there are flushes, treating the head may make the problem worse if it is not done skillfully. When there is a possibility of this occurring, it is best to use points on the arms and legs. Also, sometimes the headaches are caused by stiff shoulders; in such cases, the stiff shoulders should be treated. Finally, the underlying pattern itself must be addressed. For instance, if the headache is associated with a pattern of Spleen deficiency, points on the abdomen should also be used. TABLE 20-3 lists points that can be used to address these issues.

Table 20-3	Branch Treatment Points for Headaches and Related Symptoms
Location	**Points**
ARMS AND LEGS	Headaches: LI-4, LI-11, ST-44, SI-4, BL-62, GB-41 Heavy headedness: ST-42, PC-9 Flushes: BL-58, PC-3, LR-5
HEAD	BL-10, GB-4 to GB-6, GB-20, **GV-15, GV-17, GV-20,** GV-21, **GV-22,** GV-23
ABDOMEN	ST-21, ST-25, CV-4, CV-12 to CV-14
BACK	SI-14, BL-11, BL-42, GB-21, GV-11

Case History

PATIENT: 50-year-old woman

CHIEF COMPLAINT: This patient had a long history of suffering from headaches, vomiting, and diarrhea on a monthly basis.

VISUAL: She was thin and pale; her tongue was moist and looked anemic.

SYMPTOMS: She habitually suffered from soft stools and little appetite. She had chills in both the hands and feet. The headaches did not coincide with her menstrual periods, which were regular. She had no thirst, and when she felt nauseous, saliva would build up in her mouth. Her urine appeared to lessen when she had her headaches.

PULSE: The overall pulse was sunken, rough, deficient, and a little bit slow. The left proximal pulse was deficient, although the left distal and medial pulses were not so bad. The right distal pulse was not so deficient, but the right medial pulse was deficient.

ABDOMEN: There was an overall weakness and softness about the abdomen with no resistance or tightness anywhere. The flesh itself also felt weak and feeble.

TREATMENT: In the initial stages, I decided to treat her for Spleen deficiency/yang deficiency/cold, but any slightly deeper needling always made her headaches and vomiting worse, after which it took three to four days to recover. To be honest, I was not sure whether the acupuncture was helping her and whether the recovery period was a natural phenomenon.

I reconsidered the abdominal diagnosis and the pulse and decided to treat her for Spleen deficiency/Kidney deficiency/cold where the root treatment simply consisted of tonifying KI-3. Next, I concluded that her headaches were probably caused by heat stuck in the yang brightness meridian, despite the lack of abdominal and pulse signs to back up this guess. To treat this problem, I very lightly shunted ST-44. I was also very careful with the abdomen and back and used only contact needling to tonify the areas where the protective qi was deficient. With this treatment, the headaches and vomiting ceased after one session. I continued treating her using this strategy for a year, and she had no further recurrence of the headaches.

20.4 SEIZURE DISORDERS

Diagnosis

Seizure disorders—also known as epilepsy—are chronic conditions characterized by some alteration in consciousness, often in combination with uncontrolled bodily movements. Traditional medicine primarily deals with grand mal seizures that are characterized by attacks during which the patient loses consciousness and suffers whole body muscular spasms. In premodern texts, seizures fall under a variety of rubrics including withdrawal-mania (癲狂 *ten kyō/diān kuáng*), mania-withdrawal (狂癲 *kyō ten/kuáng diān*), and fright wind or childhood convulsions (驚風 *kyō fū/jīng fēng*). The character 狂 (*kyō/kuáng*) means run amuck, go insane, and mania; the reason why this character is included in the term for seizures is probably because the pathology is considered to be similar in these various conditions. In addition, in some cases of seizure disorders, the mental faculties of the patient are adversely affected, which is another possible reason why the character is used. In *Guide to Etiology*, the very highly regarded Edo period practitioner, Okamoto Ippo, opposed the lumping together of these pathologies and stated that, according to the approach outlined in *Basic Questions*, mania and seizure disorders should be regarded as separate entities.

However, I believe that dividing seizures into mania (狂 *kyō/kuáng*), withdrawal (癲 *ten/diān*), and convulsions (癇 *kan/xián*) is not entirely without merit because they all share similar pathologies. Indeed, in *Guide to Etiology*, Okamoto observes that all three of these occur because of the combination of phlegm, thin mucus, and heat. Mania is said to be due to a large amount of heat, giving a yang excess pattern. Relative to mania, withdrawal is thought to be more closely associated with deficiency heat, rather than excess heat. In Chapter 20 of the *Classic of Difficulties*, mania is described as redoubled yang (重陽 *chō yō/chóng yáng*) and withdrawal as redoubled yin (重陰 *chō in/chóng yīn*). Heat is said to be at the root of withdrawal, while the branch problem is phlegm. And in Chapter 59, phlegm is said to be at the root of convulsions, while the branch problem is heat.

From the above we can deduce that the mania discussed in the classical texts corresponds to what modern medicine calls manic disease. In any case, we learn from the classics that:

- Withdrawal and convulsions are caused by phlegm and heat.
- Withdrawal and convulsions have more deficiency heat than mania.
- Heat plays a bigger role in withdrawal than in convulsions.

As far as patterns are concerned, withdrawal is caused by either Spleen deficiency/Liver excess/heat or Lung deficiency/Liver excess/heat, and convulsions are caused by Liver deficiency/yin deficiency/heat. Regardless of the pattern, there is a characteristic buildup of heat that originates in the chest and migrates to the head.

In the case of Spleen deficiency/Liver excess/heat, the Liver excess heat rises to the head via the lesser yang meridian. This is surprisingly easy to cure. By contrast, a pattern of Lung deficiency/Liver excess/heat includes an element of Kidney deficiency/yin deficiency, which means that the generated heat rises to the head via the marrow. This pattern is difficult to cure. Finally, a pattern of Liver deficiency/yin deficiency/heat produces deficiency heat that rises to the head, which is relatively mild and is easy to treat.

Treatment

I have not seen enough cases of seizures to write any case histories, but I do have enough experience to list a few points that are useful, which I will describe below and in TABLE 20-4. I will also list one set of points that is recommended in important premodern texts.

The main thing to recognize about treating seizures is to check the upper back on the Governing vessel for pain on pressure. Retained needles and moxibustion should be applied at points such as GV-9, GV-11, and GV-12 that exhibit pain. For children, moxibustion should be applied at GV-12.

If the patient does not exhibit dulling of the mental faculties and experiences only mild convulsions and very brief periods of unconsciousness, apply a root treatment and follow this by retaining needles in the reactive points on the Governing vessel and back-associated points. The root treatment will often be for Liver deficiency/yin deficiency/heat, and following this protocol should result in a cure in about three years. In a few cases, following this protocol has been known to completely reverse EEG irregularities.

However, it is very difficult to cure cases where the patient has both seizures and some clouding of the mental faculties. I am actually treating one of these cases at the moment, and although the patient notices that his body feels light and he is sleeping better, the main symptoms do not appear to have changed much.

Quite a few premodern texts, such as the fourteenth-century *Yellow Emperor's Moxibustion Classic of the Bright Hall* and the sixteenth-century *Introduction to Medicine*, as well as a number of Edo era books, mention demon crying (鬼哭 *kiko ku/guǐ kū*) moxibustion to treat seizures. This is done by tying the thumbs and toes together with string and applying four cones of scarring moxibustion at SP-1 and LU-11. These books state that, because the digits are tied together, one cone can be used to burn both well points at once. A fine idea! However, there is no need to fixate on this part of the technique as one can get good results from doing the treatment one point at a time.

Table 20-4	Branch Treatment Points for Seizures
Location	Points
ARMS AND LEGS	LU-11, **BL-62**, KI-1, **KI-6**
HEAD	BL-10, GB-20, GV-20, GV-22, GV-24
SHOULDERS AND BACK	BL-18, BL-23, BL-42, BL-52, **GV-8, GV-9, GV-11, GV-12**
ABDOMEN	ST-19, LR-14, CV-14

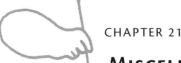

CHAPTER 21

Miscellaneous Disorders

T HE DISORDERS DISCUSSED in this chapter are those that are commonly seen in my clinic and which do not fit into the other categories discussed in Part Two. I will deal here with problems of the eyes, teeth, ears, skin, and thyroid as well as diabetes and disorders of children. It would have been nice to have a separate chapter on endocrine diseases, including thyroid problems and diabetes mellitus. Unfortunately, while hyperthyroidism and diabetes are common problems in my clinic, I do not have much experience treating other endocrine diseases. For this reason, I have included thyroid problems and diabetes mellitus here, but not other endocrine conditions. In addition, while it would have been possible to have a separate chapter on pediatric disorders, the treatment methods for children are both very simple and very similar to each other, and so I have included these problems here as well.

Diseases of the eyes, teeth, and ears sometimes require a referral to a dentist or physician. These diseases will take longer to heal if the patient has stiff shoulders; thus, if this complaint is present, it should be treated regardless of the main complaint. Diseases of the eyes, teeth, and ears can often be effectively treated with acupuncture and moxibustion, but if the acupuncture and moxibustion treatments are performed in conjunction with medical treatment, the results will be even faster.

21.1   EYE DISEASES

Diagnosis

Patients suffering from eye problems will commonly fall into one of the following traditional and modern categories: pseudomyopia (defective vision resembling myopia), presbyopia (age-related visual problems), color blindness, tired eyes, heat felt in the eyelids, cramping of the eyelids, watery eyes, floaters, bloodshot eyes, blurred vision, abnormal eye secretions, a sense of a foreign object in the eye, dazzled eyes (see Section 20.1), painful eyes, itchy eyes, the appearance of a lattice-type design in the line of vision, double vision, difficulty in focusing the eyes, and even the onset of blindness.

When you see a patient with one of these problems, it is usually best to recommend that they receive an evaluation from an eye specialist before proceeding. This is especially true if the patient's vision is worsening. The patient may receive a positive diagnosis from the ophthalmologist or may be told that there is nothing to worry about; in any case, it is worth referring the patient for an evaluation. Provided that there is no serious causative disease, symptoms such as color blindness, pseudomyopia, tired eyes, heat felt in the eyelids, cramping in the eyelids, watery eyes, bloodshot eyes, hordeolum (a suppurative inflammation of a gland in the eyelid, also called a stye), ingrown eyelashes, and itchy eyes can be cured with acupuncture and moxibustion. While people with color blindness may be able to identify all the colors in a color chart after receiving acupuncture and moxibustion treatments, I have doubts about whether this constitutes a cure by modern medical standards. In addition, depending on the severity of the problem, only a month or so of treatment may be enough to cure pseudomyopia.

More serious problems, such as conjunctivitis, keratitis, corneal ulcerations, cataracts, glaucoma, and detached retinas, are more difficult to treat. It is best if these patients are seen in conjunction with an ophthalmologist. I have had patients with glaucoma that responded poorly to measures instituted by an ophthalmologist but who nevertheless responded well to acupuncture and moxibustion. Also, acupuncture and moxibustion treatments can stabilize bleeding into the fundus of the eye.

Problems like atrophy of the optic nerve, retinitis pigmentosa, cataracts secondary to diabetes, uveitis from Behçet, and iritis are difficult to treat using both modern medicine and traditional medicine. However, if the patient knows this but still asks to be treated, then it is up to the practitioner to persevere even though it will be an uphill struggle.

In traditional medicine, the eyes are associated with the Liver. It is also said that all of the meridians are connected with the eyes. In his early eighteenth-century text *A Collection of Acupuncture and Moxibustion Treasures*, Masatomi Hongo observes:

> The eyes are the outward expression of the Liver and represent the flowering of the essence of the five yin organs. All the meridians connect to the eyes. The iris is Liver wood, the inner and outer edges of the eyes are the Heart fire, the upper and lower lids are the Spleen earth, the whites of the eyes are Lung metal, and the pupil is the essence of Kidney water. If the eyes suddenly become red, swollen, and painful, it is wind-heat of the Liver meridian; chronic dark disease is Kidney disease; difficulty in seeing far is Heart deficiency; [and] difficulty in seeing close up is a lack of Kidney water.

The state of the Liver can be discerned by observing the eyes. The Liver stores blood, and blood nourishes the eyes. It is also true that people with big eyes have a tendency toward Liver excess and those with small eyes have a tendency toward Liver deficiency/yang deficiency as well as more serious eye diseases such as detached retina.

It is also possible to get information concerning various pathologies by checking the different parts of the eye. For instance, drooping eyelids or spasms of the eyelids are often indicative of Spleen deficiency. Diseases of the eye itself, however, are usually indicative of Liver excess or Liver deficiency.

As discussed in Chapter 19, in the past, women who had just given birth were told not to use their eyes because they were already blood deficient and prolonged use of the eyes at this time would consume even more blood, ruining their eyesight. In the modern age, with the widespread use of television and computers, near-sightedness is increasing, especially among elementary school students. All of these problems relate to the overuse and consumption of blood.

In the past, people used to believe that children who suffered from night terrors and bad temper would lose their eyesight. In fact, rather than losing their eyesight, such children would develop Liver deficiency, which would result in muscular spasms and the development of strabismus or a squint. It is a fact that patients suffering from strabismus usually have a pattern of Liver deficiency, which can be cured with appropriate treatment.

As for the pulse, Toshi Yamanobe notes in *Pulse Method Handbook*:

> Eye diseases are wood and fire diseases. When the left distal pulse is flooding and rapid, this is Heart fire flaring up. When the Liver pulse is wiry and flooding, there is a preponderance of Liver fire. When both the right distal and [right] medial pulses are also wiry and flooding, this means that the power of the Liver fire is such that it scorns the metal that tries to intercede but cannot prevail, and [thus the Liver] dominates and suppresses the earth.

According to this passage, we see that eye diseases are due to heat. What we have to be concerned about is where this heat is coming from. Here it says that a flooding, rapid pulse is from the Heart fire flaring up. This pulse is floating, big, strong and, to top it all off, rapid. Because of the location of the pulse, it is clear that it reflects a dysfunction of the Small Intestine meridian; vis-à-vis eye diseases, this would mean that we are dealing with an acute problem with a large amount of inflammation. The overall pattern is that of Spleen deficiency, and the treatment should include shunting the Small Intestine as part of a Spleen deficiency/Liver excess/heat pattern. This type of patient is rarely seen today in acupuncture clinics, as the individual would normally go to an ophthalmologist first.

After the initial stage, the pulse will begin to sink and become stronger. This means that the Heart has begun to absorb the heat. When this occurs, the pattern switches into the more serious Lung deficiency/Liver excess/blood stasis.

Returning to the passage, the author notes that a left medial pulse that is wiry and flooding indicates that there is a preponderance of Liver fire, that is, a large amount of heat in the Liver. Actually, however, a flooding pulse is floating and overflowing in nature; therefore, the text is really referring to a Gallbladder pulse that is floating, excessive, and wiry. This would correspond to the pattern of Liver deficiency/Gallbladder excess or Liver excess/heat.

Also, the Liver fire can influence the Heart via the generative cycle, and the Heart in turn affects the Lungs via the controlling cycle. This corresponds to Liver deficiency/yin deficiency/heat with the heat influencing the Lung and Large Intestine meridians.

Based on this text and my own clinical experience, I would say that the patterns associated with eye diseases are those of either blood stasis (Spleen deficiency/Liver excess or Lung deficiency/Liver excess) or Liver deficiency (yin or yang deficiency). Eye problems that are based on a pattern of Lung deficiency/Liver excess/blood stasis are usually chronic and/or difficult to cure. Examples would include retinitis pigmentosa or glaucoma. On the other hand, eye problems that are based on a pattern of Spleen deficiency/Liver excess/blood stasis are much easier to cure. For instance, hordeolum and ingrown eye lashes are caused by this type of blood stasis pattern. Finally, growths that may appear on the inside of the eyes and nearly obscure the pupils can be caused by either type of blood stasis pattern.

Table 21-1	Branch Treatment Points for Eye Diseases
Problem	**Points**
BLOODSHOT EYES AND SORE EYES	**LI-11**, SI-3, PC-6, PC-7, TB-2, GB-5, GB-6, GB-16, knuckle of distal interphalangeal joint of middle finger
WATERY EYES	**LI-11**, SI-4, SI-19, **GB-20**, GV-24
EYELID INFLAMMATION	**LI-4, LI-11**, SI-3, BL-65, GB-15, GB-21, GV-20, GV-23
KERATITIS	SI-1 to SI-4, **SI-14**, TB-1, TB-3, **TB-20**, BL-18, BL-67, GB-1, GB-20, **GB-21**, GB-40
TIRED EYES	LI-11, ST-36, **BL-10, GB-20**, GV-7
CATARACTS	**LI-14, ST-36**, SI-14, **SI-19, BL-18**, BL-19, BL-43, **TB-20**
CENTRAL RETINOCHOROIDITIS	LI-4, **LI-11, LI-14, ST-36**, BL-13, BL-15, BL-17, BL-20, N-HN-44
GLAUCOMA	**LI-14**, SI-14, BL-43, **GB-20, GB-21**, knuckle of second joint of thumb and middle finger
HORDEOLUM, INGROWN EYE LASHES	**LI-2 (see text), SI-19, BL-43**, point on apex of helix of ear, point on tip of tragus of ear

Treatment

Most eye problems respond well to an appropriate root treatment plus treatment for stiff shoulders. Depending on the type of eye problem, a corresponding branch treatment will be necessary (TABLE 21-1). For pseudomyopia and color blindness, needles should be retained at LI-4, ST-1, ST-8, ST-36, BL-2, GB-1, and GB-3. Other useful points include BL-4, BL-5, BL-8, and BL-9. The needles should be retained at these points for about 20 minutes or so daily, for 15 to 30 days. This will cause the eye problem to start to improve. With color blindness, a color chart should be used to check the results of treatment after each session. Chronic pseudomyopia is more difficult to treat, and the younger the patient, the easier it will be to achieve good results.

An extra point used in the treatment of central retinochoroiditis (inflammation of the choroid and retina) is N-HN-44 (上天柱 *kami ten chū/shàng tiān zhù*), which is located 0.5 units above BL-10. For hordeolum, use moxibustion at the Sawada-style location for LI-2, that is, locate the point on the Large Intestine meridian at the edge of the crease found by bending the proximal interphalangeal joint of the index finger. For bloodshot eyes and sore eyes, use scarring moxibustion on the knuckle of the distal interphalangeal joint of the middle finger, and for glaucoma, apply scarring moxibustion on the middle of the knuckles of the second joint of the thumb and middle finger.

21.2 TOOTHACHE

Diagnosis

Treating the teeth is, of course, normally the domain of the dentist. However, acupuncture can be very effective at treating problems that sometimes resist the effects of pain killers such as stubborn toothaches, cavities, and gingivitis. Simply put, for our purposes, toothache can be considered as being caused by stiff shoulders. Therefore, if we carry out the appropriate root treatment and loosen the shoulders, the pain is usually relieved quite quickly. Having said this, there are some stubborn cases that persist in the face of acupuncture treatment.

The problem usually arises as a result of yang brightness meridian heat or cold, which typically has its origin in Spleen deficiency. We must remember, however, that other patterns can also lead to yang brightness meridian heat, and so we have to ascertain the correct pattern for each person and then shunt or tonify the yang brightness meridian. I can say, though, that toothache from Kidney deficiency is often difficult to treat.

In the *Pulse Method Handbook*, Toshi Yamanobe observes:

> Diseases of the teeth, where the right distal and medial pulses are [either] rapid and flooding or wiry and flooding, [are due to] wind attack of the Intestines and Stomach. When the proximal pulse is flooding, big, and deficient, this is Kidney deficiency. When there is toothache and the teeth are loose, this is the flaring up of fire. *Introduction to*

Medicine says that the teeth are connected with the bones and represent the exterior of the Kidneys. When the [Kidney] essence is full, the teeth will be solid, [but] when the Kidneys decline, the teeth weaken. When there is deficiency heat, the teeth will be loose. The leg yang brightness Stomach [meridian's] connecting vessel goes into the gums of the upper teeth and does not move [further, as it ends there]; cold drinking water is preferred and hot liquids are detested. The arm yang brightness Large Intestine meridian's connecting vessel goes into the gums of the lower teeth and does not stop [as it does not end there]; hot liquids are preferred and cold drinking water is detested. The *Divine Pivot* states that when cold drinking water is not detested, the leg yang brightness meridian should be used. When cold drinking water is detested, it is the arm yang brightness meridian that should be used. So it does not matter if it is the upper teeth or the lower [teeth], the treatment should be based on the like or dislike of cold and heat.

According to this passage, a Stomach meridian toothache feels better when it is cooled and worse when it is warmed; this occurs because there is more of a tendency for heat to collect in the Stomach than in the Large Intestine. I do not think we need to stick too closely to the advice given in the last part of the passage. Of course, there are cases where the toothache feels better when it is warmed, but in most cases, there is a large amount of heat in both the arm and leg yang brightness meridians. In addition, there are times when the heat can spread as far as the lesser yang meridian as well as the Governing and Conception vessels, as in cases of severe sinusitis.

Treatment

Basically speaking, if the diagnosis is correct, the root treatment is appropriate, and the stiff shoulders are made loose by the correct branch treatment, then the tooth problem should be cured. However, it is important to work diligently on the branch treatment (TABLE 21-2). The most often used point is LI-7. However, the entire area between LI-4 and LI-10 should be palpated, and scarring moxibustion should be applied to the hard, painful points. These points tend to manifest as lumps the size of grains of rice and so can be easily missed. If all goes well when the moxibustion is applied, the patient will not feel it as hot at first. The moxibustion is continued until the heat is felt, by which time the pain and swelling of the teeth should have cleared up. For gingivitis, an effective point is M-LE-9 (女膝 *jo shitsu/ nǚ xī*), an extra point found on the back of the heel in the middle of the calcaneous bone.

Table 21-2	Branch Treatment Points for Toothaches
Location	Points
ARMS AND LEGS	**LU-7**, LI-3, LI-4, LI-6, LI-7, **LI-9, LI-10**, ST-36, ST-42, **ST-44**, BL-62, **KI-2**, M-LE-9
HEAD	ST-6, ST-7, SI-5, SI-18, BL-8, TB-17, TB-20, GB-2, GB-5, GB-10, GB-12, GB-17, CV-24

21.3

EAR
DISEASES

Diagnosis

The ears are connected to the Kidneys, but from the perspective of meridian topography, they are primarily supplied by the lesser yang meridians. It is because of this that either Kidney deficiency or lesser yang meridian heat can cause ear problems. Lesser yang heat commonly comes from a pattern of Spleen deficiency/yin deficiency/heat or Spleen deficiency/Liver excess/heat. However, in acute cases, the heat will also have spread to the greater yang and yang brightness meridians, and so it is important to check for areas that exhibit pain on pressure all along these meridians, and to use these points in the treatment.

Ear problems that originate from Kidney deficiency will manifest as tinnitus, sudden deafness, or gradual hearing loss. Ear problems that originate from lesser yang meridian heat usually present as infections of either the middle or outer ear.

My elder brother (alas, now departed) actually broke his eardrum completely due to a febrile disease. We applied scarring moxibustion at BL-23, and over a relatively short time the eardrum grew back and hearing returned to that ear. This example shows that even if the case looks hopeless from a modern medical standpoint, there are times when traditional medicine may be able to help. It is important to always retain a sense of hope even when dealing with difficult diseases.

Treatment

For treatment of tinnitus and poor hearing, scarring moxibustion at BL-23 and acupuncture at TB-17, GB-11, and TB-3 is good. For outer ear infections and earache (including earaches that arise as a result of an inflammation of the parotid glands), KI-2 and LI-11 should be used. For middle ear infections, use KI-2 and apply moxibustion at a point near SP-2 on the inside of the crease formed when the big toe is bent at the first digit. Also, acupuncture at TB-17 is effective.

Table 21-3	Branch Treatment Points for Ear Diseases
Location	**Points**
ARMS AND LEGS	LI-1, LI-5, LI-6, SI-2, SI-4, SI-5, BL-65, TB-2, TB-5, TB-8, TB-9, GB-43
HEAD	SI-19, BL-8, BL-9, TB-21, TB-22, GB-2 to GB-4, GB-10, GB-12, GV-20

21.4   SKIN DISEASES

Skin problems in our society are usually treated by medical specialists. However, it is quite common for acupuncture and moxibustion to be effective when the dermatologist cannot help. Some examples are discussed below.

Diagnosis and Treatment

ATOPIC ECZEMA

Recently, atopic eczema has become the most common form of skin rash. With both traditional medicine as well as modern medicine, this condition is difficult to treat. From a traditional standpoint, the source of atopic eczema is considered to be constitutional Lung deficiency. If this condition transforms into Liver deficiency/yin deficiency/heat and the resulting heat enters the yang meridians, the upshot can be eczema. The transformation of a Lung deficient constitution into Liver deficiency represents a change that follows the controlling cycle; it is, therefore, difficult to cure. There also cases where the change may be from Lung deficiency to Kidney deficiency, resulting in a pattern of Lung deficiency/Liver excess/blood stasis.

Of course, the root treatment should be suitable and the branch treatment should consist of light stimulation. However, areas where the eczema has turned the skin black are indicative of blood stasis, and so it is often good to perform local pricking to cause a small amount of bleeding. In general, the younger the patient, the more successful the result. Patients who are approaching their twenties become Kidney deficient as a result of the side effects of any administered steroids. In these cases, moxa head needling to BL-23 is effective.

Another traditional method that I feel could be effective would be the use of the four flower disease gates (四華患門 *shi ka kan mon/sì huá huàn mén*) method of moxibustion, discussed in Chapter 14. Unfortunately, the young people of today dislike scarring moxibustion, and so I have not tried it for this condition.

ALOPECIA

This is a rather acute form of hair loss that is not related to normal balding, for which there is no effective treatment. This pattern is almost always that of Lung deficiency/Liver excess/blood stasis or Liver deficiency/yang deficiency/cold, the point being that we need to concentrate on treating the Liver and Gallbladder meridians. In addition, it is helpful to perform scarring moxibustion on the problem area, typically using five half-rice-grain sized moxa cones. Depending on the person, there are cases where once hair loss begins, it must go to completion before any regrowth can begin. However, with continued treatment, the patient can be sure that after the hair is lost, it will grow back. Finally, because of the mental and emotional aspects involved in alopecia, it is good to examine the upper part of the Governing vessel (from GV-9 to GV-12) for tenderness on pressure. Scarring moxibustion should be applied at any tender points.

Corns and Warts

Scarring moxibustion can be administered directly on the affected area. When dealing with corns, the moxibustion should be performed with the intention of burning them off. For harder warts, a larger number of cones will be needed to affect a cure. Moxibustion on SI-7 is useful for both. Fukaya, the famous moxibustion practitioner, recommended ST-41, ST-36, and SP-6 for corns. The most common root pattern in these patients is Spleen deficiency/yin deficiency/heat.

Urticaria

This condition can be a result of blood stasis, but in most cases, urticaria is thought to arise as a result of Spleen deficiency with heat in the Small Intestine meridian. LI-15 is useful for treating this problem, but the point is located nearer to the edge of the shoulder than usual. Fukaya suggested a point on the edge of the shoulder (between TB-14 and LI-15) together with TB-14. These points are also useful for other types of skin eruptions.

Frostbite

Frostbite occurs because of insufficient blood, which leads to cold and a vulnerability to environmental cold. Most of the time, the pattern is that of Liver deficiency/yang deficiency/cold. Heat perception moxibustion or thread moxibustion can be applied on the affected area with good results. If the area has darkened, pricking can be done to let out a few drops of blood.

Inflammation of the Bed Beneath the Nails

Scarring moxibustion is performed right in the middle of the nail. Fukaya recommends dividing the nail into three sections, from top to bottom. The middle of the upper section is then taken as the point for scarring moxibustion. Another method is to apply the moxa at the base of the bed of the nail. Normally, just one cone will feel hot, but if this is not the case, the burning of moxa should be continued until it is felt to be hot. It is also effective to combine this point with moxibustion at LI-4 at this time.

Boils

Boils are large, pimple-like lesions that are filled with pus. Due to the use of antibiotics and the overall improvement in nutrition, it is not so common to see these cases anymore. If, however, you do see a patient suffering from the early stages of this condition, lay a slice of garlic over the boil and apply moxa on top of it. This is done until the pain of the boil disappears. Another method is to apply thread moxa around the area of the boil. Scarring moxibustion can also be applied to points that show pain on pressure, including perhaps LI-4, LI-10, ST-36, SI-7, and BL-63. The pattern is that of Spleen deficiency or Lung deficiency with heat in the yang brightness meridian. Fukaya also says that moxibustion to the underside of the angle of the mandible (the point should be painful on pressure) will be effective. According to him, one to five cones of moxa should result in a cure.

21.5   DIABETES

Diagnosis

The traditional condition most closely linked to either type 1 or type 2 diabetes is wasting and thirsting disorder (消渇 *shō kyaku (katsu)/xiāo kě*). This disorder was first noted in *Essentials from the Golden Cabinet*, where it is described as internal heat consuming the fluids of the body, thereby leading to a strong thirst. In premodern texts, there are three divisions of diabetes:

UPPER WASTING (上消 *jo shō/shàng xiāo*): This represents the form of diabetes where the main problem manifests as heat in the upper burner. In this case, the fluids of the Lungs dry out, giving rise to heat. The symptoms commonly include dry mouth, chest pain, mouth ulcers, a feeling of being hot and irritable, and a lack of appetite (although some texts say increased appetite). The stool and urine are normal, although some texts, including the Edo period *Guide to Etiology* by Okamoto Ippo, indicate that even in these cases there is increased urination.

If heat from Kidney deficiency/yin deficiency or Liver deficiency/yin deficiency moves to the Lungs, it will dry out the fluids, causing a dry mouth. This can be regarded as Lung yin deficiency. However, we resist this designation when, in some cases, the right distal pulse is slippery—not deficient—when pressed firmly. In such cases, the Lung pulse is found to be strong even when the overall pulse is thin and weak, including the pulse at the Kidney and Liver positions. As noted above, there is a disagreement in the classics concerning the appetite and amount of urine in these patients. From my experience, it appears that patients have no real appetite but are able to finish a meal once it is begun, and that the urine is often scanty.

MIDDLE WASTING (中消 *chū shō/zhōng xiāo*): This represents the form of diabetes where the main problem is heat in the middle burner. In this case, the fluids of the Spleen are deficient and heat builds up in the Stomach. The main symptoms include dry mouth and an increase in appetite, with a paradoxical loss of weight. In addition, there is spontaneous sweating, constipation, and scanty, dark urine.

When heat from Kidney deficiency/yin deficiency moves to the Stomach, it causes (not surprisingly) Stomach heat, which gives rise to an increase in appetite. (This is discussed in Chapter 12.) If this heat penetrates even deeper than the Stomach, it will attack the Spleen, causing diabetes. However, if the Spleen receives the heat, and if it stays there, death will ensue. The heat is, therefore, normally pushed back out to the Stomach, which is important in the etiology of this disease.

The pulse also reflects this. The right middle pulse is easily felt on light pressure, but is deficient on firm pressure. Also, the left proximal Kidney pulse is (not surprisingly) deficient on firm pressure. The overall pulse is slippery or wiry and strong. When there is a large amount of heat from deficiency in the Spleen, Stomach, and Kidneys, the patient will lose weight because the fluids are drying up; this symptom indicates that the condition is serious.

LOWER WASTING (下消 *ge shō/xià xiāo*): This represents the form of diabetes where the main problem is heat in the lower burner. In this case, the fluids of the Kidneys are deficient, giving rise to a buildup of heat. The main symptoms include dry mouth and scanty urine that is difficult to pass. The limbs begin to waste away and feel hot and irritated, the face and ears display a darkish hue, and there is weight loss.

The three types of diabetes detailed above all display heat in different areas that must be removed. Although there are three locations for this heat, the main source is the Kidneys, particularly in lower and middle wasting. Kidney deficiency/yin deficiency produces the heat that spreads to the rest of the body. With upper wasting, Kidney deficiency may be responsible for the disease, but Liver deficiency/yin deficiency/heat may be the cause instead. There are also cases where diabetes can result from a disease progression related to alcohol abuse that can be viewed as Spleen deficiency/Liver excess/heat, where the fluids of the Kidneys and the Spleen are depleted.

Finally, there are cases where the heat from Kidney deficiency/yin deficiency does not spread to other parts of the organ-meridian system; instead, the heat dries up the fluids of the Kidneys. Of course, in this case, the symptoms will include a dry mouth, good appetite, and some urinary difficulty. However, the urination is often copious and frequent at night because, during the night, the yang qi moves internally, bringing even more heat to the Kidneys and Bladder, which are already overly hot. The pulse will be sunken, slippery, and tight.

Treatment

The root treatment involves quelling the deficiency heat from either Kidney or Liver deficiency. The branch treatment is also very important. For diabetes, moxa head needling at SP-8 and ST-36 is effective. At times, just SP-8 is sufficient, but at other times, it is more effective to combine it with SP-6.

Retained needling can be applied on the abdomen. On the back, moxa head needling is applied at BL-20. In addition, find the tender point somewhere between GV-6 and GV-8 and apply direct scarring moxibustion (7 moxa cones). Other points that are good for moxibustion are GV-1, GV-14, and M-BW-24 (腰眼 *yō gan/yāo yǎn*); 10 cones are sufficient. To locate GV-1 properly, choose a tender point in the area; this is used to treat heat in the Bladder. Here, in particular, it is important to use small cones, slowly introducing the heat by covering the cones with the fingers.

Some practitioners say that moxibustion is ineffective for diabetes, and indeed, words to this effect can be found in some premodern texts. However, this refers to direct scarring moxibustion with a large number of cones that result in suppuration, or moxibustion that is designed to cause suppuration in the first place. These types of moxibustion can be problematic. However, direct scarring moxibustion with 7 to 20 cones is absolutely acceptable. Other points are shown in TABLE 21-4 below, including the use of M-HN-20 (金津;玉液 *kin shin; gyoku eki/jīn jīn; yù yè*), which is located on either side of the frenulum of the tongue.

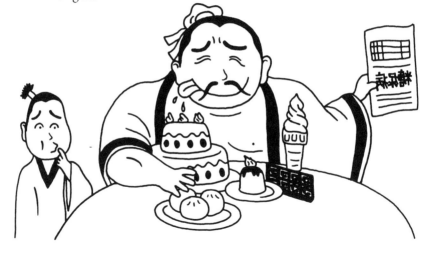

A sweet tooth leads to diabetes

Table 21-4	Branch Treatment Points for Diabetes
Location	**Points**
ARMS AND LEGS	LI-11, ST-43, SP-5, **KI-2**, PC-8, TB-1, LR-2, **LR-3**
HEAD	GV-26, CV-23, M-HN-20
ABDOMEN	ST-25, CV-2, CV-4, CV-6, **CV-12**
BACK	**BL-23**, BL-27, BL-28, BL-29, **BL-49**

Case History

PATIENT: 59-year-old female domestic worker

CHIEF COMPLAINT: This patient was diagnosed with diabetes about five years prior. At the time of her visit to the clinic, her blood sugar level was 400 units, measured two hours after meals.

VISUAL: She was a little overweight, with obvious water retention throughout her body, and marked edema in her legs. Her tongue was dry.

SYMPTOMS: She was unsteady on her feet and experienced numbness of the hands and feet on standing for any length of time. Her knees were painful to the extent that she was unable to kneel, which, for a Japanese, is the equivalent of not being able to sit in a chair for a Westerner. She suffered from stiff shoulders and clouded eyesight, although she did not have cataracts at that time. Her feet were cold with bouts of uncomfortable heat sensations. She had constipation, hot flushes, dry mouth (thirst), and difficultly urinating. She had no real desire to eat but was able to finish a meal once she had started. There was pain on the left side of the chest.

PULSE: The pulse was sunken, rough, thin, and a little rapid. Having said this, the right distal pulse was big, slippery, and excessive; the right medial pulse was rough and of average strength; the right proximal pulse was of average strength; the left distal pulse was a little strong; the left medial pulse was excessive; and the left proximal pulse was deficient.

ABDOMEN: The chest felt hot to the touch and had signs of water stoppage. There was resistance to pressure in the upper abdomen around CV-14.

TREATMENT: From the above information, I believed that the patient had Kidney deficiency with heat in the greater yin meridian that led to the diabetes. KI-7 and LU-10 were tonified and moxa head needling was applied to SP-8, ST-36, and SP-6. Needles were also retained at tender sites on both knees.

   This type of treatment was continued for three days at which point the thirst, unsteadiness on her feet, edema of the legs, and chest pain were alleviated. She also began to develop an appetite, indicating that the heat from the greater yin Spleen meridian was being pushed out into the yang brightness Stomach meridian. However, this process also led to the development of mouth ulcers. A week later, her blood sugar levels were normal, but still her mouth ulcers had not recovered. However, four days later, the ulcers improved, her appetite, stools, and urine were normal, and she began to work again.

21.6 HYPERTHYROIDISM

Diagnosis

This condition is also known as Graves' disease and is due to excessive secretion of thyroid hormones. Women get the disease more often than men, and it is unexpectedly common among patients that come for acupuncture. The type of symptoms that can be seen are swelling of the thyroid gland, abnormal protrusion of the eyeball (called exophthalmos), a tendency to palpitations and exhaustion, a roaring appetite with paradoxical weight loss, a tendency to sweat easily, and a propensity to becoming excited. Traditionally speaking, the pathology is clearly a Kidney deficiency/yin deficiency pattern with a large amount of heat from deficiency. The palpitations arise because the deficiency heat of the Kidneys causes a buildup of heat in the Heart. The increase in appetite is a result of the deficiency heat steaming up to the Stomach. The weight loss occurs because the deficiency heat causes the fluids and sweat to leave the body, and the swelling in the throat area—in this case the thyroid—arises because the deficient Kidney meridian causes the qi to lose its anchor and rise upward, gathering in the upper portion of the meridian.

The classical literature discusses two conditions: steaming bones (蒸骨 *jō kotsu/zhēng gǔ*) and stirring of fire from yin deficiency (陰虚火動 *in kyo ka dō/yīn xū huǒ dòng*). The pathology, signs, and symptoms of these conditions have much in common with hyperthyroidism.

Treatment

There is no need for any special form of treatment. The root treatment should focus on the Kidney deficiency/yin deficiency/heat pattern, with needles retained at points on the abdomen and back, and tonification of both KI-2 and CV-4. The latter point is used because it tonifies the lower burner and thus improves the anchoring, grasping function of the Kidneys. KI-2 is the fire point of the Kidney meridian; tonifying this point will cool the heat from the deficient Kidneys at the same time as it cools the Heart. Treating CV-4 will tonify the lower burner, which improves the anchoring function of the Kidneys.

21.7 DISORDERS OF CHILDREN

The most common complaint involving children is fever from an infection. The next most common complaint focuses on the upper respiratory problems that accompany the infection, such as coughing and asthma. Next in line are digestive disorders (including stomachaches, vomiting, and diarrhea) and emotional and behavioral disorders (including nervousness, overexcitability, truancy, anorexia, and overeating). Acupuncture and moxibustion are suitable for treating these conditions, including anxious or highly strung children. Acupuncture and moxibustion should not be used to treat other internal medical disorders not listed below. The ability to recognize which disorders are suitable and which are not is an important part of clinical practice.

Diagnosis

FEVERS

The most common form of infection in children is colds, but influenza and simple summer fevers also occur quite often. Other childhood diseases that begin with fever include rubella, measles, sudden skin eruptions, and chicken pox. Because they all begin with fevers, it sometimes is difficult to identify the underlying disease, but we should make an attempt to do so. A fever should be taken seriously as there is a possibility that the condition will evolve into such serious problems as pneumonia or meningitis. Acupuncture and moxibustion are more than adequate for treating, say, a summertime fever, but if there is any doubt as to the diagnosis, it is best to refer the patient to a physician. If the fever persists despite the treatment, either the technique is poor or the diagnosis is one of a serious disease.

A fever is usually indicative of Lung deficiency, but if at the same time there is loss of appetite, then the pattern is usually one of Spleen deficiency. If, in addition to a fever, the lips are pale, the ankles are cold, and there is a lack of vitality, the child should be treated for a Spleen deficiency/yang deficiency/cold pattern.

COUGHS AND ASTHMA

In some children, the fever may break, but they are left with persistent coughing or asthma. For adults, this would commonly be treated as Spleen deficiency with Lung heat. With children though, it is often indicative of Lung deficiency. If the asthma is chronic, the pattern may be Spleen deficiency or Liver deficiency. Up to the age of six, children's asthma is usually a result of Lung deficiency.

VOMITING AND DIARRHEA

Some children's diseases result in fever with vomiting and diarrhea. Because there is a real risk of dehydration, the child should be referred to a physician as soon as possible if the patient does not respond quickly to acupuncture and moxibustion. Special care should be taken if the child's lips are more pale than usual. Children are full of yang qi, but in some cases their yang qi can quickly become extremely deficient. In less serious cases, acupuncture and moxibustion are effective.

Sometimes children are treated with a suppository or enema to bring a fever down, but consequently suffer from diarrhea. In most of these cases, the pattern is that of Spleen deficiency/yin deficiency or Spleen deficiency/yang deficiency.

Nosebleeds

Children who are prone to getting nosebleeds usually have a pattern of Spleen deficiency/yin deficiency/heat. Other accompanying symptoms include stomachaches, slouching, and lack of vitality.

Nervousness and Overexcitability

The problems considered here are not connected with fever, and the patterns are determined by considering the signs and symptoms. There are a wide variety of possible basic patterns, including the following:

- Children who are irritable, restless, have a bad temper, and twitch or have convulsions often have a Liver deficiency pattern.

- Children who wake up at night crying as if in shock, try to eat inedible objects, lack an appetite, and have stomachaches, diarrhea or constipation, middle ear infections, and sinusitis or nasal inflammation should be treated for a Spleen deficiency pattern.

- Bed wetting is indicative of either Liver deficiency or Kidney deficiency. If the child is especially fat, the pattern is often Kidney deficiency.

- Children who cry at night with great sadness, have delicate skin, are prone to fevers and swollen tonsils, often have runny noses, and sometimes have headaches are considered to have a Lung deficiency pattern.

Truancy

This is starting to become more of a problem in Japan. It is relatively common in elementary and high school students, and occurs in some cases even in university students. It can be considered as a type of neurosis, but at the university level, it may be indicative of something more serious, such as schizophrenia. To be safe, it is best to refer these children to a specialist.

This problem in elementary and high school students is usually accompanied by complaints of, say, headache, stomachache, or constipation, with these symptoms being used as an excuse not to go to school. If the child succeeds in avoiding school in this way, in a short while, the child will not be getting up in the mornings and will be absent from school for long periods. The mental state of these children varies with the individual, but simply put, they are usually lacking in independence. They are unable to make decisions and act of their own accord, and because of this, they stop going to school. The other way of looking at this problem is to see that in some ways the act of refusing to go to school is a necessary stage that some children have to go through to establish the beginnings of independence.

In this way, it can be considered a sort of 'work slowdown' against parental intervention and criticism.

As far as acupuncture and moxibustion treatment is concerned, as always, we attempt to find the underlying pattern and treat it accordingly. This is actually surprisingly helpful, especially if it is combined with finding out why the child cannot become independent. The conclusion that I have come to in my practice is that the parents are constantly criticizing their children.

Normally, the mother cocoons the child in unconditional love, while the father gives the child a good telling off when he or she is bad. This is the proper yin and yang balance in the household and will encourage the normal development of independence. This balance is disrupted, however, when the mother criticizes and instructs to such a degree that the child becomes a robot. A mother may often say that she was strict with her child, but normally this really means that the child has been ordered around to such an extent that the child does not have the emotional or physical space to develop independent thinking skills. At the same time, recently, fathers have tended to be too kind and too understanding, and this is another factor in preventing the child from becoming independent.

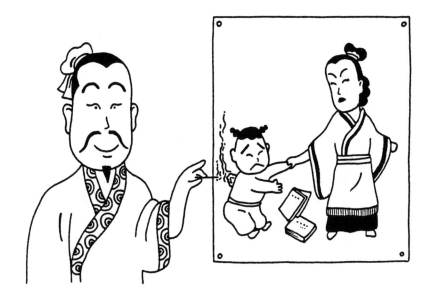

Moxibustion is good for truancy

If children grow up in this manner, they will often become adults who are overly attached to their mothers. Children that reject this try to do something about the situation but are unsure of the specific actions that should be taken, especially as they have not had the opportunity to carry out much independent action. Accordingly, in this unclear state, these children make their intent known by refusing to go to school.

In this situation, the mother should refrain completely from criticizing the child (constructive or otherwise). Although this is easier said than done, in those families where this has been achieved, the children have responded surprisingly well. If this is carried out early on in the evolution of the problem, the child will not be away from school for too long.

ANOREXIA AND OVEREATING

Anorexia is common among young pubescent girls. For whatever reason, they just cannot eat. If they attempt to force something down, they may vomit. Because of this situation, they may stop menstruating. Of course, they will lose weight and become thin, but despite this, they will be incredibly hard workers and full of energy. Their psychological state is complicated, but the condition has its roots in not wanting to grow up. Of course, if they are spoiled a little bit or are allowed to behave a little childishly at this stage, there would probably be no problem. They are also not the sort to go out and commit crimes, and thus they find themselves in a tight corner of their own making.

Overeating is also common in young pubescent girls and is a manifestation of unsatisfied desires, for instance, the denial of sexual desires. The same is probably true with boys. In some cases, marriage provides the solution to the problem, without any treatment. For those who seek treatment, no special points or approach is needed, as treating the basic pattern will prove helpful.

Treatment

For infants, contact needling will be the main method of treatment. The areas to be treated include the meridians of the arms, legs, chest, abdomen, and back. On the arms and legs, the needling is done along the course of the yin meridians but against the direction of flow of the yang meridians. On the chest and upper back, the needling is done from top to bottom while the needling on the lower abdomen and lower back is done from bottom to top. As well as performing contact needling, a root treatment is done using a *tei shin*, a thick needle often used in needling children. with a rounded end not meant for insertion but held to the point.

When the child is older and starts going to kindergarten, it is possible to use the same type of needles that are used for adults because at this age, it is necessary to insert to a level where the skin is just broken. Actually, scarring moxibustion (on a very small scale) is the best method to use on such young children, but unfortunately, unless there is some extraordinary reason for doing it, kids hate it. Children who are in upper elementary and middle school are treated using needles that are identical to those used by adults and may need to be treated by retaining needles on the back.

Contact needling involves patting and stroking with the left hand of the area to be needled. The right hand, which does the needling, does so by means of a fine, rapid vibration of the hand until the area being treated becomes red. If the skin does not become red, there is no effect. Too much redness, and the child will develop a fever. This does not mean that the needle is scraped on the skin. Rather, the redness comes about because of the combination of the thumb, index finger, and tip of the needle hitting the skin at the same time. The thumb and index finger cushion the effect of the needle so that it is not painful.

TABLE 21-5 lists points that are intended for use on older children, from upper elementary school on up. Contact needling should first be performed prior to using these points, and, as noted above, they are treated with adult-size needles. The needles should just break the skin, and only simple insertion is necessary. The points should be chosen according to the signs and symptoms, and can be used by adults as well.

Table 21-5	Branch Treatment Points for Disorders of Children
Problem	**Points**
FEVER	GV-12
COUGH AND ASTHMA	ST-9
DIARRHEA	Right lower abdominal area
CONSTIPATION	Left lower abdominal area
BED WETTING	CV-3
TRUANCY AND REFUSAL TO EAT	GV-9, GV-11, GV-12
MIDDLE EAR INFECTION AND MUMPS	KI-2, TB-17
SINUSITIS	GV-20, GV-23
CONVULSIONS	LI-2
LACK OF APPETITE	LR-13, GV-4, CV-12
TWITCHES	BL-18, GV-4, GV-12
INGUINAL HERNIA	SP-5

BIBLIOGRAPHY

▶ **Premodern Texts** (These are listed in alphabetical order by English title for reference to the main text of this book.)

Anthology of Edified Learning (啓迪集 *Kei teki shu)*, Manase Doha, 1574.

Basic Questions (素問 *So mon/Sù wèn*); part of the *Inner Classic,* probably Eastern Han.

Classic of Difficulties (難經 *Nan gyō/Nàn jīng*); anonymous, probably Eastern Han.

Classic of Nourishing Life with Acupuncture and Moxibustion
(針灸資生經 *Shin kyū shi sei kyō/Zhēn jiǔ zī shēng jīng*); Wáng Zhí-Zhōng, 1220.

Discussion of Cold Damage (傷寒論 *Shō kan ron/Shāng hán lùn*);
Zhāng Zhōng-Jǐng, 3rd century.

Discussion of the Origins and Symptoms of Disease (諸病原侯論 *Sho byō gen kō ron/
Zhū bìng yuán hòu lùn);* Cháo Yuán-Fāng, 610.

Divine Husbandman's Classic of the Materia Medica (神農本草經 *Shin nō hon zō
kyō/Shén nóng běn cǎo jīng);* anonymous, probably Eastern Han.

Divine Pivot (靈樞 *Rei sū/Líng shū*); part of the *Inner Classic,* probably Eastern Han.

Essentials from the Golden Cabinet (金匱要略 *Kin qi yo raku/Jīn guī yào luè*);
Zhāng Zhōng-Jǐng, 3rd century.

Precious Mirror of Oriental Medicine (東医宝鑑 *Dong ui bo gam/Dōng yī bǎo jiàn);*
Heo Jun, 1613.

Guide to Etiology (病因指南 *Byo in shi nan*); Okamoto Ippo, 1695.

Inner Classic (內經 *Nai kei/Nèi jīng*); anonymous, probably Eastern Han.

Introduction to Medicine (醫學入門 *I gaku nyū mon/Yī xué rù mén)*; Lǐ Tǐng, 1575.

Moxibustion Classic from the Yellow Emperor's Bright Hall (黄帝明堂灸経 *Ko tei mei do kyu kei/Huáng dì míng táng jiǔ jīng)*; anonymous, probably Song.

Principles of Acupuncture and Moxibustion (鍼灸則 *Shin kyū soku)*; Suganuma Shukei, 1767.

Pulse Classic (脈經 *Myaku kei/Mài jīng)*; Wang Shu-He, 3rd century.

Pulse Method Handbook (脈診手引草 *Myaku shin tebiki sō)*; Yamanobe Toshi, 1746.

Pulse Method Instructions (脈法指南 *Myaku ho shi nan)*; Okamoto Ippo, 1755.

Restoration of Health from the Myriad Diseases (万病回春 *Man byo kai shun/Wàn bìng huí chūn)*; Xí Tíng-Xián, 1587.

Ripples from the Way of Acupuncture (鍼道発微 *Shin dō hatsu bi)*; Ashihara Kenko, 1731.

▶ **Modern Texts** (These are listed in alphabetical order by author.)

Aikawa Naoki, *Encyclopedia of Medicine* (医学大辞典 *I gaku dai ji ten)*. Tokyo: Nan Zan Do, 1993.

Fukaya Izaburo, *Complete Book of Point Location* (取穴方のすべて *Shu ketsu ho no subete)*. Tokyo: Shinkyu Nose Kaisha, 1986.

Fukaya Izaburo, *Medical Canon of Moxibustion* (灸法医典 *Kyu ho i ten)*. Tokyo: Taniguchi Shoten, 1988.

Fukaya Izaburo, *Research on Famous Moxibustion Points* (名灸穴の研究 *Mei kyu ketsu no kenkyu)*, vols. 1 and 2. Tokyo: Shinkyu Nose Kaisha, 1978.

Fukaya Izaburo, *Selected Interpretations of Famous Family Moxibustion Methods* (名家灸選釈義 *Mei ka kyu sen shaku gi)*. Tokyo: Kan Kan Do Shuppan Sha, 1967.

Fukaya Izaburo, *Stories of Curing Diseases with Moxibustion* (お灸で病気を治した話 *Okyu de byoki wo naoshita hanashi)*, vols. 1-12. Tokyo: Shinkyu Nose Kaisha, 1958.

Bibliography

Fukaya Izaburo, *Treasury of the Practical Use of Points* (経穴活用宝典 *Kei ketsu katsu yo ho ten*). Tokyo: Shinkyu Nose Kaisha, 1984.

Fukaya Izaburo, *Treatment through Moxibustion* (灸による治療法 *Kyu ni yoru chi ryo ho*). Tokyo: Shinkyu Nose Kaisha, 1965.

Hǎo Jīn-Kǎi, *Dictionary of Extra Points for Acupuncture and Moxibustion* (鍼灸奇穴辞典 *Shin kyu ki ketsu ji ten/Zhēn jiǔ qí xuè cí diǎn*), trans. by Hirai et al. Tokyo: Fu Rin Sho Bo, 1987.

Hongo Masatomi, *Collection of Acupuncture and Moxibustion Treasures* (鍼灸重宝記 *Shin kyu cho ho ki*), commentary by Ono Bunkei. Tokyo: I Do No Nippon Sha, 1959.

Ikeda Masakazu, *Classic of Difficulties Handbook* (難経ハンドブック *Nan gyo handobukku*). Tokyo: I Do No Nippon Sha, 1983.

Ikeda Masakazu et al., *Herbal Medicine and Acupuncture and Moxibustion Looked at from an Organ-Meridian Perspective* (臓腑経絡からみた漢方と鍼灸 *Zofu keiraku kara mita kanpo to hari kyu*). Imabari, Ehime Ken. Japan: Kanpo Inyo Kai, 1994.

Ikeda Masakazu, *Learning from the Classics* (古典の学び方 *Ko ten no manabikata*). Tokyo: I Do No Nippon Sha, 1993.

Kato Motoyo, *An Explanation of Chapter 2 of the Yellow Emperor's Inner Classic: Divine Pivot* (黄帝内経霊枢, 本輸篇解説 *Ko tei nai kei rei sū hon yu hen kai setsu*). Tokyo: Keiraku Chiryo Gaku Kai, 1993.

Kimura Chuta, *Secret Selections of Acupuncture and Moxibustion* (鍼灸極秘抄 *Shin kyu kyoku hitsu sho*), commentary by Araki Hiroshi. Tokyo: Taniguchi Shoten, 1990 (originally published 1780).

Maruyama Masao, *Remarks on the Atlas of Points from the Bronze Man* (訓注, 銅人愈穴図経 *Kun chu, do jin yu ketsu xu kei*). Nagoya: Seki Bun Do, 1974.

Cháo Yuán-Fāng, *Discussion of the Origins and Symptoms of Disease* (諸病原侯論 *Sho byo gen ko ron/Zhū bìng yuán hòu lùn*), trans. and ed. by Muta Koichiro. Tokyo: Taniguchi Shoten, 1978 (originally published 610).

Naito Kitetsu and Kosoto Takeo, *Interpretation of Puzzles from the Medical Classics* (意釈医経解惑論 *I shaku i kei kai waku ron*). Tokyo: Chikuchi Shokan, 1981.

Naito Kitetsu and Kosoto Takeo, *Interpretation of the Discussion of Cold Damage* (意釈 傷寒論類編 *I shaku sho kan ron rui hen)*. Tokyo: Chikuchi Shokan, 1981.

Okabe Sodo, *Meridian Therapy with Acupuncture and Moxibustion* (鍼灸経絡治療 *Shin kyu kei raku chi ryo)*. Nagoya: Seki Bun Do, 1974.

Shirota Bunshi, *Foundations of Acupuncture and Moxibustion Therapeutics* (鍼灸治療基礎学 *Shin kyu chi ryo ki so gaku)*. Tokyo: I Do No Nippon Sha, 1975.

Ueda Hideao, *Internal Medicine* (内科学 *Nai ka gaku)*. Tokyo: Asakura Sho Ten, 1987.

Uge Son, *Essentials from the Rare Treasury* (蔵珍要編 *Zo chin yo hen)*, commentary by Ikeda Masakazu. Tokyo: I Do No Nippon Sha, 1988.

Wáng Shū-Hé, *Pulse Classic* (脈經 *Myaku kei/Mài jīng)*, trans. and ed. by Ikeda Masakazu, annot. by Kosoto Takea. Tokyo: Taniguchi Shoten, 1991 (originally published 3rd century).

Yamanobe Toshi, *Pulse Method Handbook* (脈法手引草 *Myaku ho tebiki so)*, rev. by Okabe Sodo. Tokyo: I Do No Nippon Sha, 1963.

Yokota Shohei, *Home Medicine* (家庭医学 *Ka tei i gaku)*. Tokyo: Kyow Sho In, 1993.

Point Index

BL-47, 96, 182, 186, 197
BL-48, 96, 199, 213
BL-49, 178, 182, 186, 197, 208, 270
BL-50, 178, 182, 186, 196, 208
BL-51, 186
BL-52, 113, 157, 179, 182, 190, 213, 216, 241, 258
BL-53, 109, 113, 114, 165, 220
BL-54, 16, 71, 72, 109, 113, 114, 213, 220
BL-55, 229, 252
BL-56, 113, 116, 196, 202
BL-57, 109, 113, 196, 252
BL-58, 21, 22, 26, 81, 101, 113, 116, 160, 167, 168, 185, 202, 213, 233, 234, 255
BL-59, 26, 115, 116, 185, 225, 234
BL-60, 75, 76, 82, 101, 109, 113, 115, 196, 216, 225
BL-62, 79, 82, 109, 139, 140, 178, 246, 255, 258, 264
BL-63, 7, 8, 197, 246, 268
BL-64, 101
BL-65, 113, 262, 265
BL-66, 72
BL-67, 7, 8, 139, 140, 232, 234, 262

——— C

CONCEPTION VESSEL
CV-2, 229, 236, 270
CV-3, 109, 173, 186, 213, 216, 229, 236, 277
CV-4, 31, 72, 76, 79, 82, 84, 101, 109, 130, 151, 157, 161, 164, 165, 168, 173, 178, 182, 186, 190, 191, 196, 200, 213, 216, 225, 229, 239, 246, 247, 255, 270, 272
CV-5, 31, 178, 196, 208, 213, 216, 229, 236
CV-6, 31, 129, 143, 146, 161, 178, 182, 186, 190, 196, 199, 216, 219, 220, 225, 229, 236, 252, 270
CV-7, 101, 109, 161, 190, 208, 213, 219, 225, 229, 236
CV-8, 92, 190, 197, 220, 233
CV-9, 101, 178, 181, 183, 186, 190, 199, 207, 208
CV-10, 164, 178, 182, 186
CV-11, 164, 186

CV-12, 35, 72, 73, 79, 82, 84, 92, 93, 101, 109, 129, 130, 151, 157, 160, 161, 163, 164, 165, 173, 178, 182, 183, 186, 191, 196, 199, 200, 213, 229, 246, 247, 252, 255, 270, 277
CV-13, 129, 182, 246, 252
CV-14, 35, 76, 79, 129, 157, 164, 177, 178, 183, 186, 198, 199, 237, 246, 247, 255, 258
CV-15, 92, 93, 146, 157, 163, 164, 168, 186
CV-16, 186
CV-17, 130, 163, 164, 165, 168, 182, 233, 236
CV-18, 190, 233
CV-20, 129, 130
CV-22, 97, 128, 129, 130, 135, 165
CV-23, 129, 270
CV-24, 78, 264

——— E

Earth points, 7
EXTRA POINTS
asthma point, 128, 130
dǎn náng xué, 199
gān yán diǎn, 199
guǐ dāng, 135
hè dìng, 100
helical apex, 262
hepatitis point, 199
inner GB-37, 229
insomnia point, 207
lǐ nèi tíng, 186, 233
M-BW-16, 93, 113, 196, 213
M-BW-24, 108, 110, 270
M-BW-25, 108, 109
M-BW-35, 239
M-HN-20, 270
M-HN-3, 78, 138
M-HN-9, 252
M-LE-1, 186, 233
M-LE-16, 100, 115, 157, 208
M-LE-23, 199
M-LE-27, 100
M-LE-5, 207, 208, 252
M-LE-9, 264
middle finger point, 78, 79
N-HN-44, 262
N-LE-14, 199

HERB & FORMULA INDEX:
ENGLISH & CHINESE

General Index

Practitioners, personality as factor in
treatment efficacy, xxxvii–xxxviii
Pre-Edo texts, 2
Precious Mirror of Oriental Medicine, 173
Predisposing factors, xxvii
Pregnancy conditions, 221, **231**–234
Premature ejaculation, 218, 219
Premature menstruation, 226
Pressure
response in deficiency and excess, xxxiv
in tonification and shunting, xli
Priapism, 218
Principles of Acupuncture and Moxibustion, 92,
143, 178, 244
Profuse menstruation, 229
Profuse sweating, 119
Prostatitis, in men with history of
tuberculosis, 215
Prostrating vertigo, 243
Protective qi, tonification in Lung deficiency/
yang excess/heat pattern, 7
Psychological disorders, 242–243
depression, 250–251
insomnia, 248–250, 251–253
mania, 251
obsessive compulsive disorder, 251
schizophrenia, 251
Pulmonary diseases, **143**–151
Pulmonary edema, 143, 144
Pulmonary emphysema, 143, 144
case study, 150–151
good response to acupuncture and
moxibustion, 145
Pulse Classic, 232
Pulse diagnosis, xxxi
in deficiency and excess, xxxiv
differentiation by, xxxv
emphasis in meridian therapy, 2
in patterns of Kidney deficiency, 30
in patterns of Spleen deficiency, 30
rapidity and insomnia, 248
rough pulse, 6
signs of overall yang deficiency, 176–177
Pulse Method Handbook, 87, 244, 261, 263
Pulse speed, reducing with acupuncture, 167
Pyelonephritis, 211

─── **Q**

Qi, association with Lung, xxi
Qi deficiency, cold patterns related to, xxiii
Qi painful urinary dribbling, 210
Qi stagnation, 135
in coughing and wheezing disorders, 127
role in hemorrhoids, 202
Questioning examination, xxvii–xxx

─── **R**

Rapid pulse, in insomnia, 248–249
Raynaud's disease, 224
Reactive points, changing according to
pattern, 68
Red cheeks, in Liver deficiency/yang
deficiency/cold pattern, 38
Redoubled yang, 257
Redoubled yin, 257
Respiratory diseases, 118–119
acute febrile disease, **119**–120, 122–124
coughing and wheezing, **124**–132
nasal disorders, **136**–140
pulmonary diseases, **143**–151
sore throat, **132**–136
sweating disorders, **140**–143
Retinitis pigmentosa, 262
Rheumatism
in Lung deficiency/yang deficiency/cold
patterns, 20
in Spleen deficiency/Kidney deficiency/cold
patterns, 29
Ripples from the Way of Acupuncture, 92
Root pattern, 2
Root treatment, xxvi, xxxii, 65
insufficient to affect cure, 68
non-retention of needles in, 9
in order of treatment, xxxviii
tonification and shunting in, xliv–xlv
Rotten swelling, 205
Running piglet qi, 134, 166, 168–169

─── **S**

Salads, avoiding in low blood pressure, 160

Withdrawal mania, 257
Women, association between blood and sex, 81
Women's diseases, **221**–222
  cold extremities, **222**–225
  female genital problems, **225**–231
  menopausal problems, **238**–241
  postpartum problems, **234**–238
  pregnancy and childbirth problems, **231**–234
Wrist pain, **101**
Writer's cramp, **102**
Wry neck. *See* Stiff neck

──── **X**

Xavier, Francisco, ix

──── **Y**

Yagishita Katsunosuke, x
Yanagiya, Sorei, x
Yang brightness heat, xxx
  in nasal polyps, 137
  in toothache, 263
Yang brightness meridians
  association with trigeminal nerve, 77
  facial paralysis in, 83
  and frontal headaches, 254
  pathway through nose, 138
  transfer of problems between, 11
  transmission of acute febrile disease through, 122
Yang brightness pulse, 191
Yang deficiency
  in absence of sweating, 140
  defined, 18
  inclusive of both yin and yang deficiency, 21
  of lower burner, 122
  of middle burner, 121
  spreading of cold from, xxiv
  spreading of heat from, xxiii
  stagnation caused by, 41
  of upper burner, 121
  weak voice in, xxvii
  in whiplash, 75

Yang deficiency cold pattern
  in coughing and wheezing, 125
  in low blood pressure, 159
Yang deficiency/cold patterns
  necessity of tonifying both yin and yang in, 19
  tonification and shunting in, xliv
Yang deficiency/heat patterns, 19
Yang excess heat
  association with heat/stagnation buildup, 4, 11
  tonification and shunting in, xlv
Yang meridians
  as repository of excess conditions, xix
  shunting of, 66
Yang organs, receipt of heat or cold from yin meridians, 118
Yang qi
  decrease at greater yang meridian level, 133
  forming fire at gate of vitality, 25
  of Lung, 4–5
  simultaneous depletion in yin organs and yang meridians, 18
  stagnation and pooling in excess conditions, 41
Yang qi deficiency
  cold production from, xx
  in Kidney deficiency/cold pattern, xxii
  in sore throats, 133
Yellow Emperor's Moxibustion Classic of the Bright Hall, 258
Yellow jaundice, 197
Yellow sweat, 140, 142
Yin, overabundance of, xix
Yin and yang, double deficiency of, 18
Yin deficiency
  in constipation, 193
  in early awakening, 249
  heat production from, xix
  of lower burner, 122
  of middle burner, 121
  as opposite state from Liver deficiency/yang deficiency/cold pattern, 37
  in sexual dysfunction, 217
  spreading of heat from, xxiii, 86
  of upper burner, 121
Yin deficiency heat

in chronic sweating, 141
  tonification and shunting in, xliv
Yin deficiency/heat patterns, xxii
  table, 63
Yin excess, 41, 48
  correspondence with Liver excess, xix
Yin excess heat, tonification and shunting in,
  xlv
Yin meridians
  heat transmitting through in acute febrile
    diseases, 122

receipt of heat or cold from yang organs,
  118
  tonification of, 66
Yin organs, associations with substances/
  functions, xxi
Yoshikawa, Akiko, xlviii

——— **Z**

Zhang, Jie-Bin, 146
Zhang, Zhong-Jing, xvi, 5, 166, 173, 197